PATIENT SAFETY FIRST

PATIENT SAFETY FIRST
RESPONSIVE REGULATION IN HEALTH CARE

edited by

JUDITH HEALY AND PAUL DUGDALE

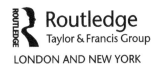

Routledge
Taylor & Francis Group

LONDON AND NEW YORK

First published 2009 by Allen & Unwin

Published 2020 by Routledge
2 Park Square, Milton Park, Abingdon, Oxon OX14 4RN
605 Third Avenue, New York, NY 10017

Routledge is an imprint of the Taylor & Francis Group, an informa business

Cataloguing-in-Publication details are available
from the National Library of Australia
www.librariesaustralia.nla.gov.au

Index by Chitra Karunanayake
Set in 10.5/13 pt ITC Garamond by Midland Typesetters, Australia

ISBN-13: 9781742370583 (pbk)

CONTENTS

FIGURES AND TABLES

FIGURES

TABLES

ACKNOWLEDGMENTS

The work for this book was supported by a grant from the Australian Research Council, the research partners being the Australian National University, the Australian Commission on Safety and Quality in Health Care, and Australian Capital Territory Health. We wish to thank the contributors for their excellent chapters and wise advice. Our special thanks go to Peter Maguire for his sterling efforts in tracking down references and organising and editing the chapters into a coherent format.

LIST OF
CONTRIBUTORS

Christopher Baggoley (BVSc (Hons), BM, BS, B SocAdmin, FACEM) is the Chief Executive of the Australian Commission on Safety and Quality in Health Care. He was previously an Executive Director of Public Health and Clinical Coordination, Chief Medical Officer with the South Australian Department of Health and Professor of Emergency Medicine. He is a Fellow of the Australasian College for Emergency Medicine, and has been a member or chair of many national committees, including the Board of the National Institute of Clinical Studies from 2004-07.

Bruce Barraclough (AO, MBBS, FRACS, DDU, FACS, FAICD, Hon. FRCS (Eng), Hon. FRCS (Ed), Hon. FCSHK, Hon. FRCST) is Associate Dean (Clinical Strategy) University of Western Sydney Medical School, Honorary Professor, University of Sydney Faculty of Medicine, Board Chair, New South Wales Clinical Excellence Commission and President and Chair of the Executive Board of the International Society for Quality in Health Care (ISQua). He was formerly Chair of the Australian Council for Safety and Quality in Health Care and President of the Royal Australasian College of Surgeons.

Jenny Berrill (BA App Sc, MHA, FCHSE, MRCNA) is a Lecturer in the School of Management, College of Business and Economics, Australian National University, Canberra. She has 30 years' experience in clinical services, government and academia. She is the Executive Director of

ProACT, has conducted work for governments, health-profession groups and consumer-interest groups, and has been a member of national committees including those concerned with the safety and quality of health care.

Jeffrey Braithwaite (PhD, FAIM, FCHSE) is Foundation Director of the Institute of Health Innovation, Director of the Centre for Clinical Governance Research and Professor in the School of Public Health and Community Medicine, University of New South Wales. He has an international reputation in leadership and organisational behaviour in health settings. His research examines the changing nature of health systems, particularly patient safety and the structure and culture of organisations. He has published multiple times in the *British Medical Journal, The Lancet, Social Science and Medicine* and other prestigious journals. Jeffrey has received numerous national and international awards including UNSW Vice-Chancellor's awards for teaching and for research papers.

John Braithwaite (PhD) is a Federation Fellow in the Regulatory Institutions Network at the Australian National University, Canberra. He has published widely on responsive regulation and restorative justice. He has been a member of the Economic Planning Advisory Council, a part-time Commissioner with the Trade Practices Commission, and a member of the Council on Business Regulation. John's books have won many prizes. His responsive regulation ideas are updated in Braithwaite et al., *Regulating Aged Care: Ritualism and the New Pyramid* (Edward Elgar, 2007).

Heather Buchan (MBChB, MSc, FAFPHM) was foundation Chief Executive Officer of the National Institute of Clinical Studies—now part of the National Health and Medical Research Council. She has worked in New Zealand, the United Kingdom and Australia in the hospital, academic and government sectors. Heather is the Vice Chair of the Guidelines International Network and has a specific interest in the translation of evidence into clinical practice.

Steve Clarke (BA, PhD) is a Research Fellow in the Program on the Ethics of the New Biosciences, James Martin 21st Century School and Faculty of Philosophy at the University of Oxford. He is on leave from the Centre for Applied Philosophy and Public Ethics in Australia, where he is a Senior Research Fellow. He holds a PhD in Philosophy from Monash University and has previously held appointments at the University of Melbourne, the University of Cape Town and La Trobe University. Steve has published in such journals as the *British Journal for the Philosophy of Science*, *Journal of Medicine and Philosophy*, *Philosophical Psychology* and the *Journal of Risk Research*. He is co-editor, with Justin Oakley, of *Informed Consent and Clinician Accountability: The Ethics of Report Cards on Surgeon Performance* (Cambridge University Press, 2007).

Angus Corbett (BA, LLB, LLM) is a Visiting Fellow in the Centre for Clinical Governance Research in Health, Faculty of Medicine and Associate Professor, Faculty of Law at the University of Technology, Sydney.

Stephen Duckett (PhD, DSc, FASSA) is President and Chief Executive Officer of Alberta Health Services, Canada. His previous positions were Chief Executive, Centre for Health Improvement, Queensland Health, Professor of Health Policy and Dean of the Faculty of Health Sciences at La Trobe University, and Secretary of the Australian Government Department of Human Services and Health from 1994–96. He has also held various operational and policy positions in the Victorian Department of Health and Community Services. An economist, he has published widely on health sector issues, including *The Australian Health Care System* (Oxford University Press, 2007).

Paul Dugdale (BMBS, MA, MPH, PLD, FAFPHM) is Director of Chronic Disease Management for Australian Capital Territory Health and Director of the Australian National University Centre for Health Stewardship. He is a public health physician with first-hand governance experience in the health sector, including as ACT Chief Health Officer, Director of General Practice Finance in the Commonwealth Department of Health and Medical Superintendent of Liverpool Hospital (NSW). His book *Doing Health Policy in Australia* (Allen & Unwin) was published in 2008.

Kathy Eagar (MA, PhD, FAFRM (Hon)) is Director of the Centre for Health Service Development at the University of Wollongong. She has over 30 years' experience in Australian health and community services as a clinician, senior manager and health academic. She has authored over 350 articles, papers and reports on management, quality outcomes, information systems and funding, including, with P. Garret and V. Lin, *Health Planning: Australian Perspectives* (Allen & Unwin, 2001).

Ian Freckelton (BA Hons, LLB, PhD, FACLM (Hon)) is a Senior Counsel in Crockett Chambers in Melbourne. He also holds a professorial position in law, forensic medicine and forensic psychology at Monash University. He is a lawyer member of the Mental Health Review and Disciplinary Appeals Boards in Victoria, and the Independent Review Panel that hears appeals from decisions by health practitioner boards in Victoria. He was a long-time member of Victoria's Medical and Psychologists' Registration Boards. He is the editor of the *Journal of Law and Medicine*. His publications in the medico-legal area include, with Kerry Petersen (eds), *Disputes and Dilemmas in Health Law* (Federation Press, 2006), *Regulating Health Practitioners* (Federation Press, 2006) and, with David Ranson, *Death Investigation and the Coroner's Inquest* (Oxford University Press, 2006).

Judith Healy (BA, MSW, PhD) is Associate Professor in the Regulatory Institutions Network, Australian National University. She has worked in Australia, the United States and Europe for universities, policy think tanks and the European Observatory on Health Systems and Policies. Her research interests include health sector regulation and the comparative analysis of health systems. Her books include, with Martin McKee (eds), *Hospitals in a Changing Europe* (Open University Press, 2002) and, also with Martin McKee (eds), *Health Care: Responding to Diversity* (Oxford University Press, 2004).

David Hirsch (BA, LLB, BCL) is a Barrister in Selborne Chambers, Sydney. He has seventeen years' experience specialising in medical negligence litigation. He is the former head of the medical negligence department of a leading national Australian law firm and now practises exclusively as a specialist barrister in medical negligence cases. He has handled many of the leading Australian cases in this field, lectured at the University of Sydney and written many articles in both medical and legal publications. He is currently the chair of the Medical Negligence Special Interest Group of the Australian Lawyers Alliance and sits on a committee of the New South Wales Clinical Excellence Commission.

Julie Johnson (MSPH, PhD) is Associate Professor in the Faculty of Medicine and Deputy Director Centre for Clinical Governance Research in Health at the University of New South Wales. Her career interests involve building collaborative relationships to improve the quality and safety of health care through research, teaching and clinical improvement. She has a master's degree in public health from the University of North Carolina and a PhD in evaluative clinical sciences from Dartmouth College in Hanover, New Hampshire.

Niall Johnson (PhD) joined the Australian Commission on Safety and Quality in Health Care in 2007, having previously worked with organisations as diverse as Médecins Sans Frontières, News Limited and Hewlett-Packard. He has degrees from Australia, Canada and the United Kingdom. His publication record includes monographs, edited collections and articles in journals including *Nature Medicine*, *Lancet Infectious Diseases*, *Proceedings of the Royal Society* and the *Bulletin of the History of Medicine*.

Judy Lumby (AM, RN, BA, MHPEd, PhD) held a Clinical Chair in Nursing and has been Dean of Nursing in two universities, and an Executive Director of the College of Nursing. Her research has focused on patients' experiences of illness and disease. Her publications include, with Debbie Picone, *Clinical Challenges* (Churchill Livingston, 2000) and *Who Cares? The Changing Health Care System* (Allen & Unwin, 2001). Her latest book is *The Gift: Grandmothers and Grandchildren Today* (Pluto Press, 2007). In 2008 she was awarded an AM for her services to nursing education, professional organisations and the community. She is an Emeritus Professor at the University of Technology, Sydney, an Adjunct Professor at both the University of Western Sydney and the University of Adelaide, and Director of the Joanna Briggs Foundation.

Malcolm Masso (RN, MNA, MPH) is a Senior Research Fellow at the Centre for Health Service Development, University of Wollongong. Prior to joining the Centre, he worked for over 25 years in the health system as a clinician and manager, including fifteen years of executive responsibility for clinical services in both large and small hospitals in rural and metropolitan areas.

Justin Oakley (BA, PhD) is Director of the Centre for Human Bioethics at Monash University. He is the editor, with Steve Clarke, of *Informed Consent and Clinician Accountability: The Ethics of Report Cards on*

Surgeon Performance (Cambridge University Press, 2007) and *Bioethics* (Ashgate, 2009), and is author of *Morality and the Emotions* (Routledge, 1993) and, with Dean Cocking, *Virtue Ethics and Professional Roles* (Cambridge University Press, 2001). He recently led an NHMRC-funded project on the ethics of providing patients with surgeon-specific performance data as part of the informed consent process.

William B. Runciman (MBBCh, FANZCA, FJFICM, FHKCA, FRCA, PhD) is Professor of Patient Safety and Healthcare Human Factors at the University of South Australia, and was Foundation Professor of Anaesthesia and Intensive Care at the University of Adelaide. He is President of the Australian Patient Safety Foundation, a member of the International Patient Safety Classification Group, and Co-chair of the Research Methods and Measures Group of the World Alliance for Patient Safety, World Health Organization. He has published some 200 scientific papers and chapters. His most recent book is, with Alan Merry and Merrilyn Walton, *Safety and Ethics in Healthcare: A Guide to Getting it Right* (Ashgate, 2007).

Peter Sprivulis (MBBS, PhD, FACEM, FACHI) is Clinical Associate Professor of Emergency Medicine at the University of Western Australia, Clinical Epidemiologist and Health Informatician. He is a Harkness Fellow in Healthcare Policy and currently advises the National E-Health Transitional Authority on planning national e-health services to improve the quality of health care in Australia. Peter has internationally recognised expertise in health care improvement, demand management and patient safety, and works clinically at Fremantle Hospital Emergency Department, Western Australia.

David Studdert (LLB, ScD, MPH) is a Federation Fellow at the University of Melbourne and a Professor in the Law School and School of Population Health. He joined the faculty in 2007 from the Harvard School of Public Health, where he was Associate Professor of Law and Public Health. He previously held positions as a policy analyst at RAND (Santa Monica, USA), a policy advisor to the Victorian Minister for Health, and a practising lawyer. His research focuses on policy issues at the intersection of the legal and health care systems, with recent projects addressing compensation system reform, disputes over informed consent and disclosure of medical injury. He has authored more than 120 articles in leading international medical, health policy and law journals.

Joanne F. Travaglia (MEd) is a Research Fellow, Centre for Clinical Governance Research in Health, Faculty of Medicine, University of New South Wales. She has a background in social work, health services management and policy, and medical sociology. Her particular interests are in patient safety and vulnerability in both patients and staff. She has published in journals including the *International Journal for Quality in Health Care, Quality and Safety in Healthcare* and *Social Science and Medicine*. She has co-authored articles, chapters and monographs on incident reporting, root cause analyses, patient safety inquiries and clinician attitudes to patient safety.

Kieran Walshe (BSc, Dip HSM, PhD) is Professor and Co-Director of the Centre for Public Policy and Management at Manchester Business School. His particular interests are in public services regulation, the performance of public services, and policy evaluation and learning. He writes regularly for journals including the *British Medical Journal, Health Service Journal, Health Affairs, Milbank Quarterly* and *Quality and Safety in Healthcare*. He acted as an expert for the Bristol Royal Infirmary Inquiry, and advises the National Audit Office on health care issues. He is a member of the Council for Healthcare Regulatory Excellence, and is the Research Director of the Department of Health's service delivery and organisation research program. His books include *Regulating Healthcare: A Prescription for Improvement?* (Open University Press, 2003), with R. Boaden, *Patient Safety: Research into Practice* (Open University Press, 2005) and, with Judith Smith, *Healthcare Management* (Open University Press, 2006).

Heather Wellington (MBBS, LLB) is a medical practitioner and lawyer with a background in health services management and health care policy. She is a consultant with the national law firm Phillips Fox, and an Honorary Senior Lecturer at Monash University Department of Epidemiology and Preventive Medicine. She was a member of the Australian Council for Safety and Quality in Health Care. She is Chair of the Board of Directors for the Peter MacCallum Cancer Centre, a City of Greater Geelong councillor, a director of the Geelong Medical and Hospital Benefits Association, a director of the Victorian Division of the National Heart Foundation, a director of Barwon Water and a director of the Infertility Treatment Authority.

1

REGULATORY STRATEGIES FOR SAFER PATIENT HEALTH CARE

Judith Healy and Paul Dugdale

REGULATING PATIENT SAFETY

Health care can be risky for patients. Public inquiries continue to reveal unsafe practices in busy modern hospitals, surveys report that around one in ten patients experiences 'things that go wrong'— that is, they suffer an adverse event during their hospital stay—and more people die each year in health care accidents than in road accidents. Realisation is dawning that medical errors are common events. Large numbers of adverse events do not necessarily mean that doctors and nurses are making more errors than in the past, but rather that there are now more opportunities for things to go wrong. Technological advances have substantially expanded the reach of health care, and more people undergo medical and surgical treatments; however, greater opportunities for intervention also increase the potential for harm. The Hippocratic injunction, 'first, do no harm', thus has new relevance for modern medicine, and patients now are less reassured by the mantra 'Trust me, I'm a doctor'.

Health care governance has been undergoing substantial change since the beginning of the twenty-first century. Many countries, including Australia, have set up new regulatory bodies and are strengthening both internal regulation (by the professions and health industry) and external regulation (by the state and the public) in order to ensure better and

1

safer health care (McLoughlin et al. 2001).This is a major regulatory shift. Historically, clinical performance in the health sector (to the limited extent that it *was* regulated) was handled by the medical profession and not subjected to external scrutiny (Chief Medical Officer 2006). While most other sectors of the economy were brought under the purview of 'the new regulatory state' in the 1980s (Osborne and Gaebler 1992), the state's regulatory response to the health sector has been somewhat belated. First, the state traditionally has not sought to govern the medical profession but rather to ensure that medicine governed itself (Osborne 1993). Second, the medical profession has strongly opposed external regulation as antithetical to medical professionalism. Third, medical practitioners have a very narrow and negative view of regulation as being about inspections and rules.

We take a much broader view of regulation in this book. We take it to mean governing the flow of events (Ayres and Braithwaite 1992).The chapters are framed within the responsive regulation model and seek to both describe and prescribe health sector governance. Responsive regulation involves multiple regulatory actors and multiple mechanisms, beginning with persuasion, but with the capacity to range upwards to punishment for the most recalcitrant (Braithwaite 2002; Braithwaite et al. 2007).The contributors all argue that better regulation in the health sector is warranted in order to improve the safety of health care for patients— although their views about how best to do this differ somewhat. The nuanced and participative approach of responsive regulation is proposed here as an appropriate model, since it proceeds on the basis that health professionals, after all, seek to do good and not harm.

This review of patient safety regulatory strategies is timely. A flood of initiatives is currently being proposed. These promise solutions in reducing well-known risks to patient safety. For example, the Patient Safety Alliance has endorsed five priority practices, dubbed 'the High 5s'. These are standardised protocols to prevent errors in the following areas: patient care handover, correct site/correct procedure/correct person surgery, medication continuity, high-concentration drugs, and effective hand hygiene (World Health Organization 2007). About a dozen other evidence-based patient safety practices have also been recommended, arising from systematic reviews of the research literature (Shojania et al. 2001; Leape and Davis 2005).

The first point is that many of the recommended patient safety practices are clinical interventions—such as prescribing anti-clotting drugs before surgery—rather than more upstream regulatory interventions. This book addresses the issue of which regulatory strategies are most effective in ensuring that patient safety practices, such as risk-reducing drug prescriptions, are actually carried out. The second point is that patient safety research must also look beyond the confines of evidence-based clinical medicine. Health systems research encompasses a variety of methods, since many issues are not amenable to classic scientific double-blind control trials and also involve political and cultural considerations (World Health Organization 2004). The chapters in this book thus consider complex regulatory issues from different points of view, including the legal tradition of reasoned argument. The third point is that since many studies come from the United States and United Kingdom, we must consider whether research findings can be generalised to the Australian policy context.

The following chapters by leading patient safety experts discuss key regulatory strategies underway in Australia that are intended to make health care better and safer for patients. They address the following questions:

- How is a particular regulatory strategy intended to impact upon patient safety?
- What reform proposals and debates are underway in Australia and internationally?
- Is there evidence the strategy will improve the safety and quality of patient care?

THINGS THAT GO WRONG

Malcolm Sparrow (2000) argues that the central purpose of regulation is the abatement or control of risks to society, while the essence of the regulatory craft is to 'pick important problems and fix them'. Are risks to the safety of patients significant enough to warrant regulatory intervention? One way to gauge the significance of the patient safety problem is to measure the frequency of adverse events. Medical language uses somewhat euphemistic terms, such as iatrogenic (doctor-caused) injury and nosocomial (hospital-acquired) infections. Pending a taxonomy being agreed by the World Health Organization, the following is a useful definition of an adverse event: 'An event that results in unintended harm to the patient by an act of commission or omission rather than by the underlying disease or condition of the patient.' (Institute of Medicine 2004: 327)

The Quality in Australian Health Care Study (QAHCS) conducted in 1995 still provides the most comprehensive estimate of the scale of adverse events in Australian public hospitals (Runciman et al. 2000; Wilson and Van Der Weyden 2005). A re-analysis of the data for comparability with overseas studies found that adverse events occur in 10.6 per cent of annual hospital admissions, with 51 per cent of these events considered preventable; 1.7 per cent of admissions experienced serious disability resulting from an adverse event; and 0.3 per cent of patients died from an adverse event (Thomas et al. 2000). Studies in other countries, including the United States (Brennan et al. 1991; Thomas et al. 2000), Canada (Baker et al. 2004) and Britain (Vincent et al. 2001), report that between 4 and 12 per cent of hospital patients experience adverse events. While there is a compelling humanitarian reason for reducing adverse events, there is also an economic rationale, since several studies have estimated that adverse events account for over 15 per cent of hospital budgets, mainly because patients end up staying much longer in hospital (Runciman and Moller 2001; Ehsani et al. 2006). Patient safety, therefore, has been revealed to be a major and costly problem in modern hospitals around the world.

Extrapolating the QAHCS findings to 2003-04 Australian public hospital admissions (Australian Institute of Health and Welfare 2006) suggests an annual hospital toll of 6300 preventable deaths from adverse events. The 'jumbo jet' analogy (based on 416 passengers in a Boeing 747) is that 6300 hospital deaths is equivalent to the number of lives lost in fifteen plane crashes. The lack of public outcry about the magnitude of the hospital toll attests to the power of the medical mystique, and also shows that ignorance is bliss, since few state health departments report publicly on the number of adverse events occurring in their hospitals.

Adverse events can be classified in many ways, but the main point here is that an enormous variety of things can go wrong—which makes it difficult to address the multifarious causes. For example, the QAHCS review of adverse events in Australian hospitals identified 518 principal categories of harm to patients, of which the top ten accounted for only 25 per cent of all adverse events (Runciman and Moller 2001). The causes of adverse events are much debated, with a distinction frequently drawn between people error and system error. Of course, different causes suggest different solutions, depending on whether the proximate cause was illegible medication labelling or a lapse in concentration by an exhausted intern. For example, a national medication alert was issued after fatalities where vincristine was mistakenly injected into the spine instead of into a vein, with contributing factors being confusing storage and labelling, and inexperienced staff (Australian Council for Safety and Quality in Health Care 2005).

Regulatory rhetoric in the health sector generally avoids 'naming, blaming and shaming'. The idea is to promote a 'safety culture', not 'a blame culture', in order to encourage learning from near-misses and adverse events, and so prevent future occurrences. James Reason's work is influential and salutary in pointing out that errors usually have intertwined and multiple causes, so a high-risk organisation such as a hospital should engineer a series of safeguards to prevent the confluence of factors that allows an error to occur (Reason 2000). The case of wrong-site surgery (shown in Box 1.1) illustrates a series of errors that are understandable individually, but which together were disastrous for the patient and distressing for the doctor.

Box 1.1 In the matter of Dr A

Event description

In November 2002, Patient S was seen by Dr A and diagnosed with cancer of the left breast. In December 2002, Dr A assisted the surgical registrar in performing a right total mastectomy. Prior to the surgery, Dr A had failed to correctly complete the patient's consent form and the hospital admission request form, and did not have the patient's medical records in the operating theatre.

Contributing factors

Patient S was an elderly woman who suffered from dementia and spoke little English. The patient's daughter attended the first consultation but the patient was admitted to hospital from the nursing home by her son-in-law. Dr A was very busy on the day of the surgery, completed the admission forms without consulting the patient's medical record, and entered R as shorthand for 'right mastectomy' instead of entering 'left mastectomy'. The patient was not brought to the hospital's pre-admission clinic and thus did not go through the usual hospital checking procedure.

What action followed

After the error was discovered, Dr A spoke to the family and performed the left mastectomy that evening. The patient recovered with no evidence of further cancer (as at December 2003). Dr A instituted several safety

---

5

> changes to his surgical checking procedure. The hospital instituted a correct patient/site/procedure protocol. The Medical Tribunal of NSW, at its hearing in 2006, reprimanded Dr A and ordered him to pay 70 per cent of the costs of the complainant (Medical Tribunal of New South Wales 2006).

Widespread patient safety problems and associated regulatory failures are uncovered during public inquiries into 'medical scandals'. For example, the cases of Dr Patel in Queensland and Dr Reeves in New South Wales, widely reported in the Australia media, have produced pressures for regulatory reform. An inquiry into public hospitals in Queensland (Davies Report 2005) was triggered by a nurse who, after repeated complaints were ignored by hospital managers, complained to a politician about an incompetent surgeon, Dr Jayant Patel, at the Bundaberg Hospital. Dubbed 'Dr Death' in extensive media coverage, a series of inquiries led to major administrative reforms in the Queensland Health Department and criminal proceedings against Dr Patel (Thomas 2007). The case of a gynaecologist and obstetrician, Dr Graham Reeves, dubbed the 'Butcher of Bega' by the newspapers, has strengthened calls for national medical registration, thorough checks of credentials by employers and a change in New South Wales law, whereby doctors now are legally required to report medical malpractice by colleagues (Hohenboken 2008).

The accumulation of reports about substandard practice and malpractice means that 'leaving it to the doctors' is no longer acceptable to either the state or the public. For example, a series of medical scandals in Britain led the editor of the *British Medical Journal* to declare that the era of regulatory reliance on the medical profession was over: 'all changed, changed utterly' (Smith 1998). New regulatory bodies have been established in England to monitor hospitals and other health services, and the medical governance of doctors is in the process of being transformed under the banner of restoring public trust and ensuring patient safety (Secretary of State for Health 2007).

RESPONSIVE REGULATION

The case for strengthening the regulation of health care is generally accepted. Given the context of the extensive web of existing regulations, the central issue is what regulatory strategies are likely to be effective. Many strategies can be pursued within the existing statutes, but some

6

will require new law or new use of existing law. Others will require new bodies to pursue them, or new standards to be agreed upon. Without a sense of strategy, reform will merely add complexity. This book essentially proposes that the strategy of responsive regulation be taken up to guide both regulatory reform and regulatory practice into the future.

Responsive regulation takes the context, culture and conduct of those being regulated into account (Braithwaite 2002). This is appropriate in the health sector, given its powerful professional cultures of specialised knowledge, its ethical base and its tradition of service to the community (Healy and Braithwaite 2006). Regulatory strategies can be categorised as types of policy instruments (Gunningham and Grabosky 1998), and these are further developed below in relation to the health sector:

- *Voluntarism* is based on an individual or organisation undertaking to do the right thing without any coercion (e.g. a doctor can choose whether to adopt clinical guidelines).
- *Self-regulation* is where an organised group regulates the behaviour of its members (e.g. hospitals agree on industry-level accreditation standards, and medical boards promulgate codes of ethics).
- *Economic instruments* involve supply-side funding sanctions or incentives for providers (e.g. a performance bonus), and demand-side measures that give more power to consumers (e.g. consumer choice of doctor).
- *Co-regulation* involves a partnership between external and internal regulators (e.g. statutory medical tribunals involve the state and the medical profession).
- *Meta-regulation* involves an external regulatory body monitoring the internal regulators to ensure they are regulating satisfactorily (e.g. the Australian Government under the Australian Health Care Agreements could monitor whether the states regulate agreed performance standards in their public hospitals).
- *Command and control* involves enforcement by government or its agents (e.g. imposing sanctions for lack of compliance with licensing and registration laws).

Responsive regulation argues that most regulatory activity should occur at the base of the regulatory pyramid—for example, by encouraging voluntary compliance with agreed standards, and by trying soft words before hard words—the idea being to give cheaper and more respectful options a chance to work first. However, regulators must have the capacity to escalate sanctions in the minority of situations where persuasion fails. The threat of enforcement is a powerful motivator in reinforcing voluntary efforts to improve performance. The pyramid thus offers a way to classify and think about regulatory mechanisms, to identify regulatory gaps and overlaps, and to design a comprehensive regulatory framework (Braithwaite et al. 2005). The strategies and mechanisms discussed throughout this book can be located in such a regulatory pyramid (see Figure 1.1). The diagram does not cover the whole proliferation of regulatory mechanisms, and some mechanisms may be 'soft' or 'hard', depending on their level of authority.

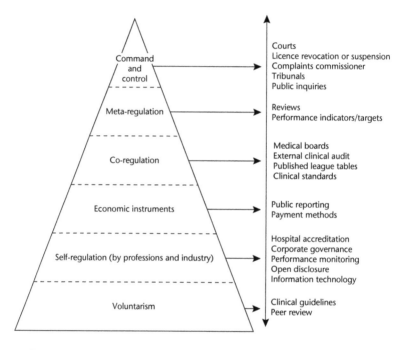

Figure 1.1 Responsive regulation pyramid of strategies and examples of patient safety mechanisms

Source: Healy and Braithwaite (2006): 557

The regulation of clinical performance in the health sector has traditionally occurred at the base of the regulatory pyramid, relying upon voluntary efforts to provide good quality health care on the part of professionals, and upon self-regulation by professional and industry groups. Continuing safety and quality problems show that soft regulation is not enough. Self-regulation by professional and industry groups is being supplemented by co-regulation in partnerships between the state and civil society, and by meta-regulation where authorities monitor whether internal regulation by health departments, professional groups and industry bodies is satisfactory. Continued failures in internal regulation may provoke escalation to command and control, including judicial-style investigations, mandatory standards enforceable through law, and patients seeking recourse through the courts.

A responsive regulator invokes multiple mechanisms since one regulatory mechanism is seldom sufficient; each has its strengths and weaknesses. A two-pyramid model, building on sanctions and strengths, makes clear that rewards motivate just as well as punishments (Braith-waite et al. 2007). However, the application of multiple supports and multiple sanctions requires regulatory sophistication, especially as mechanisms must complement, not conflict. Thus responsive regulators must be smart regulators (Gunningham and Grabosky 1998). They must be flexible in mixing and matching regulatory mechanisms, agile in moving up or down a regulatory pyramid, and innovative in crafting regulatory responses from among an array of supports and sanctions.

TRENDS IN HEALTH SECTOR GOVERNANCE: WHO WATCHES DOCTORS AND HOSPITALS?

Multiple regulators, as well as multiple mechanisms, are a feature of complex regulatory fields—and the complex Australian health sector is particularly difficult to govern (Healy et al. 2006; Duckett 2007). The Australian health sector exemplifies decentred regulation, with the concept, as proposed by Julia Black (2002), defined by five characteristics: complexity, fragmentation, interdependencies, overlapping public and private spheres, and ungovernability. The Australian health field is *complex*, since the many regulators and myriad of regulatees make it difficult to trace regulatory cause and effect. It is also *fragmented*, since power and knowledge are dispersed across public and private spheres and levels of government, so that no one actor possesses all the capacity required to formulate and implement a policy. There are *interdependencies*, since responding to any problem requires action by several actors. There is considerable *overlap* in regulatory activities across levels of government and public and private sectors. Finally, the Australian health care field is often regarded as *ungovernable*, with continual tension between the Australian Government and the states in a federal system of government. As well as this, powerful medical groups often oppose government intervention, while state health departments can be reluctant to demand compliance from prestigious hospitals and doctors.

These decentred characteristics present a regulatory challenge. A responsive regulator in a complex field seeks to engage others in networked governance, since no one regulator acting alone can encompass all aspects of a field or expect to have a substantial impact (Burris et al. 2005). Networked governance involves regulatory conversations in order to arrive at shared views on principles and practices. Regulatory constellations thus form over time as actors gravitate together, develop shared ways of thinking and link separate mechanisms into a web of controls (Jordana and Sancho 2004). An effective governance network takes time to form among scattered regulatory actors, although networks are beginning to form among the different actors in the Australian health sector that are responsible for regulating different types of goods and services: drugs and devices, GP practices, hospitals and other health care facilities, and professionals.

In sketching a policy context for this book, the following history outlines regulatory strategies in relation to general practice, hospitals, professionals and pharmaceuticals (see Table 1.1).

Table 1.1 Examples of regulatory mechanisms

Area	Mechanism (regulator)	Examples
Drugs, devices and procedures	Health technology assessments (national bodies)	Therapeutic Goods Administration approves safety; Pharmaceutical Benefits Advisory Committee (since 1980s) recommends on cost-effective drugs; Medical Services Advisory Committee (since 1988) recommends procedures for Medicare schedule;
GP practices	Accreditation (profession and industry)	Royal College of General Practitioners sets standards; industry bodies (set up from 1997) accredit; Divisions of General Practice funded since the 1990s;
	Professional development	Membership of the Royal College of General Practitioners requires continuing training;

Public hospitals	Legislation (state)	Legislation in each state could regulate safety and quality;
	Budget (state)	Commonwealth and state funds, state administers payment;
	Accreditation (NGO)	NGO established in 1974 sets standards and accredits;
	Administration (state)	Most states run public hospitals so have regulatory powers e.g., to require hospitals to participate in adverse event reporting;
	Management	Hospitals, as employers, implement patient safety practices e.g., credentialling, open disclosure, root cause analyses;
Professionals	Registration (state)	state medical boards—to be a national registration authority;
	Professional development (colleges)	Colleges run professional development programs, mostly voluntary;
	Discipline (states)	Patients can complain to state health care complaints commissioners or professional boards;
	Performance (state laws, peer review)	Health practitioner legislation dates from the nineteenth century, with professional conduct standards strengthened since the 1990s;
	Tort law	Patients take malpractice complaints to court under common law;
	Inquiries (coroner)	State Coroner may inquire into deaths involving medical error.

The *voluntarism* strategy preferred by professionals, who strongly defend their claim to professional autonomy, is being strengthened through mechanisms of persuasion, such as information dissemination and quality assurance activities. Clinical guidelines are increasingly a key regulatory mechanism, although some argue that guidelines should be made standards that carry force (see Chapter 9). Peer review is another key mechanism that is based mostly upon voluntary participation. Peer pressure on professionals for improved practice (at least in hospitals) previously came from team observations on the ward or in the operating theatre, but more pressure now comes from formal peer review and comparisons of patient outcomes data.

Self-regulation by the professions historically has been the main regulatory approach. Medical regulators date back to the nineteenth century, when the medical profession achieved state protection over its title and field of practice and statutory medical boards were established. These boards guard entry to the professions and, under their legislation, set standards, provide guidance and take disciplinary action in egregious cases. In the voluntarist tradition, practitioners are expected, but not required, to keep their knowledge and skills up to date. Registration boards in some countries, and for some parts of the medical profession in some states of Australia, require regular recertification of competence and 'fitness to practise'. Colleges strictly control access to membership and all encourage—though most do not require—continuing professional development.

General practice has been reformed in Australia over the last decade, mostly by encouraging the 6000 or so general practices to self-regulate. For example, from the 1990s the Australian Government has funded Divisions of General Practice to encourage quality assurance activities by peers, while the Royal College of General Practitioners requires members to regularly update their training. The accreditation of GP practices and hospitals is based upon self-regulation by NGOs controlled by the medical profession and industry.

Health departments in the Australian states are tightening their internal regulation of public hospitals, not least because most states (Victoria is an exception—see Chapter 5) have abolished autonomous hospital boards and brought hospitals back under ministerial control. As employers, hospitals exert considerable control over the practice of hospital health care. Many patient safety mechanisms must be put in place in hospitals, where accountability is diffuse and management proceeds through committees, not lines of command.

Market instruments are little used to regulate clinical performance in the Australian health sector, in contrast to pay for performance schemes in the United States and the United Kingdom. As health care is mainly government funded, governments potentially have the power to use various payment mechanisms to regulate doctors and hospitals. However, market principles are applied to regulation, such as the need to argue on economic grounds for any regulatory change, and the need to scrutinise proposals in terms of impact upon efficiency and constraints upon competition. Consumers have powers of exit or voice (Hirschman 1970). Sometimes patients can exit (by going to another doctor or hospital), and increasingly they are raising their voices (by complaining to professional boards and complaints commissioners).

General practice is the exception. The Practice Incentives Program provides financial incentives for accreditation and a range of quality-oriented activities, and the Medicare Benefits Scheme pays a higher benefit to GPs who participate in continuing medical education. These measures have attracted very high participation levels among general practitioners and enjoy the support of most parts of the medical profession. They show that such economic incentives can be built into the regulatory mix in Australia in a powerful way, and can be expected to work well in other parts of the medical profession.

Increasingly, *co-regulation* with the state is invoked in order to strengthen regulation. Most state government health departments have set up a penumbra of advisory committees with members from the professions and health industry. However, industry and professional groups are less trusted to regulate members and peers. For example, some states have transferred disciplinary decisions from medical boards to independent medical tribunals.

Meta-regulators have been established in many countries—notably in the United Kingdom, given its National Health Service—but Australia generally prefers advisory bodies. The Australian Commission for Safety Quality in Health Care was set up in 2006 as an advisory body to the Australian Conference of Health Ministers (similar to its precursor council established in 2000). The Council of Australian Governments (COAG) is taking more interest in health care governance in a federal system of government. For example, COAG in 2007 agreed to establish a national registration scheme to cover nine health professions subject to statutory registration in all jurisdictions: medicine, nursing, physiotherapy, dentistry, pharmacy, optometry, chiropractic, osteopathy and psychology (Council of Australian Governments 2007). Some state governments, notably New South Wales and Queensland, have strengthened oversight of health care by establishing statutory bodies, including building upon or supplementing the statutory complaints commissioners.

Command and control, or enforcement, is little used in the health sector except in egregious cases. Compared with the United States, Australia has not passed a large or coherent body of patient safety law, although many state laws might be applied to patient safety. For example, legislation pertaining to professional conduct was strengthened in the 1990s. Aggrieved patients also can seek recourse in tort law if they are willing to take malpractice complaints to the courts—although the impact upon patient safety generally is arguable.

The regulation of pharmaceuticals is not covered in this book except to note that Australia is a world leader in this area (Jackson 2007). The point made here is that the Australian Government, which funds the Pharmaceutical Benefits Scheme (PBS), regulates the safety and quality of drugs and devices through command and control, and economic instruments. In contrast to medical goods, health services and professionals generally are not regulated from the top of the regulatory pyramid.

This overview of trends illustrates the interconnected nature of regulatory mechanisms. An intervention in one area thus can cause perturbation throughout a web of regulatory controls, and unintended ripples may have a significant impact.

THE CHAPTERS

The contributors discuss regulatory mechanisms being tried in Australia and internationally, and examine what is known about their impact upon patient safety. They identify promising paths for improving the safety and quality of health care for patients. The chapters, organised within the responsive regulation pyramid, begin with voluntary strategies and proceed to enforcement strategies. These discussions of regulatory experiences illustrate increasing external intervention by the state to strengthen health sector accountability and restore public trust, a growing demand from the state and the public for transparency, and an exploration of creative ways to reduce risks to patient safety. The chapters also show that health care regulation is an interdisciplinary enterprise that draws upon legal, economic, political, administrative and cultural regulatory instruments, with the chapters being written by lawyers, economists, sociologists, nurses and medical practitioners.

John Braithwaite (Chapter 2) sets the scene by discussing the many options available to a health care regulator, drawing upon both a sanctions-based and a strengths-based pyramid, with examples drawn from his major study of regulation in the nursing home industry in Australia, the United Kingdom and the United States. Braithwaite argues that there is no need to rely on a single and powerful regulator to make responsive regulation work in a knowledge society. A persuasive and innovative practitioner can 'lead from behind' by enlisting colleagues and superiors into a network of governance—as did Nurse Response in his hypothetical example.

Bruce Barraclough and his fellow authors (Chapter 3) outline the array of improvement strategies underway in many countries, especially where governments and international organisations regard patient safety as a 'public value', as did the Council of Europe in its comprehensive recommendations in 2006. While the emphasis differs across countries, seven strategies are being applied internationally to improve the quality and safety of health care for patients: accreditation, pay for performance, information, education, leadership, the law, and systems redesign around patient-centred care.

Heather Buchan, Niall Johnson and Christopher Baggoley (Chapter 4) discuss the considerable and voluntary efforts of groups of Australian clinicians in seeking to improve the quality of clinical practice. Research collaboratives are popular, although there is little research so far on their effectiveness. Australia has been a leader in establishing clinical registers (databases of health-related information on individuals) that monitor and evaluate treatment outcomes. Clinical guidelines are being developed in many areas, and efforts are being made to increase their modest uptake and so improve patient outcomes.

Heather Wellington and Paul Dugdale (Chapter 5) discuss the difficulties of managing hospitals, with their professional subcultures, entrenched traditions and the market forces that make hospital managers tread warily when attempting to regulate the performance of doctors. There are also state-based differences in how hospitals are governed in the context of different public sector cultures.

Stephen Duckett (Chapter 6) outlines the efforts in Queensland Health to roll out policy changes across the state in the wake of scathing criticisms by public inquiries of the management of Queensland's hospitals. Whatever the faults of a huge unitary bureaucracy where line management stretches from the Director-General down to a clerk in a hospital admissions office, central control means that changes can be put in motion. Queensland Health has sought to change its clinical governance arrangements, leadership behaviour and workplace culture. The values underpinning these changes are accountability, transparency and participation.

Kieran Walshe (Chapter 7) discusses the perennial tensions between the interests of professionals and the interests of the public, with reforms internationally leaning unequivocally towards the public interest. The governance of professionals is being overhauled, in the context of an expanding number of occupational groups seeking recognition from the state, greater professional mobility between countries, and workforce reforms that are changing the skill mix and redesigning work roles and functions. The United Kingdom offers a fascinating case study due to its recent far-reaching reforms to the regulation of the professions.

Ian Freckelton (Chapter 8) provides a Senior Counsel's legal view on contemporary developments in the jurisprudence of the law around legal entities such as medical boards, tribunals, ombudsmen and coroners. In particular, he tracks the shift from investigations based on establishing fault and meting out discipline, towards other approaches aimed at improving performance of the practitioner and even the health system. While these newer approaches may retain an adversarial legal character, they have an important role to play within a responsive regulatory network, and show a stronger connection to the various levels of such networks than the older, disciplinary style of legal regulation of health professionals.

William Runciman and Judy Lumby (Chapter 9) continue the case for using clinical standards, and argue that they can offer both force and practical support for implementation as a routine. This chapter provides a useful list of the clinical practice guidelines agreed by the top advisory bodies of the United States, United Kingdom and Australia, which show how much potential there is for biological impact on population health if regulation is used to drive better quality care.

Justin Oakley and Steve Clarke (Chapter 10) discuss the practice and ethics of public reporting on surgical practice, including success and death rates. In a sense, this is about allowing the evidence on practice excellence and problem practice to see the light of day and illuminate choice by patients, clinical governance by managers and continuous improvement by the professionals concerned. Part of the value of the chapter is the careful presentation of the arguments against publication of surgical report cards, including the unintended consequences for patients and professionals that can result.

David Studdert (Chapter 11) discusses open disclosure of medical injury more generally. This can be a confusing area of law at the intersection of professional pride and fear, malpractice insurance and litigation. The chapter provides a very clear rundown of the arguments, evidence and architecture of laws around open disclosure, including how they mesh with other regulatory developments.

As a practising lawyer, David Hirsch (Chapter 12) rounds off the collection of legal chapters. He makes a lucid argument in defence of litigation by patients against doctors and hospitals, and reminds us about some of the basics in society concerning what people can and should not do to each other, and the importance of mechanisms to redress wrongdoing. The chapter also outlines some of the logic of litigation law that should be better understood in the professional community.

Jenny Berrill and Judith Healy (Chapter 13) address the theory and practice of hospital regulation through accreditation and like approaches. They provide a taxonomy of the constellation of regulatory mechanisms applied to hospitals, and a discussion of current trends toward improving the responsiveness of hospital regulation.

Peter Sprivulis (Chapter 14) discusses current and planned developments in electronic health information systems (e-health), showing how they work as part of the regulatory framework for health services. The chapter provides a number of illustrations of how e-health initiatives create value—improved clinical care—through broad-based regulatory strategies, developed through consensus, but given force in their implementation.

The final chapter, by Malcolm Masso and Kathy Eagar, looks at the role of public inquiries in improving safety and quality of care. Such inquiries are necessarily bound up with the partisan politics of the day wherever they are conducted, but often identify problems and solutions of far wider import and application. However, their effectiveness in bringing about practical local improvements in health service safety and quality requires a sustained, and ideally bipartisan, political commitment to health service improvement, which is easily overshadowed in the current political environment.

TRUST, TRANSPARENCY AND CREATIVITY

These chapters document the array of regulatory reforms that are underway in the health sector. Health policy debates have gained renewed vigour with Australia's change of national government in late 2007—the first in eleven years. Drawing on Kingdon's (1984) model, three streams are converging that have pushed patient safety forward on the government policy agenda: the problem stream (recognition of a significant problem), the politics stream (active advocates for change) and the policy stream (policy solutions being available). Shakespeare said it more succinctly in *Julius Caesar*: 'There is a tide in the affairs of men ...' These chapters offer lessons for formulating and implementing patient safety regulatory reforms, and some common themes emerge in relation to trust, transparency and creativity.

The first theme is *trust*. The erosion of trust in the willingness of professional and industry bodies to regulate their members has prompted calls for greater external accountability to the state and the public. The chapters in this book document the greater accountability now expected from professionals and health care provider organisations. First, regulators want to be able to trust those they regulate—and this is a key issue in the regulation of health professionals. Responsive regulation begins from the assumption that most people are trustworthy most of the time. Regulators sometimes encounter ill-will, of course, and must find ways of dealing with those who refuse to comply with reasonable protocols, preferably before they become a hazard to their patients. To be responsive, a regulator needs to understand the professional and organisational cultures involved. Professionals and services also protest that they are over-worked and under-resourced, so regulation must avoid imposing an unreasonable burden. This book provides insight into the human drama of health care gone wrong, whether in a courtroom or a professional tribunal, or in the management of hospital doctors.

Second, regulatees are more likely to trust and respond positively to regulators if they are able to participate in regulatory decisions. Increasingly, health practitioners are trained to identify patient safety risks and solutions, and are involved in trialling whether an intervention works as expected. For example, regulators and practitioners together can better decide whether to embark on a 'big-bang' reform or to proceed at the usual glacial pace.

The main rationale for patient safety reform, however, is that members of the public want to trust their doctors and hospitals. A former president of the UK General Medical Council, in arguing the case for more effective professional regulation, has expressed the general public sentiment well:

'All patients want good doctors they can trust.'(Irvine 2007: 256)

Transparency is the second theme, and the Australian health sector has been very slow to embrace transparency as a regulatory principle. There is increasing pressure for more transparency in internal regulatory decisions, such as open disclosure to patients of adverse events, publication of medical tribunal reports, and public reporting on the performance of hospitals and doctors. Australian health regulators and health providers generally leave patients in the dark when it comes to regulatory decisions, since traditionally such deliberations—including disciplinary determinations about doctors—have been regarded as 'secret doctors' business' (Healy et al. 2008). Medical governance in many countries is being pushed to be more transparent and hence more accountable:'The trend is for medical regulatory bodies to demonstrate more transparency in their processes and ways of working and to become more accountable to external authorities.' (Chief Medical Officer 2006: 112)

The final theme is *creativity*. Transparency is important if we are to learn from creativity. The concept of 'democratic experimentalism' argues that transparency is a pragmatic choice for managers in the information age, since it enables them to learn from innovative experiments underway elsewhere (Dorf and Sabel 1998). Comparisons that draw on the diversity of experience across hospitals and across the Australian states should be seen in positive terms, as a learning opportunity. The first point is that regulatory schemes must be careful not to stifle creativity and aspirations to achieve ongoing improvement. As John Braithwaite argues persuasively in Chapter 2, many of the improvements in safety and quality depend upon the daily decisions made by health care professionals. Lipsky's (1980) findings hold as true for doctors and nurses as they do for public sector workers: decisions are made in the daily practice of street-level bureaucrats rather than through operational circulars issued by head office. While hospital management sets the framework, signs the contracts and employs the workforce, it cannot tightly control what happens in the myriad of rapid care decisions that are made on a patient case-by-case basis by health professionals. Creativity might be termed cunning, of course, and this can have positive or negative expression. Oakley and Clarke (Chapter 10) discuss the many examples of practitioners and managers 'gaming the system' in relation to the public reporting of performance indicators. Some medical practitioners are experts in maximising their earnings through the byzantine regulations of the Medicare schedule.

The second point is that it is often surprising how policies are applied. Health professionals are very creative in applying schemes in ways that the people who designed them had not expected. Further, health system policies are context dependent, and a scheme that works in one place might not function well in another. This presents a major challenge to standardisation as a patient safety strategy. A set of practice guidelines developed in one hospital may not work in another. Regulatory guidelines also need to be continually reinvented, given rapid changes—such as new technology—in the health care environment. A related point is that the practice of health care is changing rapidly, and health systems are never static. Regulatory frameworks and strategies therefore must have the capacity for continual adaptation and reinvention.

CONCLUSION

The goal of improving health is a powerful motivator in human affairs. It drives a significant portion of scientific endeavour, public expenditure and commercial enterprise. The importance of this book lies in the somewhat unfashionable recognition of the importance of the administrative arts in creating and delivering value through health improvement. This is particularly important because of the scale, politics and essential dangerousness of health care. Within the administrative arts, regulation is concerned with the operation of power and influence, so will always be contentious and subject to reform and innovation. We hope that this book provides some insight into what regulatory reform is important and how it can be progressed, and that it will contribute to the evolution of a more responsive regulatory environment for the provision of health care in the coming years.

REFERENCES

Australian Council for Safety and Quality in Health Care (2005), 'High risk medication alert: Vincristine',<www.health.gov.au/internet/safety/publishing. nsf/Content/vincristine>, accessed 10 February 2009

Australian Institute of Health and Welfare 2006, *Australia's Health 2006*, Australian Institute of Health and Welfare, Canberra

Ayres, I. and Braithwaite, J. 1992, *Responsive Regulation: Transcending the Regulation Debate*, Oxford University Press, Oxford

Baker, G., Norton, P., Flintoft, V., Blais, R., Brown, A., Cox, J., Etchells, E., Ghali, W., Hebert, P., Majumdar, S., O'Beirne, M., Palacios-Derflingher, L., Reid, R.J., Sheps, S. and Tamblyn, R. 2004, 'The Canadian Adverse Events Study: The incidence of adverse events among hospital patients in Canada', *Canadian Medical Association Journal*, vol. 170, no. 11, pp. 1678–86

Black, J. 2002, 'Critical reflections on regulation', *Australian Journal of Legal Philosophy*, vol. 27, pp. 1–35

Braithwaite, J. 2002, *Restorative Justice and Responsive Regulation*, Oxford University Press, Oxford

Braithwaite, J., Healy, J. and Dwan, K. 2005, *The Governance of Health Care Safety and Quality*, Commonwealth of Australia, Canberra

Braithwaite, J., Makkai, T. and Braithwaite, V. 2007, *Regulating Aged Care: Ritualism and the New Pyramid*, Edward Elgar, Cheltenham

Brennan, T., Leape, L., Laird, N., Hebert, L., Localio, A., Lawthers, A., Newhouse, J., Weiler, P. and Hiatt, H. 1991, 'Incidence of adverse events and negligence in hospitalized patients', *New England Journal of Medicine*, vol. 324, no. 6, pp. 370-6

Burris, S., Drahos, P. and Shearing, C. 2005, 'Nodal governance', *Australian Journal of Legal Philosophy*, vol. 30, pp. 30-58

Chief Medical Officer 2006, *Good Doctors: Safer Patients: Proposals to Strengthen the System to Assure and Improve the Performance of Doctors and to Protect the Safety of Patients*, Department of Health, London

Council of Australian Governments (COAG) 2007, *Council of Australian Governments Meeting Communique*, COAG, Canberra

Davies Report 2005, *Queensland Public Hospitals Commission of Inquiry Report*, State of Queensland, Brisbane

Dorf, M. and Sabel, C. 1998, 'A constitution of democratic experimentalism', *Columbia Law Review*, vol. 98, no. 2, pp. 267-473

Duckett, S. 2007, *The Australian Health Care System*, Oxford University Press, Melbourne

Ehsani, J., Jackson, T. and Duckett, S. 2006, 'The incidence and cost of adverse events in Victorian hospitals 2003-04', *Medical Journal of Australia*, vol. 184, no. 11, pp. 551-5

Gunningham, N. and Grabosky, P. 1998, *Smart Regulation: Designing Environmental Policy*, Clarendon Press, Oxford

Healy, J. and Braithwaite, J. 2006, 'Designing safer health care through responsive regulation', *Medical Journal of Australia*, vol. 184, no. 10, pp. S56-9

Healy, J., Maffi, C. and Dugdale, P. 2008, 'A national medical register: Balancing public transparency and professional privacy', *Medical Journal of Australia*, vol. 188, no. 4, pp. 247-9

Healy, J., Sharman, E. and Lokuge, B. 2006, 'Australia: Health system review', *Health Systems in Transition*, vol. 8, no. 5, pp. 1-155

Hirschman, A. 1970, *Exit, Voice and Loyalty: Responses to Decline in Firms, Organizations and States*, Harvard University Press, Cambridge, MA

Hohenboken, A. 2008, 'Charges urged for "Butcher of Bega" Graham Reeves', *The Australian*, 31 July

Institute of Medicine 2004, *Patient Safety: Achieving a New Standard of Care*, Institute of Medicine, The National Academies Press, Washington, DC

Irvine, D. 2007, 'Everyone is entitled to a good doctor', *Medical Journal of Australia*, vol. 186, no. 5, pp. 256-61

Jackson, T. 2007, 'Health technology assessment in Australia: challenges ahead', *Medical Journal of Australia*, vol. 187, no. 5, pp. 262–4

Jordana, J. and Sancho, D. 2004, 'Regulatory designs, institutional constellations and the study of the regulatory state', in *The Politics of Regulation: Institutions and Regulatory Reforms for the Age of Governance*, eds J. Jordana and D. Levi-Faur, Edward Elgar, Cheltenham, UK, pp. 296–320

Kingdon, J. 1984, *Agendas, Alternatives and Public Policies*, Little Brown and Co, Boston

Leape, L. and Davis, K. 2005, 'To err is human; to fail to improve is unconscionable', *The Commonwealth Fund: From the President*, New York

Lipsky, M. 1980, *Street-Level Bureaucracy: Dilemmas of the Individual in Public Services*, Russell Sage Foundation, New York

McLoughlin, V., Leatherman, S., Fletcher, M. and Wyn Owen, J. 2001, 'Improving performance using indicators: Recent experience in the United States, the United Kingdom, and Australia', *International Journal for Quality in Health Care*, vol. 13, no. 6, pp. 455–62

Medical Tribunal of New South Wales, 2006, *In the Matter of Dr A.*, No. 400131/05, <www.nswmb.org.au/index.pl?page=127>, accessed 15 June 2008

Osborne, D. and Gaebler, T. 1992, *Reinventing Government: How the Entrepreneurial Spirit is Transforming the Public Sector*, Addison-Wesley, Boston

Osborne, T. 1993, 'History of the human sciences', *Economy and Society*, vol. 22, no. 3, pp. 345–56

Reason, J. 2000, 'Human error: Models and management', *British Medical Journal*, vol. 320, no. 7237, pp. 768–70

Runciman, W. and Moller, J. 2001, *Iatrogenic Injury in Australia*, Australian Patient Safety Foundation, Adelaide

Runciman, W., Webb, R., Phelps, S., Thomas, E., Sexton, E., Studdent, D. and Brennan, T. 2000, 'A comparison of iatrogenic injury studies in Australia and the USA. II: Reviewer behaviour and quality of care', *International Journal of Quality in Health Care*, vol. 12, no. 5, pp. 379–88

Secretary of State for Health 2007, *Trust, Assurance and Safety—The Regulation of Health Professionals in the 21st Century*, The Stationery Office, London

Shojania, K., Duncan, B., McDonald, K. and Wachter, R. 2001, *Making Health Care Safer: A Critical Analysis of Patient Safety Practices*, Agency for Healthcare Research and Quality, Rockville, MD

Smith, R. 1998, 'All changed, changed utterly', *British Medical Journal*, vol. 316, no. 7149, pp. 1917–18

Sparrow, M. 2000, *The Regulatory Craft: Controlling Risks, Solving Problems and Managing Compliance*, The Brookings Institution, Washington, DC

Thomas, E.J., Studdert, D.M., Runciman, W.B., Webb, R., Sexton, E., Wilson, R., Gibberd, R., Harrison, B. and Brennan, T. 2000, 'A comparison of iatrogenic injury studies in Australia and the USA I: context, methods, casemix, population, patient and hospital characteristics', *International Journal for Quality in Health Care*, vol. 12, no. 5, pp. 371-8

Thomas, H. 2007, *Sick to Death*, Allen & Unwin, Sydney

Vincent, C., Neale, G. and Woloshynowych, M. 2001, 'Adverse events in British hospitals: Preliminary retrospective record review', *British Medical Journal*, vol. 7285, no. 322, pp. 517-19

Wilson, R.M. and Van Der Weyden, M. 2005, 'The safety of Australian healthcare: 10 years after QAHCS', *Medical Journal of Australia*, vol. 182, no. 6, pp. 260-1

World Health Organization 2004, *World Report on Knowledge for Better Health: Strengthening Health Systems*, World Health Organization, Geneva

World Health Organization World Alliance for Patient Safety 2007, *Patient Safety Solutions*, <www.who.int/patientsafety/solutions/en>, accessed 2 May 2008

2

LEADING FROM BEHIND WITH PLURAL REGULATION

John Braithwaite

One of the concerns often expressed about responsive regulation applied to health (Braithwaite et al. 2005) is that no single regulator is responsible for the Australian health system. So who is to make the regulatory pyramid described by Healy and Dugdale in Chapter 1 work? This chapter shows how decentred regulation of health safety (Black 2002) does not necessarily involve a crisis of ungovernability, only of top-down governability. A nurse's eye view of this challenge is explored. It is conceived as a challenge for multi-level governance that works through nodes which decisively coordinate improvement.

A NURSE'S EYE VIEW OF RESPONSIVE REGULATION

Nurse Response is not a nurse manager. She is an ordinary nurse recently assigned to work with Dr Good and Nurse Deed. The Good–Deed team is generally conscientious, competent and caring with patients. But Nurse Response notices immediately on joining the pair that they have been quite sloppy in their compliance with an important protocol. Nurse Response decides to respond with support to assist compliance. After a procedure completed somewhat sloppily with regard to the protocol, and after Dr Good fails to record things she should, according to the protocol, Nurse Response says: 'If you don't mind, I'll write this into the patient's notes because I'm a bit of a stickler for the protocol. I don't mind doing it because I know you are so busy, Dr Good. It's just that my experiences have convinced me if we all follow this protocol all the time, every once in a blue moon it will save a life. So I feel uncomfortable not doing it.'

The next time our brave nurse works with the Good–Deed team on this procedure, the sloppiness is gone. An exemplary job is done and Dr Good completes all aspects of protocol record-keeping herself. As they wash up, Nurse Response says to Good and Deed that she really admired aspects of how well they completed the procedure. She also says she really likes working with them because they show her professional respect even though they are more medically knowledgeable than her.

Nurse Response leads from behind

At a subsequent care planning meeting with Good, Deed and many others, Nurse Response says she is pleased to see that, across both floors on which she works, compliance with this protocol is improving. Again she explains why she cares about it. She asks whether the team could keep statistics on protocol compliance to show whether they are capable of moving it up from the current level of compliance, which she guesses to be 70 per cent, to 100 per cent. Can they also plot incidents of the kind of infection the protocol is designed to prevent? They agree. A year later, compliance has moved from 70 to 100 per cent and incidence of infection has fallen. Dr Good writes a little memo on this outcome, which management circulates around the entire hospital. Soon, almost everyone in the hospital is taking the protocol seriously. A hospital-wide study documents an association between a move to 98 per cent compliance over the next few years with reduction in the incidence of infection, but also with an unexpected benefit not previously documented. Through this unexpected benefit, Dr Brilliant from the hospital's management team sees a way that the protocol can be both simplified and improved. Dr Brilliant writes all this up and publishes in a journal which is read by Inspector Rex from the Health Department. Rex gets the improved, simplified protocol implemented, as recommended by Brilliant. He emails all hospitals in the state a copy of Brilliant's paper. This is part of the campaign Rex shares with Nurse Response to improve compliance with this protocol. Triple-loop learning (Parker 2002) is occurring here—from the Good–Deed team to all the teams on their two floors, to the entire hospital, to the whole hospital system.

Nurse Response is only a little cog in the hospital machine, but she knows she has 'led from behind'[1]—and, of course, she looks on with pride at these developments. Nurse Response then organises her senior colleagues to support the nomination of Dr Brilliant for an Order of Australia. She makes a special plea that the citation their peers will read in the Australia Day morning newspapers says 'For contributions to health quality and safety' rather than the more usual contributions to a traditional discipline of medicine. She wants the nation to recognise the lives that can be saved by the leadership Brilliant has shown for safety and quality, rather than Brilliant's official positions in the college and profession. Perhaps a citation quite like this has never occurred for an Order of Australia. This is not a true story! It is one that illustrates the possibility, not the probability, that even the most junior cog in the medical machine can lead from behind at all levels of the pyramid of supports (also described as a strengths-building pyramid) in Figure 2.1 (below). Before we get misty-eyed about our hero's triumphs, albeit not taking the credit, a darker phase of her professional life is about to unfold.

Nurse Response is restructured and punished

Unfortunately, Nurse Response is caught up in one of the perennial hospital restructures of her CEO, Mr Shuffle. She arrives at work to be told she has been reassigned to work with Dr Bad and Nurse Seed. Bad thinks the protocol is just another Shuffle conspiracy to make their professional lives a bureaucratic misery. When Nurse Response tries to support him in completing the protocol, he humiliates her in front of colleagues for 'wasting time on paperwork and bureaucratic make-work' when she should be concentrating on delivering nursing care. She tries again and again to reason in evidence-based ways about the benefits of the protocol. Each time, she is put down. Ultimately, she draws a deep breath and complains about Bad–Seed protocol compliance to their supervisor, Dr No. No tells her that Bad is a hospital hero for standing up to Shuffle's silly systems. Who is she to question such an experienced clinician?

Our hero is a determined woman. Shaking with trepidation, she fronts Mr Shuffle's office to discuss the Bad–Seed non-compliance and what Dr No said in response to her complaint. Shuffle chews her out, railing against junior staff who bring problems that should be sorted in the ward and points to his priority, the next restructure pasted on computer printouts around his office wall. Over drinks and tears that night, Dr Good and Nurse Deed counsel Nurse Response to let go. There is nothing more she can do. She rejects their advice, deciding to bide her time and hope that perhaps one day Dr Good will be promoted into Dr No's job. But Response also has fine detective skills that open an opportunity earlier than she expected. These skills enable her to connect a case of blatant protocol non-compliance to an adverse event that costs a patient their life. Dr No has managed to cover the tracks of this connection so that the patient's family never discovers why their loved one died. She writes a brief of evidence on the adverse event and its non-recording, but Mr Shuffle seems to lose it in the pile of paper in his in-tray. During the month when she hears nothing back from Shuffle's office, Dr Bad trumps up a case of professional negligence against Nurse Response. She is pilloried by her peers for it. Then she takes her complaint to the Health Department, who sits on it after being told by Shuffle that Nurse Response is only making this complaint because the hospital is taking disciplinary action against her for negligence. Nurse Response then meets with the family of the deceased patient. Their solicitor commences a suit against the hospital and conducts a press conference on the circumstances of the death. The Minister for Health sees it on television and carpets Shuffle for failing to heed the well-known research of Dr Brilliant. Shuffle then publicly apologises for the adverse event, demotes Dr No, replacing him with Dr Good, settles with the family and leads compliance reform. Shuffle survives long enough to persist with revenge against Nurse Response for her alleged negligence. She commits suicide. Dr Brilliant does not attend her funeral because he is busy preparing a plenary address for a health safety and quality conference.

Nurse Response as a practitioner of networked governance

Sadly, your author is no Dickens. The point of my tale is to show that a Dickensian lens helps us to see the full range of opportunities and risks a little person confronts in moving up both a pyramid of sanctions and a pyramid of supports (see Figure 2.1). We could actually move lower down the health system hierarchy and illustrate how a cleaner or a patient might move up both pyramids of supports and of sanctions. Yes, a cleaner or a patient can educatively support a doctor by pointing out the doctor has forgotten to sterilise something that might cause infection. And they can complain and trigger legal and regulatory enforcement action in the way Nurse Response did. Of course, it is true that as we move up the health system hierarchy from nurse to nurse manager to senior doctor to hospital CEO to health department CEO, we shift to players with greater capacity to regulate responsively in a way that makes a difference.

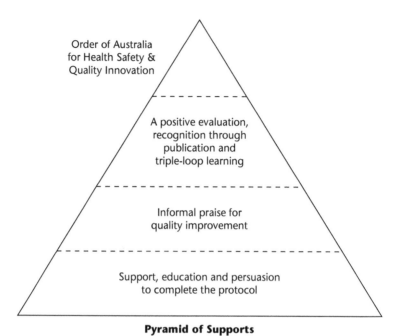

Order of Australia
for Health Safety &
Quality Innovation

A positive evaluation,
recognition through
publication and
triple-loop learning

Informal praise for
quality improvement

Support, education and persuasion
to complete the protocol

Pyramid of Supports

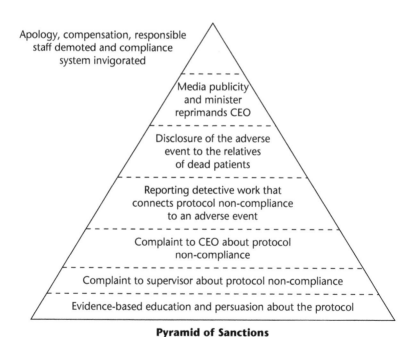

Apology, compensation, responsible
staff demoted and compliance
system invigorated

Media publicity
and minister
reprimands CEO

Disclosure of the adverse
event to the relatives
of dead patients

Reporting detective work that
connects protocol non-compliance
to an adverse event

Complaint to CEO about protocol
non-compliance

Complaint to supervisor about protocol non-compliance

Evidence-based education and persuasion about the protocol

Pyramid of Sanctions

Figure 2.1 How Nurse Response networks up pyramids of supports and sanctions

RESPONSIVE REGULATION AND NETWORKED GOVERNANCE

Responsive regulation calls for the networked governance of health care safety and quality. Nurse Response can no more do it on her own than can the Minister for Health. Nugget Coombs exercised more effective power for social change in his life than any Australian prime minister, by 'leading from behind'. He accomplished that by enrolling people both below and above him in the hierarchy of Australian governance. Miraculously, Nelson Mandela managed to lead from behind in a prison cell for 27 years. Change occurs through both the weak enrolling the strong (Latour 1986, 1987), and the strong enrolling weaker players, who then become bridges to the enrolment of different kinds of strength. The 'strength of weak ties' (Granovetter 1974) is a key to social change. This means, for example, that a single person who has weak ties to two separate tightly interwoven networks of power can couple those two networks for a project or social change. Intriguingly, Dupont (2006: 53) found in a study of networks of security in Montreal that 52 per cent of the bridges that linked together different organisational actors, such as police departments, private security firms, university security departments, professional associations, political actors, intelligence agencies and government departments, were single individuals. For 81 per cent of links, the contact points were three or fewer individuals. In the real world of networked governance, as in the fictional world of Nurse Response, weak single actors can forge the links that can escalate networked private–public action for change.

This is why the pyramid of networked escalation, adapted from the work of present and former ANU colleagues Peter Drahos, Scott Burris and Clifford Shearing (see Drahos 2004; Burris et al. 2005), is an important idea for thinking about how to improve safety and quality. Figure 2.2 captures the idea that, instead of escalating from less to more intrusive or punitive interventions as we fail to get improvement through evidence-based dialogue at the base of the pyramid, we can escalate by enrolling more and more powerful players into the dialogue until we get the movement desired. The ways of escalating are limited only by the networking imaginations of the Nurse Responses and Dr Goods of this world. This means there is no 'cookbook' for how to do responsive regulation well, and no corporate plan that the Mr Shuffles of this world can lay down to guarantee improvement. It is an accomplishment of problem-focused and strength-based networking more than structure-oriented reorganisation. Creative perseverance delivers it. Rootless, reiterative restructuring is unlikely to do so.

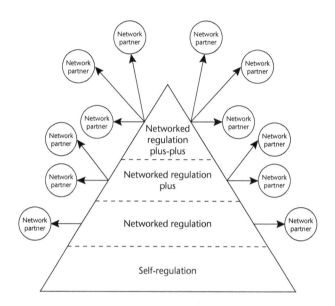

Figure 2.2 A pyramid of networked escalation

Source: Adapted from Drahos (2004).

I do not mean to suggest that strategic planning does not matter. I do mean to say, following Castells (1996), that strategic planning of agencies like health departments matters much less than it did in the heyday of Fordist production, when better top-down ordering of chaotic production systems could deliver large improvements. Organisations like hospitals have long since accrued some benefits of basic Fordist production line reforms, which see things done in a systematic way—like clean sheets routinely put on beds and the correct pills delivered on trolleys to the correct patients. The biggest further improvements may now come from governance at ad hoc nodes where networks of action are pulled together—like Nurse Response using a care planning meeting to advance her protocol project. They will also come from leadership from behind, as Mandela put it, rather than from the top.

Yes, strategic planning still matters—but in a highly qualified way. There is no point in the health department developing a strategic plan to do X when the powerful medical colleges and the Australian Nursing Federation have plans to deliver not-X. Health safety and quality improves as an interactive accomplishment of the actions of many types of organisations—professions, pharmaceutical companies, hospitals, laundries, university teachers and researchers, general practices, health departments, self-regulatory organisations, consumer watchdogs in civil society, the Australian Competition and Consumer Commission, the Ombudsman, and so on. Les Metcalfe's (1994) insight about the era of networked governance is that each of the key organisational actors focused on solving a particular problem must do their strategic planning in a way that is responsive to the strategic planning of other organisational actors focused on that problem. Clever corporate plans are crafted to align with other corporate plans, whether complementary or competitive. Smart planning creates synergies so that the combined effects of strategic plans to solve a problem are greater than the sum of the effects of the separate plans.

The galaxy of organisational players impinging on a particular problem is constantly changing in a knowledge economy where technological change puts new players on the scene with dazzling frequency. This is why responsive regulators must constantly be assembling new nodes of governance that work for a while in coordinating new improvements to health safety and quality. For example, 30 years ago it was rarely necessary to include software developers in nodes of governance to improve health safety and quality; today it often is. Sometimes developers of hand-held digital record-keeping hardware even have a place.

No environment brings more professions and more complex new technologies together in one space than a modern hospital. Patients are also more intractable subjects of these technologies than, say, the physical subjects of Silicon Valley innovation. Patients get up when told to lie down, lie down when told to get up, get upset when told to be calm, spit out pills and swallow hidden bottles of alcohol. Most of all, they simply do not understand or forget to do things as part of their therapeutic journey, especially if they are old, as many patients are. It follows that improved outcomes are fundamentally a feat of persuasion and understanding at all levels. Nodal governance is about bringing strategic players together at a relevant site of deliberation—around a bed, in a minister's office, at an international conference—to caress and cajole engagement with the project of health improvement.

Practitioners at all levels must show leadership to diagnose how and where today's blockages to achieving safety and quality are occurring. Only leadership from below can achieve this when the blockage is at the level of patient resistance. When the blockage is at lower and middling levels of health system hierarchies, blockages can often be removed by widening the circle. RegNet empirical research in health care and in other domains shows this is one of the things that master practitioners of regulation do (Braithwaite et al. 2007). When a government inspector sits down with employees of an organisation to fix a problem of non-compliance, they are quite often dismissed. Employees dig their heels in and the problem is not fixed. Instead of escalating up a regulatory pyramid immediately in response to such defiance—perhaps by prosecuting them—the smart regulator (Gunningham and Grabosky 1998) will often adjourn the meeting, give their defiance a chance to cool and encourage them to come back with new lateral thinking to fix the problem. If they do not, the node of governance can be reconvened with their boss in the circle. If their boss is an even tougher nut, even more resistantly defiant (Braithwaite 2009) than their subordinates, then the circle can be widened again to include the boss's boss, then the boss's boss's boss. Like our hero, Nurse Response, we might need to widen the circle right up to the chairman of the board, as has been documented in cases in the regulatory literature (Fisse and Braithwaite 1993: 230–7), or even the minister, before we find an actor willing to consider the evidence base.

If we widen the circle of dialogue right up to the top of the executive chain, without eliciting evidence-based responsiveness to protecting the community, then the ethics of responsive regulation require us to escalate. Escalation may even have to be up through the judicial branch of governance in search of the judge who will apply the law to the evidence about risks to the community. We might conceive recourse to the legal system as an ethical duty of our profession if we are ethically committed to being an evidence-based health professional. In real cases, like that of Dr Patel at Bundaberg Hospital, and as in the fictional case of Nurse Response, there are brave nurses, like Toni Hoffman, who refuse to be fobbed off by their CEO. For those who are not health professionals—for victims, their families, crusading public-interest lawyers or health consumer activists—there is no ethical duty to widen the circle of dialogue and escalate up the enforcement pyramid when patient safety is jeopardised. But when non-professionals do pursue their concerns, they are ethical heroes.

Likewise, patients have no ethical duty to forgive a health professional who meets with them and admits their mistake. But when patients do forgive in those circumstances, they are also ethical heroes because that forgiveness plays a part in encouraging other doctors who make mistakes to admit them and learn from them. A well-designed pyramid of supports will, from time to time, celebrate in a very public way the forgiveness of patients, just as it will celebrate the health professional who admits their mistake and crafts a systemic change to prevent recurrence.

PARADOXES OF BLAME CULTURES AND LEARNING CULTURES

Punishment has an important role in responsive regulation. Rarely—very rarely—is that importance about punishing mistakes. Punishing good people for doing bad things deters them from admitting their mistakes. This prevents us from learning how our systems fail to prevent good people from doing bad things. The key role of punishment in responsive regulation is about punishing the refusal to learn from mistakes by covering them up. A punitive response is especially likely to be the best tool to secure patient safety when a mistake is made, *and* it is wilfully covered up, *and* its perpetrators are wilfully blind to its root causes, *and then* the same terrible mistake is made again. Obviously, punishment is the enemy of a learning culture when it punishes admitting to mistakes. Punishment is the friend of a learning culture when it punishes covering up of mistakes (especially when covering up thwarts solutions and causes recurrent human suffering). In this sense, responsive regulation rejects the simple normative dichotomy that a learning culture is good and a blame culture is bad. In our Dickensian tragedy, Dr Good did not need to be blamed when he failed to comply with the protocol. It was better to persuade him into compliance in the way Nurse Response did. But it was appropriate that Dr Bad, Dr No and Mr Shuffle were all blamed for their cover-up and complicity in their repeated and wilful non-compliance with the standards of evidence-based health care. That is not to say we should deny them opportunities to redeem themselves. The evidence of the power of redemption is compelling in the organisational compliance literature. It is often the case that if you want to find the organisation with the most sophisticated compliance systems in respect of a given problem, you seek out the organisation that has been in the deepest trouble with regulatory authorities in recent times with respect to that problem (Fisse and Braithwaite 1983).

It is dangerous to see the punishment of health safety breaches as always counterproductive, simply because most safety problems are caused by bad systems rather than bad people. When we make terrible mistakes, most of us are bad enough to want to prevent those mistakes from becoming known by our professional peers. This normal human response to shame is a problem that is hard to solve without a capacity to punish. We will never uncover bad systems if professionals conceal the mistakes that reveal those bad systems. Rather, we must cultivate professional cultures that reward disclosure of near-misses and other mistakes. And when professional cultures fail to do so, and allow cover-up to fester, the law must trample over professional self-regulation to punish the cover-up. Most of the time, a professional culture of pride in learning from openness can do the regulatory work. But the contention of responsive regulation theory is that this is more likely when the consequence of professions failing to prevent cover-up will be a loss of professional autonomy. A promising regulatory solution is likely to be a non-punitive, restorative, learning culture where mistakes are admitted, combined with heavy organisational and personal penalties for cover-ups, and where a whistleblower within the organisation who reports the cover-up gets 25–35 per cent of the fine (Braithwaite 2008: Chapter 3). The whistleblower share of the fine compensates them for the likelihood that they will resign from the organisation to look for a new job, given the evidence of how miserable the lives of whistleblowers become in the organisations they have exposed.

WHY EXPANDING STRENGTHS IS EVEN MORE IMPORTANT THAN FIXING PROBLEMS

Malcolm Sparrow (2000) seems right in his belief that master practitioners of 'the regulatory craft' can achieve great things even when working inside all manner of dysfunctional regulatory governance structures. This is because his key to success is simple and amenable to ad hoc leadership. It is to 'pick the most important problems and fix them'. Sadly, most regulatory organisations are more interested in accomplishments like 'audits completed' and 'procedures manual updated' than in Sparrow's simpler prescription.

Yet it is also true that, as we learn to become better professionals, more problems get fixed by dint of that enhanced professionalism. We may prefer to be operated on by an outstanding surgeon embedded in an appalling regulatory system than by an ordinary surgeon supervised by outstanding regulation. But health care is a collective accomplishment. When the problem that needs to be fixed is a health professional who is weak at a particular task, education and training to turn this weakness into a strength are not necessarily the best fix. Often we will do better to reallocate duties so this person spends more of their time doing things that are their strengths, while someone else expands their duty statement to cover the weakness with their strengths. An example is the evidence that we are more likely to die if our heart surgery is performed by a surgeon who does not do a lot of heart surgery (Porter and Teisberg 2004). It is better to reallocate surgery so that surgeons and hospitals that operate on only a small number of hearts each year operate on none and expand the reach of those who are already strong at heart surgery.

Let us assume I am right—that, important as it is to fix weaknesses, health safety and quality improvement come more from expanding strengths. In the face of this, it seems insufficient for regulatory strategy simply to be careful not to crush strengths in the process of regulating risks. When regulatory strategy can encourage the expansion of strengths, this will often eliminate risks it might otherwise have to regulate. This is one reason why regulatory standards that require continuous improvement are a good idea (Braithwaite et al. 2007). Not only do we have a lot of evidence that regulation is counterproductive when it discourages building on strengths, but there is also evidence that inspectors who adopt the very simple, cheap practice of making a point of praising improvement accomplish marked increases in quality of care outcomes (Makkai and Braithwaite 1993; Braithwaite et al. 2007: 110–17). So it is not an option for health regulators not to get involved with the growth of strengths. Regulators must be integral to a health system's commitment to continuous improvement secured largely through building upon strengths. They can reward improvement by taking the strengths-based pyramid in Figure 2.1 seriously. And they must call to account health professionals who stop learning, and who are content that their current level of skill at their craft is good enough.

MANY AND CHANGING STRATEGIES

In a knowledge economy, new technologies and social contexts create both new problems and new opportunities for improvement at an ever-quickening rate. I also have argued that the individual and organisational actors who can help control risks and expand opportunities have become ever more variegated. It will now be argued that a knowledge economy engenders a proliferation of strategies through which regulation might be made effective. This is true in a direct sense. Hospitals increasingly have equivalents to aircraft systems that beep to remind professionals to do specific things to prevent human systems from crashing, and that, like the aircraft black box, create a record after the event of how the crash unfolded biologically. But available regulatory strategies proliferate much more because of the interactions among the lengthening list of actors involved in modern health care. Even at the small-organisation, low-tech end of health, Braithwaite et al. (2007: 306–7) concluded inductively from their fieldwork on nursing home regulation that the following range of mechanisms were often productively used by inspectors (see Table 2.1).

Table 2.1 Strategies that improved compliance in certain contexts observed in a study of nursing home inspections

Strategy	Support/ sanction	Process
Praises	Support	Congratulates improvement
Reminds	Support	Taps staff member on shoulder to remind of forgotten obligation
Commits	Support	Persuades someone that compliance would benefit residents
Shows	Support	Shows how to comply where person does not know how to do it
Fixes	Support	Inspector fixes something (e.g. releases restrained resident)
Educates	Support	Provides in-service training on the spot
Asks question	Support	Asking the right questions causes professional to accept responsibility to put something right immediately
Proposes correction	Support	Asking the right questions brings about a long-term plan that accepts responsibility
Stimulates problem-solving	Support	Asking the right questions stimulates problem-solving conversations
Proposes analysis	Support	Asking the right questions induces an insightful root-cause analysis
Triggers improvement	Support	Asking the right questions reveals the benefits of commitment to continuous improvement
Triggers consultancy	Support	Asking the right questions persuades the facility to hire a consultant
Builds self-efficacy	Support	Helps management and staff to see their own strengths

Triple-loop learning	Support	Spreads learning to other parts of facility and to other facilities
Awards and grants	Support	Nominates the facility or staff for an award or grant
Empowers	Support	Empowers pro-compliance staff by requiring a mix of strategies
Enlists third party	Support	Enlists third parties in reinforcing compliance (e.g. residents' council, relatives, other providers, advocacy group, lawyer, shareholder, media)
Triggers pre-emption	Sanction	Facility fixes problems before inspection to pre-empt any sanction
Wears down	Sanction	Keeps coming back until facility wants closure to end inspections
Signals escalation capability	Sanction	Displays capability to escalate sanctions up regulatory pyramid
Shames	Sanction	Disapproves non-compliance
Changes resource allocation	Sanction	Penalty withheld on condition resource allocation is changed
Deters	Sanction	Imposes a penalty
Exposes	Sanction	Reports non-compliance on public website or facility noticeboard, inducing either reputational or market discipline, or both
Protects future residents	Sanction	Bans new admissions until problem is fixed
Management change	Sanction	Triggers management replacement or facility sale by signalling escalation up regulatory pyramid
Incapacitates individual	Sanction	Reports professional to licensing body that withdraws/suspends licence
Incapacitates facility	Sanction	Withdraws/suspends licence for facility

Source: Adapted from Braithwaite et al. (2007): 306–7.

A diverse and changing cast of actors, problems, opportunities and strategies in a sense means that governing nodally is the only way we can govern (Wood and Shearing 2007). We cannot govern health care by a procedures manual. As new players come on to the field and create opportunities to build new strengths and be tripped up by new problems, smart regulators assemble the particular set of players capable of grasping contextually attuned strategies to the emerging problems and opportunities. If an attempt to put together a node of governance bungles a bundle of regulatory strategies, they reassemble a more fruitful node of players who contemplate more fertile strategies. For example, late twentieth century diplomacy to prevent war grasped the possibility that different nodes of peacemaking might even operate simultaneously. So if foreign ministers are faltering at reaching agreement on how to forge peace, those same ministers might encourage third-party mediation. NGOs like Just Peace bring civil society actors and lower-level officials from the warring nations together in a different place and encourage them to follow a different strategy (such as step-by-step confidence-building as opposed to nothing-is-agreed-until-everything-is-agreed negotiation). This kind of simultaneous second-track diplomacy, even third-track diplomacy, is now common.

In such a world, regulatory culture becomes less a rulebook and more a storybook (Shearing and Ericson 1991). Master practitioners of regulation learn how to be creative entrepreneurs of problem-fixing and strengths-expanding by attending to stories of how other master practitioners fixed some other problem. Carol Heimer (1997) observes that: 'We would not have great symphony orchestras if conductors focused only on keeping musicians from playing out of tune.' Nor would they succeed with a procedures manual on how to conduct. When great musicians play together, they infuse one another with sensibilities about how to reach new heights with their music. In this sense, perhaps a jazz ensemble is a better metaphor for how excellence is accomplished. 'Man,' retells the jazz musician, 'and then he just came in with dang dang de dang.' Excellence in steering health systems is also more likely to come from a plurality of players learning from stories of health system management about how to lead from behind to remove risks and improve quality. As Table 2.1 begins to illustrate, the diversity of scripts available to them as they swap stories may not be less than those available in jazz improvisation.

Part of what the strengths-based pyramid is about is institutionalising storytelling about how leaders pulled safety and quality up through new ceilings. As crass as the Academy Awards are, they are about much more than cleavage and red carpets. They bring together the master practitioners of the profession to tune into stories. What was so great about this actor that she should receive a lifetime achievement award? What inspired the director of this winning film to cast it in such a bold fashion? It is institutionalised storytelling about achievements to a gathering of filmmaking folk. Nursing home regulation has perhaps been better at publicising and spotlighting the travellers along this path to improved safety and quality than the regulation of hospitals or general practice (Braithwaite et al. 2007).

Another way of putting the problem with a rulebook manual mentality is that it can prevent professionals from thinking. This is by no means inevitably the case. A good example is Judith Healy's (2008) work on the *Correct Patient, Correct Site, Correct Procedure Protocol*, which reminds surgeons to check that they are about to operate on the correct site of the correct patient. But we know that we need to limit rules and protocols lest professionals become so overwhelmed by their number that they ignore them, or else ritualistically tick boxes (Braithwaite et al. 2007: 219–304). Nuclear power plant safety used to be regarded as such a huge regulatory risk that large numbers of detailed rules needed to be strictly enforced. Yet the Commission of Inquiry into the Three Mile Island nuclear reactor disaster revealed the problem was that nuclear power plant operators had become rule-following automatons (Rees 1994). They were so imbued with a culture of getting all the rules in compliance that they lacked systemic wisdom about their nuclear plant. When something out of the ordinary happened (like an impending meltdown!) they were incapable of thinking through where the safety system might have broken down. Instead they kept running through lists of rules to see whether they had slipped up in complying with one of them. Their ability to think systemically and diagnostically was smothered in an avalanche of rules. That is a significant risk against which health and safety experts must guard constantly.

CONCLUSION

Responsive regulation does not need a single regulator to make a regulatory pyramid work. This is because the best responsive regulation in a knowledge society is an accomplishment of networked governance. It would be a bad thing if there were a single regulator—whether a state or non-state regulator—responsible for patient safety. Flux and complexity mean we should want individual patients to be regulators of patient safety, just as we want individual nurses, doctors and managers to steer safety. We should want professions, colleges, self-regulatory organisations, government health departments, the World Health Organization, medical device manufacturer associations, private hospitals associations, the Australian Commission of Safety and Quality in Health Care, the Australian Consumers Association and many others to be players in patient safety regulation. The world has passed the point where it is possible for a single top-down rule of state law to achieve an objective like health safety.

This is not to deny problems of regulatory redundancy and costly duplication. It is to see virtue in redundant engagement where different actors bring different strengths into the regulatory circle from their disparate ways of seeing and learning. Fertile coordination of redundancy can come from nodal governance. It can come from widening circles of deliberation when narrower ones fail, and from tripling loops of learning. Strategic planning still has a place in coordination. But it must be strategic planning where organisations respond to the strategic planning of other organisations.

The fundamental ambition of responsive regulation remains to drive regulation down to the base of pyramids of supports and sanctions, where help, education and persuasion do most of the work. Steering health systems so they expand strengths is more important than steering them to prevent problems. Stronger clinical skills will save more lives than stronger strategic safety audits. Yet we can have both. And we can face squarely the reality that each can crowd out the other. A blizzard of rules can smother clinical excellence. Bitter experience shows that an arrogant clinician can make a basic error, like wrong-side surgery, after dismissing pettifogging protocols to prevent mistakes he says he has never made in decades of practice. Part of continuous improvement in health care is continuous improvement in the parsimony of protocols. Another is continuous improvement in their strategic potency. Both have the best chance of coming from nodes of governance that get the right players around the table for an evidence-based conversation. Good regulatory research can show when extra sets of controls improve safety and when they cumulatively reduce safety.

Perhaps top-down Mr Shuffles have been too much in charge of health governance debates. Perhaps we need more prominence for the Dr Sciences of patient safety evaluation and for leaders from behind, from every level of health hierarchies. Nodal governance can secure more innovative and adaptive paths to continuous improvement without creating an accountability crisis (see Braithwaite 2008). We remain responsible for our own health. Our doctor remains accountable for the treatment she prescribes. The hospital remains accountable for the safety systems it puts in place for its patients. The parliament remains accountable for the laws under which we might sue hospitals. Only in much more limited senses should we hold nodes of governance accountable for their regulatory failures. Sheeting home accountability in any strong sense to nodes of governance makes about as much sense as holding the medical profession accountable for a public health problem, like the level of obesity in a society. Problems like obesity may be amenable to solution through evidence-based nodal governance, but we remain accountable for our own fat.

So we cannot restructure health bureaucracies at one point in time to deliver improvements in patient safety that will endure for long. We cannot implement a 'cookbook' regulatory strategy. We cannot write a rulebook that will dramatically improve the regulation of patient safety. We are likely to find that storybooks of continuous improvement in health safety and quality are more important than rulebooks. Scientists of health regulation can test the evidence base on this from other sectors. Finally, we can be evidence based about how to create a learning culture in health systems. When we do that, one of the paradoxes we might discover is that to improve systems by nurturing a culture of learning from mistakes, we will need a blame culture that deters cover-up of mistakes (combined with a profession and a society that rewards honesty about mistakes). In all this, Australia has a long way to go, a lot of experimentation to venture, and stories of failure and excellence to share.

REFERENCES

Black, J. 2002, 'Critical reflections on regulation', *Australian Journal of Legal Philosophy*, vol. 27, pp. 1–3

Braithwaite, J. 2008, *Regulatory Capitalism: How it Works, Ideas for Making it Work Better*, Edward Elgar, Cheltenham

Braithwaite, J., Healy, J. and Dwan, K. 2005, *The Governance of Health Care Safety and Quality*, Commonwealth of Australia, Canberra

Braithwaite, J., Makkai, T. and Braithwaite, V. 2007, *Regulating Aged Care: Ritualism and the New Pyramid*, Edward Elgar, Cheltenham

Braithwaite, V. 2009, *Defiance in Taxation and Governance: Resisting and Dismissing Authority in a Democracy*, Edward Elgar, Cheltenham

Burris, S., Drahos, P. and Shearing, C. 2005, 'Nodal governance', *Australian Journal of Legal Philosophy*, vol. 30, pp. 30–58

Castells, M. 1996, *The Information Age: Economy, Society and Culture, Volume 1: The Rise of The Network Society*, Blackwell, Oxford

Coombs, H.C. 1983, *Trial Balance: Issues of My Working Life*, Sun Books Papermac, Melbourne

Drahos, P. 2004, 'Securing the future of intellectual property: Intellectual property owners and their nodally co-ordinated enforcement pyramid', *Case Western Reserve Journal of International Law*, vol. 36, no. 1, pp. 53–78

Dupont, B. 2006, 'Mapping security networks: from metaphorical concept to empirical model', in *Fighting Crime Together: The Challenges of Policing and Security Networks*, eds J. Fleming and J. Wood, UNSW Press, Sydney, pp. 35–59

Fisse, B. and Braithwaite, J. 1983, *The Impact of Publicity on Corporate Offenders*, State University of New York Press, Albany, NY

Granovetter, M.S. 1974, 'The strength of weak ties', *American Journal of Sociology*, vol. 78, no. 6, pp. 1360–80

Gunningham, N. and Grabosky, P. 1998, *Smart Regulation: Designing Environmental Policy*, Clarendon Press, Oxford

Healy, J. 2008, *Safe Surgery in Australian Hospitals: Implementation of the Correct Patient, Correct Site, Correct Procedure Protocol*, Report to the Australian Commission for Safety and Quality in Health Care, Canberra

Heimer, C. 1997, *Legislating Responsibility*, American Bar Foundation Working Paper, no. 9711, American Bar Foundation, Chicago

Latour, B. 1986, 'The powers of association', in *Power, Action and Belief: A New Sociology of Knowledge?*, Sociological Review Monograph No. 32, ed. J. Law, Routledge and Kegan Paul, London, pp. 264–80

——1987, *Science in Action*, Open University Press, Milton Keynes

Makkai, T. and Braithwaite, J. 1993, 'Praise, pride and corporate compliance', *International Journal of the Sociology of Law*, vol. 21, pp. 73–91

Metcalfe, L. 1994, 'The weakest links: building organisational networks for multi-level regulation', in *Regulatory Co-operation for an Interdependent World*, Organisation for Economic Co-operation and Development (OECD), Paris, pp. 49–71

Parker, C. 2002, *The Open Corporation*, Cambridge University Press, Cambridge

Porter, M.E. and Teisberg, E.O. 2004, 'Redefining competition in health care', *Harvard Business Review*, vol. 82, no. 6, pp. 64–77

Rees, J.V. 1994, *Hostages of Each Other: The Transformation of Nuclear Safety Since Three Mile Island*, University of Chicago Press, Chicago

Shearing, C. and Ericson, R.V. 1991, 'Culture as figurative action', *British Journal of Sociology*, vol. 42, no. 4, pp. 481–506

Sparrow, M. 2000, *The Regulatory Craft: Controlling Risks, Solving Problems and Managing Compliance*, The Brookings Institution, Washington, DC

Wood, J. and Shearing, C. 2007, *Imagining Security*, Willan, Portland, OR

NOTES

1   I have told dozens of people over the years that Nugget Coombs, one of Australia's greatest public servants and activists, and an ANU colleague, used to say that he tried to 'lead from behind'. On choosing this title for the paper, however, assiduous library searches have failed to turn up any documentary evidence of Coombs saying this, though many Coombs utterances consistent with it were found. Part of this philosophy was getting on with the job backstage while politicians were busy fighting over credit. It also meant getting more done by enrolling the enthusiasm of a host of different frontstage leaders appropriate to different projects. In our story, Nurse Response allows Dr Brilliant to get the credit for promoting her project and he is the one who gives plenary speeches at health safety and quality conferences on it. In his autobiographical *Trial Balance*, Coombs (1983: 141) quotes Lao Tzu: 'Working yet not taking credit. Leading yet not dominating. This is the Primal Virtue.' Yet after all these years of telling people what Nugget Coombs used to say about leadership, I found Nelson Mandela actually did use this expression: 'It is better to lead from behind and to put others in front, especially when you celebrate victory when nice things occur. You take the front line when there is danger. Then people will appreciate your leadership.' (<http://thinkexist.com>, accessed 14 September 2008)

3

INTERNATIONAL TRENDS IN PATIENT SAFETY GOVERNANCE

Bruce Barraclough, Jeffrey Braithwaite, Joanne F. Travaglia, Julie Johnson and Angus Corbett

Claudia H has been diagnosed with cancer. Today is her first visit to Methodist Hospital since her diagnosis, to begin treatment. She knows from a close friend and from her extensive search on the internet that others have described radiotherapy as 'going down to the fires of hell' because of the experience of the treatment, but also because most radiation oncology bunkers are in the basement of hospitals. Prior to today's visit, Claudia completed the admission process online, was given a parking number for the visit and was asked about her choice of music. Claudia arrives at Methodist and she chooses to let the valet parking attendant park her car since this is her first visit and she is feeling particularly anxious. A volunteer is waiting, greets Claudia and takes her across the campus to radiation oncology. Claudia makes a mental note that it isn't in the basement as she was expecting, but is on the first floor of the hospital. As Claudia is registering, she is relieved that she is not asked to repeat the admission process but she is asked whether anything has changed. She is given an iPod with her choice of music to listen to while undergoing treatment. Claudia is reminded that her visit to the oncologist is scheduled after radiotherapy and, if there is a time gap between therapy and the consultation, she will have an opportunity for a massage. Overall, her care is being provided in a safety-conscious, patient-focused, quality-oriented environment.

44

If it is accepted that care that is as safe as possible is part of the creation of public value in the 'experience economy' (Pine and Gilmore 1999), the outcome of effective patient safety governance could be measured by the experience of patients having the very best evidence-based care available to them. The gap between what patients feel they should receive from their health care experience and what they actually receive from that care is a gap that remains to be filled. By providing a positive experience for patients while they are receiving accepted best care, all the dimensions of health care quality are potentially improved. These include safety, appropriateness, access, patient-centredness, efficiency and effectiveness (Pine and Gilmore 1999; Hindle et al. 2005). This chapter outlines the way in which a range of strategies, including accreditation, pay for performance, data as information, education, leadership, champions and teams, and legal drivers act together under the umbrella of patient safety governance to reduce errors and improve safety in, and create public value from, health care. Ultimately, we want health services to provide the kind of positive experience Claudia H received. But most health systems fall short of this ideal.

INTRODUCTION

Growing international concerns about patient safety in recent decades have led to the development and implementation of a basket of improvement strategies, activities and initiatives (Braithwaite and Travaglia 2008; Hindle et al. 2005; Runciman et al. 2006). These act as economic, legal, educational, organisational, ethical or professional drivers for change. Collectively, these measures can be labelled *patient safety governance*. Patient safety governance has an important aim: to provide ways to ensure that health care professionals and organisations are accountable for, and actively involved in, improving the safety of their services and ameliorating risks of adverse events. This aim is part of the broader goal of health care providers in creating public value—that is, to ensure positive patient experiences and meet societal expectations. This suggests that public value is centrally concerned with meeting individual and collective requirements for safe health systems, but it begs a deeper question: What is the nature of 'public value' in the context of providing safe health services to patients, and in terms of the governance of those services? This needs further explanation.

In his book *Creating Public Value*, Mark Moore (1997) identifies private value as the generation of profit through the production of products and services. He argues that public value is more ambiguous. It is largely achieved by meeting the desires and perceptions of individuals expressed through representative governments, by means such as the development and institution of policy, sponsoring and arranging care, or directly funding services. Such activity aims to deliver public goods and services in ways that meet both individual and collective wants and needs.

Patient safety is an important dimension of quality that is valued by patients and their families (Vincent 2006). In this sense, the provision of safe health services is one way in which authorising environments in health care, including governments, can create public value. Moore (1997) suggests that, in the creation of public value, the *authorising environment* needs to ensure that there is adequate *operational capacity* to produce the required goods and services. On this basis, governments and other decision-makers—that is, the authorising environments in the health care system—have a responsibility to enhance the operational capacity of the system to deliver improvements in patient safety.

The authorising environment at the highest level needs to establish the operational capacity to meet individual patients' and the community's needs and desires through ordered and productive arrangements, with management success predicated on successfully arranging, training and motivating staff, applying policies and rules fairly, organising services in efficient ways and producing effective outcomes. At the same time, new programs to meet emerging needs have to be planned and delivered, and therefore attracting or redeploying resources is a key management task (Moore 1997). In health care, patient-centredness is another key deliverable in terms of public value. However, the rise of consumerism is not particularly reflected in health care because the usual experience of the health system often fails to match the desires and needs of the community, unlike Claudia H's hospital encounters.

Modern health care delivery arrangements can be understood as complex adaptive systems—that is, as 'a collection of individual agents with freedom to act in ways that that are not always totally predictable and whose activities are interconnected so that one agent's actions change the context for other agents' (Plsek and Greenhalgh 2001: 625). Such systems are very challenging to both understand and manage. In complex health systems, people at different levels may simultaneously be part of the authorising environment and the operational capacity— for example, the nurse in charge of a ward or the doctor leading a clinical unit. Typically, however, we think of the Australian health system's authorising environment as the bureaucracy or political arm of government, and the operational capacity as the providers of acute, primary and community care.

There are many examples of how authorising environments attempt to influence operational capacity to address patient safety concerns. A case in point is the 2006 Council of Europe recommendation of the Committee of Ministers (see Box 3.1) to member states on the management of patient safety and prevention of adverse events in health care (Council of Europe Committee of Ministers 2006). It addresses policy issues for national implementation and international collaboration. Much of the background work for articulating these initiatives has been undertaken by the World Alliance for Patient Safety (World Health Organization World Alliance for Patient Safety 2008; Perneger 2008).

Box 3.1 Council of Europe recommendation Rec(2006)7 of the Committee of Ministers

Recommendation Rec(2006)7 of the Committee of Ministers to member states on management of patient safety and prevention of adverse events in health care. The Committee of Ministers, under the terms of Article 15.b of the Statute of the Council of Europe . . . Recommends that governments of member states, according to their competencies:

i. ensure that *patient safety is the cornerstone* of all relevant health policies, in particular policies to improve quality;

ii. develop a coherent and comprehensive *patient-safety policy framework* which:

    a. promotes a culture of safety at all levels of health care;

    b. takes a proactive and preventive approach in designing health systems for patient safety;

    c. makes patient safety a leadership and management priority;

    d. emphasises the importance of learning from patient-safety incidents;

iii. promote the development of a *reporting system* for patient-safety incidents in order to enhance patient safety by learning from such incidents; this system should:

    a. be non-punitive and fair in purpose;

    b. be independent of other regulatory processes;

    c. be designed in such a way as to encourage health-care providers and health-care personnel to report safety incidents (for instance, wherever possible, reporting should be voluntary, anonymous and confidential);

---

    d. set out a system for collecting and analysing reports of adverse events locally and, when the need arises, aggregated at a regional or national level, with the aim of improving patient safety; for this purpose, resources must be specifically allocated;

    e. involve both private and public sectors;

    f. facilitate the involvement of patients, their relatives and all other informal caregivers in all aspects of activities relating to patient safety, including reporting of patient-safety incidents.

iv. review the role of other *existing data sources*, such as patient complaints and compensation systems, clinical databases and monitoring systems as a complementary source of information on patient safety;

v. promote the development of *educational programmes* for all relevant health-care personnel, including managers, to improve the understanding of clinical decision making, safety, risk management and appropriate approaches in the case of a patient-safety incident;

vi. develop reliable and valid *indicators of patient safety* for various health-care settings that can be used to identify safety problems, evaluate the effectiveness of interventions aimed at improving safety, and facilitate international comparisons;

vii. *co-operate internationally* to build a platform for the mutual exchange of experience and knowledge of all aspects of health-care safety, including:

    a. the proactive design of safe health-care systems;

    b. the reporting of patient-safety incidents, and learning from the incidents and from the reporting;

    c. methods to standardise health-care processes;

    d. methods of risk identification and management;

    e. the development of standardised patient-safety indicators;

    f. the development of a standard nomenclature/taxonomy for patient safety and safety of care processes;

    g. methods of involving patients and caregivers in order to improve safety;

    h. the content of training programmes and methods to implement a safety culture to influence people's attitudes (both patients and personnel);

viii. promote *research* on patient safety;

ix. produce *regular reports* on actions taken nationally to improve patient safety;

x.   to this end, whenever feasible, *carry out the measures* presented in the appendix to this recommendation;

xi. translate this document and develop adequate *local implementation strategies*; health-care organisations, professional bodies and educational institutions should be made aware of the existence of this recommendation and be encouraged to follow the methods suggested so that the key elements can be put into everyday practice.

Note: Italics added
Source: Council of Europe Committee of Ministers (2006).

The ministers envisage a patient-centred, systematic approach to patient safety. The expectation is that patients, clinicians and managers will become actively involved in preventing errors. To achieve this expectation, the recommendations support the effective use of enabling mechanisms such as: information and data (including incident reports and patient complaints); consistent safety and error terminology; education (through educational institutions, professional bodies and services); and human factors analysis. As well as these and other strategies, the ministers note that additional factors which influence services' ability to prevent errors will need to be addressed. These include adequate resources, the standardisation of procedures, good communication and documentation, safe handovers, and appropriate working environments (Council of Europe Committee of Ministers 2006).

DRIVERS FOR PATIENT SAFETY GOVERNANCE

Patient safety is governed by a variety of initiatives, but different health systems seem to favour some measures over others, either by explicit choice or because of accidents of history. Governance in the United Kingdom, for example, is largely the responsibility of peak NHS agencies and commissions. In contrast, Australia takes a more voluntaristic approach in which accreditation is more prominent. As a way to explore some of the drivers for patient safety governance that are at work internationally, we asked anonymous participants (N=16) from sixteen countries at the 26th International Society for Quality in Health Care (ISQua) meeting in Copenhagen in October 2008 to label on a world map the dominant mechanisms by which patient safety was enabled in countries they represented.

Most of the 16 respondents were female (75 per cent) and working in a health service or system (60 per cent), with 50 per cent of respondents working as CEOs, directors or associate directors of quality, safety or accreditation organisations, or hospitals. They had, on average, been with their current organisation for just over eight years and within the health industry for just under 24 years. No one had been in the health industry for less than five years. The majority of respondents had either a medical (30 per cent) or nursing (30 per cent) qualification, with the most common postgraduate qualification a Masters degree (38 per cent). Of those who responded, 35 per cent had a clinical role, 75 per cent held managerial responsibilities, and 90 per cent had a quality and safety role in their current position. Respondents clearly had significant experience within health systems, predominantly within traditional disciplines but with a range of disciplines, roles, positions and levels of experience represented.

In Table 3.1 we present their responses to our question. According to participants, what were the main patient safety drivers in sixteen countries? We asked for the main driver, but some participants gave us two. The drivers fall into four categories: safety and quality policies (government, public and organisational), accreditation and regulation, market forces (including legal drivers such as litigation, and competition between health services), and research.

Although the participants from the sixteen countries identified a main driver for patient safety in this ISQua research, it is clear that every health system uses a mix of initiatives by which to govern patient safety. These are intended to effect improvements within health services, organisations, teams and amongst individual clinicians. Broadening our participants' perspectives in Table 3.2, we compiled a list of many typical measures drawn from the clinical governance and patient safety literature.

Our review shows some key drivers and strategies by which to govern patient safety. The list is not exhaustive, but it shows there are many strategies available to those with the task of tackling patient safety. The range becomes clear when we see that most of the drivers identified by the ISQua conference participants fell into only one of the seven categories of drivers and strategies: that of systems requirements. Outside of this category, quality and improvement and safety can be driven by accountability requirements (such as clinical and corporate governance), quality improvement and information strategies, risk and performance management at both the service and clinician levels, and a consumer- or patient-focused approach.

Table 3.1 The dominant mechanism enabling patient safety in sixteen countries

Country	Govt/ public policy	Accreditation	Regulation	Legal drivers	Organisation policy	Competition	To Err is Human report	Reputation
Australia	✓							
Belgium			✓					
Canada		✓						
Denmark				✓				
Germany	✓							
Ireland			✓					
Israel					✓	✓		
Italy	✓							
Jordan	✓		✓	✓				✓
Slovenia	✓		✓					
Switzerland	✓		✓					
Taiwan		✓						
Netherlands		✓						
UK				✓				
USA	✓			✓			✓	
Yemen	✓							

Table 3.2 Drivers and strategies used to address patient safety

Drivers	Strategies
Accountability	Clinical governance
	Corporate governance
	Governing boards and bodies
	Ethics committees
	Qualified privilege
	Accountability
	Public reports
Quality improvement	Quality improvement
	Quality assurance
	Audits
	Clinical indicators
	Clinical effectiveness
	Evidence-based practice
	Safety improvement programs
	Leadership, teamwork, culture change
	Safety culture
Risk management	Clinical and risk management
	Critical incidents
	Incident reporting and analysis
	Safety management
Quality information	Disclosure
	Knowledge management
	Patient consent
	Patient information
	Public interest
	Patient documentation and coding
	Information technology
Performance management	Education, training and learning
	Competence
	Credentialling
	Complaints
	Pay for performance
Systems requirements	Policy
	Regulation, certification and licensing
	Accreditation
	Standards

Drivers	Strategies
	Catalytic agencies, bodies and committees
	Research and analytical techniques
	Legal responses, including litigation
Consumers	Patient experience
	Consumerism and patient empowerment
	Patient journey
	Patient-centred care
	Complaints and compensation
	Patient safety charters

Source: Travaglia and Braithwaite (2007); Hindle et al. (2005).

KEY TRENDS

Having provided a listing of the kinds of activities available in governing patient safety, we turn to a consideration of trends. Some of the problems in identifying international trends in this area of endeavour are that the literature is highly fragmented (e.g. in reports, policy documents, medical journals and health services publications) and reform is fast paced and uneven. However, we reviewed much of this literature and discerned seven trends in patient safety governance. These trends speak to the multi-level, multi-stakeholder approach undertaken by health systems. Table 3.3 summarises the trends we have assessed as important from our review of the literature. We address each in turn.

Table 3.3 Trends in patient safety governance

Trend	Focus
Accreditation	Application of standards
Pay for performance/non-payment for producing errors	Provision of incentives and disincentives
Data as information	Aid decisions
Education	Train, teach and increase capacity
Leadership, champions, teams	Improve provision, collaboration, communication, implementation
Legal drivers, supporting catalytic agencies	Create environment, policy support, systems change
Patients' experience in getting the best-value care	Endpoint

Accreditation

The intent of accreditation of health services is to continuously improve the safety and quality of care, typically by surveying activities and outcomes against standards. Health care organisations are invariably surveyed against standards developed by health professionals, policy-makers and researchers, and most accreditation programs have an education and performance measurement component.

Accreditation of health services is not new. It commenced in a formal way in 1917 with the American College of Surgeons' standardisation program, with Ernest Amory Codman (1869-1940) taking an active role (Codman 1924). There were five initial standards:

1. There will be an organised medical staff.
2. That membership of this staff be limited to licensed physicians who are competent and of worthy character and who are professionally ethical.
3. That the staff develop rules and regulations governing professional work in the hospital.
4. Each patient will have a comprehensive medical record.
5. That diagnostic and therapeutic facilities are under competent supervision and include at least laboratory and x-ray departments.

Codman's hospital standardisation report indicated that 692 hospitals with over 100 beds had been surveyed and 89 met the standards (Codman 1914, 1918-20). Even now, some 91 years later, most health systems would wish that all hospitals complied with these initial standards. These standards, to a considerable degree, cleverly presaged the modern concept of clinical governance.

Accreditation programs and standards in individual countries can now be subjected to external review by a program put in place by ISQua. ISQua has a four-year cycle involving assessment tools and guidance, supported development, education and training, self-assessment and documentation review, onsite pre-survey review, independent peer assessment or onsite survey with a full report and recommendations for improvement. Accreditation is the formal recognition of achievement. Accreditation is a process, not an event. Many countries have fully fledged accreditation systems for acute, primary and community care, as well as specialised accreditation systems to meet particular needs, such as for laboratory services and diagnostic facilities.

To mid-2008, twenty sets of standards, two training programs and seven accreditation organisations have been accredited by ISQua in sixteen countries. The ISQua Accreditation Council that oversees this work has thirteen members (from Australia, Canada, Denmark, France, India, Ireland, Japan, Jordan, Malaysia, the Netherlands, Spain, the United Kingdom and the United States) and there are four observers from the World Health Organization, the World Bank, the World Organization of National Colleges, Academies and Academic Associations of General Practitioners/Family Physicians (WONCA) and the International Hospital Federation (International Society for Quality in Health Care 2007).

Pay for performance and non-payment for producing errors

In *Crossing the Quality Chasm: A New Health System for the 21st Century*, the US Institute of Medicine recognised that payment systems were an important governance mechanism for improving the quality of health care (Institute of Medicine 2001). In 2007, the Institute further developed this strategy when it recommended the adoption of a form of pay for performance in Medicare (Institute of Medicine 2007: Recommendation 1). This report argued that:

> The objective of aligning incentives through pay for performance— paying providers for higher-quality care as measured by selected standards and procedures—is to create payment incentives that will:
>
> - Encourage the most rapid feasible performance improvement by all providers.
> - Support innovation and constructive change throughout the health care system.
> - Promote better outcomes of care, especially through coordination of care across provider settings and time. (Institute of Medicine 2007: 3)

The Centers for Medicare and Medicaid have adopted a form of pay for performance by denying payment for certain 'hospital-acquired conditions', including a list of 'never-ever' events (Centers for Medicare and Medicaid 2008). This decision to deny some payments for some hospital-acquired conditions responds to the problem that hospitals have been able to pass on the costs associated with the occurrence of preventable adverse events (Mello et al. 2007).

Other countries have adopted, or are adopting, forms of pay for performance. Perhaps the most important of these was the introduction in the United Kingdom in 2004 of a new contract for pay for performance. The House of Commons recently conducted a review of the operation of these contracts (House of Commons Committee of Public Accounts 2008). Other international experiments and pilot projects have the broad aim of making 'value-based' payments for health care (Rosenthal 2008). These schemes include episode payment systems where a health care provider accepts a specified amount for a particular condition. Other experiments allow health care providers to share savings with those responsible for making payments, where the health care providers accept guidelines or processes for providing care (for a review of some trials of value-based payment systems, see Rosenthal 2008).The biggest challenge facing the effective implementation of pay for performance, or more broadly of 'value-based' payment schemes, is the difficulty on agreeing on the goals that these schemes are designed to achieve (for a review of the range of goals which may inform pay for performance schemes see Sage 2006).

Data as information

Errors and adverse events occur as a result of inaccurate or missing data and information, which can lead to poor decisions (Kohn et al. 2000; Runciman et al. 2006). Much effort has been expended internationally to improve the quality of data and information available to clinicians, managers and policy-makers.The overall goal is to turn poor data into good information, which in turn provides effective knowledge and wisdom about patients and organisational aspects of care that can be actioned.

The American Health Information Management Association established ten characteristics for data against which effectiveness can be measured (American Health Information Management Association 1998). These are presented in Box 3.2.

Box 3.2 Ten characteristics of data quality

Accuracy: ensure data are the correct values, valid, and attached to the correct patient record.
Accessibility: data items should be easily obtainable and legal to access with strong protections and controls built into the process.
Comprehensiveness: all required data items are included. Ensure that the entire scope of the data is collected and document intentional limitations.
Consistency: the value of the data should be reliable and the same across applications.

Currency: the data should be up to date.

Definition: clear definitions should be provided so that current and future data users will know what the data mean. Each data element should have clear meaning and acceptable values.

Granularity: the attributes and values of data should be defined at the correct level of detail.

Precision: data values should be just large enough to support the application or process.

Relevancy: the data are meaningful to the performance of the process or application for which they are collected.

Timeliness: timeliness is determined by how the data are being used and their context.

Source: American Health Information Management Association (1998).

Various initiatives are being pursued internationally to give effect to the goal of improving patient safety through effective data. These include developing electronic health records, collecting and managing information about adverse events and near-misses, and creating effective aggregated data sets on clinical and organisational matters of key concern (Runciman et al. 2006; Braithwaite et al. 2008; Callen et al. 2007).

Education

Since its inception, the patient safety movement, via various reports and inquiries, has argued for education about safety and quality (Kohn et al. 2000; Department of Health 2001). This takes the form of multiple initiatives—undergraduate, postgraduate, continuing professional, workplace training, and formal and informal learning—designed to develop conceptual understanding, knowledge and skills in creating safe environments, applying specific techniques, reporting adverse events and near-misses, and using data to manage risk and harm. But as Runciman et al. (2006) note, what distinguishes health care from other fields is that not only is the distinction between education and service delivery blurred, but its trainees often 'bear the brunt of service delivery' in particularly high-risk situations, such as acute and after-hours care (Runciman et al. 2006: 69).

Several significant issues arise from this situation. Individual educational strategies form only part of a wider set of patient safety governance measures. Education can support and enhance these measures, but it cannot substitute for them. This is largely because 'individual approaches [to education] fail to recognise that medicine is largely practised as part of a group or team embedded within a complex organisational structure' (Ferlie and Shortell 2001: 284-5). Skills training may improve trainees' and clinicians' technical abilities, but improvements in safety and quality are more often dependent on individuals' and teams' knowledge about and attitudes towards these issues—factors which are shaped by professional and organisational cultures (Douglas et al. 2001) rather than training.

Ferlie and Shortell (2001) note that health care is conducted within teams. The traditional individualised approach to health professional education works against the preparation of health professionals for interprofessional practice, a point identified by several submissions to the Australian Productivity Commission's review of the health work-force (Productivity Commission 2005). Interprofessional education and practice, including the development of competencies in teamwork, collaboration, communication, ethics and conflict resolution, are fundamental to the effective and safe provision of health care (Braithwaite and Travaglia 2005). The development of these competencies, particularly at an undergraduate level, require a revamping of educational structures as well as content (Productivity Commission 2005).

Where education and training do occur, it is still unclear what is to be included in such training—especially at the undergraduate level. Much of what has been incorporated to date has been idiosyncratic and driven largely by individual educators, and by professional or organisational perspectives and needs. A review of the literature on patient safety education identified little systematic evidence for either educational content or process (Australian Council for Safety and Quality in Health Care 2006; Walton and Elliott 2006). The World Health Organization's World Alliance for Patient Safety is currently developing a standardised, international curriculum on patient safety to address this issue. Once released, this will likely take time to find its way into curricula.

The principle of accountability requires more of health systems and services than a requirement for mandatory training. Øvretviet and Klazinga go on to note that 'with rapid changes in knowledge and technique, the professional quality can no longer be assured by merely awarding diplomas and titles after training' (Øvretviet and Klazinga 2008: 23). People have to participate in education and training, but then their performance needs to be managed over time. The performance management of health professionals in providing safer care needs to take into account a range of instructional, regulatory, organisational and workforce issues. A synthesis of some key considerations in creating such an environment is provided in Box 3.3. In short, education and training provide baseline competencies, then performance needs to be managed and ongoing opportunities provided for career-long education and training to meet various individuals' and teams' needs.

Box 3.3 Performance management and education of health professionals within a patient safety governance framework

Training
Quality, safety, interprofessionalism and patient-centred care in professional curricula, professional development and workplace training

Registration
National register of professionals established
Regulation of undergraduate and postgraduate training
Re-validation and credentialling of professionals
New safety and quality professional roles created

Standards
Quality and safety integrated into professional competency standards
Quality and safety standards established in health care professions, organisations and cultures

Disciplinary measures
Legislation and regulation of professional misconduct enforced
Responses made to misconduct of professionals
Information-sharing across states and countries about professionals convicted of misconduct

Performance management
Ongoing performance management of health professionals
Peer- and self-review encouraged
New knowledge through evidence-based practice and guidelines
Working conditions that facilitate learning and a safety culture
Workforce planning recognising limitations of clinicians and new graduates
Adequate supervision of new graduates
Policies for task-substitution across professions developed

> *Patients*
> Patients/clients, families and carers informed fully, treated respectfully and made part of the care team
>
> *Sources:* Modified from Øvretviet and Klazinga (2008); see also Aaron and Headrick (2002); Greiner and Knebel (2003); Hindle et al. (2005); Hindle et al. (2006); Productivity Commission (2005); Braithwaite and Travaglia (2005).

Leadership, champions, teams

Leadership has emerged as a key theme in the rapidly growing movement to improve patient safety. Leading an organisation that is committed to providing safer care requires creating a 'learning' organisation (Senge 1990). Common traps in thinking about error, such as blaming individuals and blaming the bureaucracy of the organisation, are overly simplistic mental models for complex systems issues. Leaders must address the systemic issues that are at work within their organisations to allow individual and organisational learning to occur.

Leadership is not about applying a collection of tools and techniques to those being led; it involves integrating the learning disciplines throughout the organisation—vision, values, and purpose; systems thinking; and mental models (Senge 1990). When defining leadership in terms of creating a learning organisation, the role of the leader is to take responsibility for learning, as a designer of the learning process, a steward of the vision and a teacher, by fostering the learning throughout the organisation (Senge 1990).

Traditionally, the emphasis on leadership has focused mainly on the level of top executives—chief executives and operating officers, directors and boards of management (Mycek 2001; Sprenger 2001). While recognising the importance of senior leadership's role in improving patient safety, it is also important to address the role of all members of the caregiving team, including the patient and their family. This caregiving unit can be referred to as a 'clinical microsystem' (Nelson et al. 1998; Mohr 2000; Mohr and Batalden 2002). It is misleading to think that leadership is only provided by a few highly positioned people in the organisation. Bolman and Deal (1997) suggest that leaders can make or catalyse events, but events can also be the catalyst that makes leaders emerge. This is evident in highly functioning microsystems, where there are formal leaders—those assigned a leadership role—and informal leaders or champions—those well-respected opinion leaders to whom others naturally look, and importantly, on-the-spot leaders—those people who step up when leadership is required.

Table 3.4 builds on the research about high-performing clinical microsystems (Mohr 2000) to provide specific actions that can be further explored (Mohr et al. 2002). This list provides an organising framework and a place to start applying patient safety concepts to microsystems.

Table 3.4 Relating microsystem characteristics to patient safety

Microsystem characteristics	Steps leaders can take to improve patient safety
Leadership	Define the quality and safety vision of the organisation
	Identify existing constraints within the organisation
	Allocate resources for planning, implementation, monitoring and evaluation
	Build in microsystem's participation and input to planning
	Align organisational quality and safety goals
	Engage the board in conversations about progress towards safety goals
	Promote and recognise prompt truth-telling about errors or hazards
	Certify helpful changes to improve safety
Organisational support	Work with clinicians to identify patient safety issues and make changes
	Put the necessary resources and tools into the hands of individuals
Staff focus	Assess current safety culture
	Identify the gap between current culture and safety vision
	Plan cultural interventions
	Conduct periodic assessments of culture
	Celebrate examples of desired behaviour (e.g. acknowledgment of an error)

Table 3.4 Relating microsystem characteristics to patient safety *(continued)*

Microsystem characteristics	Steps leaders can take to improve patient safety
Education and training	Develop patient safety curriculum Provide training and education of key clinical and management leaders Develop a core of staff with patient safety skills
Interdependence of the care team	Build Plan–Do–Study–Act improvement cycles into debriefings Use daily huddles to debrief and to celebrate identifying errors
Patient focus	Establish patient and family partnerships Support disclosure and truth around medical error
Community and market focus	Analyse safety issues in community and partner with external groups to reduce risks to population
Performance results	Develop key safety measures Create feedback mechanisms to share results with microsystems
Process improvement	Identify patient safety priorities based on assessment of key safety measures Address the work that will be required at the microsystem level
Information and information technology	Enhance error reporting systems Build safety concepts into information flow (e.g. checklists, reminder systems)

Negative publicity about medical errors brings the issue of patient safety to the attention of the board members, directors and top management of health care delivery systems. Those in charge are ultimately responsible for patient safety because they credential physicians and approve policies and procedures related to safety and risk. With the mounting scrutiny resulting from the focus on patient safety, policy-makers and executives are increasingly asking what their organisations are doing about patient safety. Senior staff can be especially helpful through active participation in committees that oversee quality and risk work in the organisation. Those in charge need to fully realise that they must come to understand the thorny issues surrounding patient safety and provide leadership to address them. They must be both alert and well equipped to provide leadership for change.

Box 3.4 Questions policy-makers, directors and board members should ask

1. What initiatives have been undertaken by the organisation to assess the safety of its patient care environment?
2. How is improving patient safety addressed in the organisation's mission statement?
3. Does the organisation have an overall approach to and plan for patient safety?
4. Does the patient safety plan include senior-level leadership, defined objectives, personnel and a sufficient budget to accomplish its goals?
5. Should the organisation create a position of chief safety officer in the executive management group?
6. What is the organisation doing to create a culture of safety?
7. What is the plan for regular patient safety progress reports to the executive committee and board of directors?

Source: Classen (2000).

Legal drivers, supporting agencies

One of the primary themes of this book is that health care relies on decentred forms of regulation. One of the features of decentred regulatory systems is that they make use of forms of networked governance. This involves regulatory conversations between regulatory actors in order to arrive at shared views on principles and practices. As discussed in Chapter 1, regulatory constellations form over time as actors gravitate together, develop shared ways of thinking and link their separate mechanisms together into a web of controls.

An important trend in the governance of safety is the recognition by governments of the importance of networking the stakeholders involved in delivering health in order to develop a 'web of controls'. The recent Council of Europe Recommendation on management of patient safety discussed earlier is indicative of this trend (Perneger 2008: 305). This Recommendation identifies the importance of achieving a number of goals, including:

- developing reporting systems for patient safety incidents;
- reviewing and enhancing sources of data concerning the quality and safety of health care;

- promoting educational programs for all relevant health care personnel;
- developing reliable and valid indicators of patient safety;
- developing mechanisms to encourage international cooperation;
- promoting research on patient safety;
- producing reports on progress in improving patient safety (Perneger 2008: 305–6).

Different health care systems will achieve these goals in different ways, but the pathways followed in particular health care systems involve forms of networked governance. In public health care systems there is reliance on public regulatory bodies to provide guidance and to assist in developing networks. Typically, these bodies have the role of facilitating the development of networks and do not have the formal power to enforce particular regulatory requirements. For example, in the United Kingdom the National Institute of Health and Clinical Excellence 'is the independent organisation responsible for providing national guidance on the promotion of good health and the prevention and treatment of ill health' (National Institute for Health and Clinical Excellence 2008).

In Australia, the Clinical Excellence Commission in New South Wales has a similar basket of functions (Clinical Excellence Commission 2008). In private health care systems, a variety of bodies perform these networking functions. In the United States, the Institute of Medicine 'provides independent, objective, evidence-based advice to policymakers, health professionals, the private sector, and the public. The mission of the Institute of Medicine embraces the health of people everywhere.' (Institute of Medicine 2008b). As part of its mission, the IOM links a very wide range of public and private bodies that are concerned with improving the safety and quality of health care (Institute of Medicine 2008a).

It is evident that multiple agencies are springing up across the world, designed to support or mandate behaviours and attitudes predicated on creating safe systems for patients. This trend is destined to continue along with the proliferation of legal instruments designed to influence providers to constitute safe care.

Patients' experience in getting the best-value care

The story told at the beginning of the chapter describes some of the principles underpinning the experience economy being introduced to health care that are found at Methodist Hospital in Houston, Texas,

United States (Methodist Hospital System 2008). In 2008, Methodist is ranked number 10 on *Fortune* magazine's list of the '100 best companies to work for' (*Fortune* 2008), and is named by *US News and World Report* as one of 'America's Best Hospitals' (*US News and World Report* 2008). It is designated a 'magnet hospital' for excellence in nursing. Awards like these have highlighted that Methodist has high staff retention rates and few problems with recruiting high-quality staff, as well as grateful patients who generally receive the care and the outcomes they desire.

Methodist leaders indicate a positive bottom line from this activity. The cost of care delivered in this way is within the usual insurance reimbursement levels, and Methodist requires its clinicians to follow evidence-based, best-practice care. The hospital assessment is that there is now almost zero downtime on radiotherapy machines due to patients being late and a similar beneficial improvement in use of doctor time. This is because patients do not have difficulty parking, and do not get lost and frustrated, bothered or angry when trying to find the radio-therapy service. The patient–doctor and patient–staff interaction generally is more positive. The questions asked by patients are more appropriately focused because of the websites offered. Compliance is improved with fewer adverse events, and doctors and other staff are happier in their work. Satisfied patients and improved staff morale are clearly related.

The real story from Methodist is that: 'Service is important but this goes much further. It individualizes the service to a particular patient and creates a "wow" moment that people will remember' (Khawaja 2008). To create this experience for patients, Randy Kirk, project specialist for the Methodist Experience, works with individuals in each department to help them craft an environment that fits the care they give a patient. Methodist has a set of values that governs all of the actions of physicians and employees—the I CARE values. *Integrity, Compassion, Accountability, Respect* and *Excellence* form the bedrock of all activities. The Methodist Experience is built upon those values and offers a new way of providing health care with the goal of creating a culture of personalised service and satisfaction for patients, but also of engaging employees and physicians to live these values on the job. To work with the Methodist Experience, staff members go through a training program. 'We hope the Methodist Experience will enable us to become as skilled at the science of personalization as we are in the science of medicine.' (Khawaja 2008).

No doubt this sounds like utopia to some providers and patients, but perhaps this may become the standard in the future? This example indicates that when it is normal for care to be well organised, thoughtfully delivered and designed to provide a positive patient experience, the key factors in effective patient safety governance will have been delivered.

CONCLUSION

There is a great deal of effort underway internationally to improve how patient safety is being governed and realised. We have traced developments through our own research, that of others, and various authoritative reports in selected countries. We have argued, following Moore (1997), that patient safety is a public value that needs to be, and is being, actively created by various means. Those in charge in the authorising environment, and those responsible for providing care, are jointly accountable for this. We have charted a path that shows that, as part of the experience economy, patients are seeking the very best goods and services. We have shown that this path is being supported by many strategies designed to improve the operational capacity of health care providers to deliver safer health care services. But what we have not been able to show is that the implementation of these strategies has resulted in demonstrable improvements in levels of patient safety and quality of experience, apart from exceptional examples such as Methodist Hospital. There is still much to be achieved.

Participants in our ISQua study of sixteen countries suggested that differing mechanisms can be identified as dominating and driving the patient safety agenda internationally. Nevertheless, each health system seems to have recourse to a mix of initiatives for tackling patient safety. We identified many commonly recurring strategies, and seven key trends which are popular internationally. While we discussed each in turn, we are cautious about what blend is optimal. The context, aims and history of each health system are different, and what works in one country, and the way that any mix of measures might be applied, differs as well.

That being said, seven prominent strategies which many health systems are pursuing have been highlighted: accreditation, pay for performance and its corollary, non-payment for producing errors, changing data into information, providing education, emphasising leadership, champions and teams, creating legal drivers and supporting agencies to catalyse change, and building services which provide superb patient experiences. The next stage will be to adduce evidence that efforts to improve on these seven fronts are demonstrating progress. We believe that when this occurs we will be able to say with a degree of confidence that patient safety governance is on the right track.

REFERENCES

Aaron, D.C. and Headrick, L.A. 2002, 'Educating physicians to improve care and safety is no accident: It requires a systematic approach', *Quality and Safety in Health Care*, vol. 11, no. 2, pp. 168–73

American Health Information Management Association 1998, *Data Quality Management Model*, American Health Information Management Association, Chicago

Australian Council for Safety and Quality in Health Care 2006, *National Patient Safety Education Framework Bibliography*, Australian Council for Safety and Quality in Health Care, Canberra

Bolman, L. and Deal, T. 1997, *Reframing Organizations: Artistry, Choice, and Leadership*, Jossey Bass, San Francisco

Braithwaite, J. and Travaglia, J. 2005, *Interprofessional Learning And Clinical Education: An Overview of the Literature*, ACT Health, Canberra

—— 2008, 'An overview of clinical governance policies, practices and initiatives', *Australian Health Review*, vol. 32, no. 1, pp. 10–22

Braithwaite, J., Westbrook, M. and Travaglia, J. 2008, 'Attitudes toward the large-scale implementation of an incident reporting system', *International Journal of Quality in Health Care*, vol. 20, no. 3, pp. 184–91

Callen, J., Westbrook, J.I. and Braithwaite, J. 2007, 'Cultures in hospitals and their influence on, and attitudes to, and satisfaction with, the use of clinical information systems', *Social Science and Medicine*, vol. 65, no. 3, pp. 635–9

Centers for Medicare and Medicaid 2008, 'CMS improves patient safety for Medicare and Medicaid by addressing "never events"', Centers for Medicare and Medicaid, Washington, D.C. <www.cms.hhs.gov/apps/media/press/factsheet.asp>, accessed 15 October 2008

Classen, D. 2000, 'Patient safety, thy name is quality', *Trustee*, vol. 53, no. 9, pp. 12–15

Clinical Excellence Commission 2008, *About the Clinical Excellence Commission*. <www.cec.health.nsw.gov.au/about.html>, accessed 15 October 2008

Codman, E.A. 1914, *A Study in Hospital Efficiency as Demonstrated by the Case Report of the First Two Years of a Private Hospital*, Thomas Todd, Boston

—— 1918-20, *A Study in Hospital Efficiency. As Demonstrated by the Case Report of the First Five Years of a Private Hospital*, Thomas Todd, Boston

—— 1924, 'Committee for the standardization of hospitals: Minimum standards for hospitals', *Bulletin of the American College of Surgeons*, vol. 8, no. 4.

Council of Europe Committee of Ministers. 2006, Recommendation *Rec (2006)7 of the Committee of Ministers to Member States on Management of Patient Safety and Prevention of Adverse Events in Health Care*, Council of Europe, Geneva. <http://zope251.cbo.hosting.amaze.nl/guidelines/guideline1/Hoofdstuk1>, accessed 29 January 2009

Department of Health 2001, *The Report of the Public Inquiry into Children's Heart Surgery at the Bristol Royal Infirmary 1984-1995: Learning from Bristol*, Stationery Office, London

Douglas, N., Robinson, J. and Fahy, K. 2001, *Inquiry into Obstetric and Gynaecological Services at King Edward Memorial Hospital 1990-2000*, Health Department of Western Australia, Perth

Ferlie, E.B. and Shortell, S.M. 2001, 'Improving the quality of health care in the United Kingdom and the United States: A framework for change', *The Milbank Quarterly*, vol. 79, no. 2, pp. 281-315

Fortune 2008, 'Methodist Hospital System: What makes it so great?, *Fortune* magazine, <http://money.cnn.com/magazines/fortune/bestcompanies/Snap shots/10.html>, accessed 13 October 2008

Greiner, A.C. and Knebel, E. 2003, *Health Professions Education: A Bridge to Quality*, Institute of Medicine, National Academies Press, Washington, DC <http://books.nap.edu/catalog.php?record_id=10681>, accessed 27 January 2009

Hindle, D., Braithwaite, J. and Iedema, R. 2005, *Patient Safety Research: A Review of the Technical Literature*, Centre for Clinical Governance Research, University of New South Wales, Sydney

Hindle, D., Braithwaite, J., Travaglia, J. and Iedema, R. 2006, *Patient Safety: A Comparative Analysis of Eight Inquiries in Six Countries*, Centre for Clinical Governance Research, University of New South Wales, Sydney

House of Commons Committee of Public Accounts 2008, *NHS Pay Modernisation: New Contracts for General Practice Services in England*, Forty-first Report of Session 2007-08

Institute of Medicine 2001, 'Aligning payment policies with quality improve-ment', in *Crossing the Quality Chasm: A New Health System for the 21st Century*, Institute of Medicine, Washington, DC

—— 2007, *Rewarding Provider Performance: Aligning Incentives in Medi-care (Pathways to Quality Health Care Series)*, Institute of Medicine, Washington, DC

—— 2008a, *Links to Related Organizations*, <www.iom.edu/CMS/8089/14796. aspx>, accessed 15 October 2008

—— 2008b, *Mission*, <www.iom.edu>, accessed 15 October 2008

International Society for Quality in Health Care 2007, *General Information*, International Society for Quality in Health Care, Melbourne, <www.isqua. org/isquaPapers/General.html>, accessed 13 October 2008

Khawaja, R. 2008, *Methodist International*, Methodist Hospital, Houston, TX. Personal communication to B. Barraclough, received November 2008

Kohn, L.T., Corrigan, J.M. and Donaldson, M.S. eds 2000, *To Err is Human: Building a Safer Health System*, National Academies Press, Washington, DC

Mello, M., Studdert, D.E., Thomas, E., Yoon, C. and Brennan, T. 2007, 'Who pays for medical errors? An analysis of adverse event costs, the medical liability system, and incentives for patient safety improvement', *Journal of Empirical Legal Studies*, vol. 4, no. 4, pp. 835–60

Methodist Hospital System 2008, *Methodist Hospital System: Leading Medicine*, Methodist Hospital System, Houston, <www.methodisthealth.com/tmhs/ home.do>, accessed 13 October 2008

Mohr, J. 2000, *Forming, Operating, and Improving Microsystems of Care*, Center for the Evaluative Clinical Sciences, Dartmouth College, Hanover

Mohr, J., Abelson, H. and Barach, P. 2002, 'Creating effective leadership for improving patient safety', *Quality Management in Health Care*, vol. 11, no. 1, pp. 69–78

Mohr, J.J. and Batalden, P.B. 2002, 'Improving safety at the front lines: The role of clinical microsystems', *Quality and Safety in Health Care*, vol. 11, no. 1, pp. 45–50

Moore, M.H. 1997, *Creating Public Value: Strategic Management in Government*, Harvard University Press, Cambridge, MA

Mycek, S. 2001, 'Patient safety—it starts with the Board', *Trustee*, vol. 54, no. 5, pp. 8–12

National Institute for Health and Clinical Excellence 2008, *About NICE*, <www. nice.org.uk/aboutnice/about_nice.jsp>, accessed 15 October 2008

Nelson, E.C., Batalden, P.B., Mohr, J.J. and Plume, S.K. 1998, 'Building a quality future', *Frontiers of Health Services Management*, vol. 15, no. 1, pp. 3–32

Øvretviet, J. and Klazinga, N. 2008, *Guidance on Developing Quality and Safety Strategies with a Health System Approach*, World Health Organization, Copenhagen

Perneger, T. 2008, 'The Council of Europe recommendation Rec(2006)7 on management of patient safety and prevention of adverse events in health care', *International Journal for Quality in Health Care*, vol. 20, no. 5, pp. 305–7

Pine, B.J. and Gilmore, J. 1999, *The Experience Economy: Work is Theatre and Every Business a Stage*, Harvard Business School Press, Boston

Plsek, P.E. and Greenhalgh, T. 2001, 'Complexity science: the challenge of complexity in health care', *British Medical Journal*, vol. 323, no. 7313, pp. 625-8

Productivity Commission 2005, *Australia's Health Workforce*, Australian Government Productivity Commission, Canberra, <www.pc.gov.au/study/healthworkforce/positionpaper/healthworkforce.pdf>, accessed 20 June 2008

Rosenthal, R. 2008, 'Beyond pay for performance—emerging models of provider-payment reform', *New England Journal of Medicine*, vol. 359, no. 12, pp. 1197-1200

Runciman, W.B., Merry, A. and Walton, M. 2006, *Safety and Ethics in Healthcare: A Guide to Getting it Right*, Oxford University Press, Oxford

Sage, W.M. 2006, 'McDonald-Merrill-Ketcham Lecture: Pay for performance: will it work in theory?', *Indiana Health Law Review*, vol. 3, no. 2, pp. 305-24

Senge, P. 1990, *The Fifth Discipline*, Doubleday, New York

Sprenger, G. 2001, 'Sharing responsibility for health system safety', *American Journal of Health System Pharmacy*, vol. 58, no. 1, pp. 988-9

Travaglia, J. and Braithwaite, J. 2007, *Clinical Governance, Safety and Quality: An Overview of the Literature*, Centre for Clinical Governance Research, University of New South Wales, Sydney

US News and World Report 2008, *America's Best Hospitals*, US World News and World Report, Washington, DC, <www.usnews.com/listings/hospital/6741960>, accessed 13 October 2008

Vincent, C. ed. 2006, *Patient Safety*, Elsevier, Edinburgh

Walton, M. and Elliott, S. 2006, 'Improving patient safety and quality: How can education help?', *Medical Journal of Australia*, vol. 184, no. 10, suppl., pp. S60-4

World Health Organization World Alliance for Patient Safety 2008, *Forward Program 2008-2009*, World Health Organization, Geneva, <http://who.int/patientsafety/information_centre/reports/Alliance_Forward_Programme_2008.pdf>, 13 October 2008

4

VOLUNTARY INITIATIVES BY CLINICIANS

Heather Buchan, Niall Johnson and Christopher Baggoley

INTRODUCTION

Efforts by health professionals to voluntarily improve safety and quality of care need to be seen in terms of how care delivery has evolved over the past several decades. Health care and health care systems became more and more complex in the final half of the twentieth century. Investment in health and medical research led to an enormous expansion in knowledge and innovation. The range and types of interventions delivered by health care professionals increased in number, complexity and risk, often requiring a coordinated effort from a multidisciplinary team. During this time, and largely because of these changes, concerns about the delivery, safety and quality of health care also grew.

Starting in the 1970s, health service researchers repeatedly documented wide variations in practice and medical care, unexplained by underlying mortality or morbidity of the population (Wennberg and Gittelsohn 1973; McPherson et al. 1982). This focus on appropriateness of care was matched by concerns about the extent to which effective care was being delivered (Cochrane 1989). Internationally, these circumstances and concerns fuelled the development of clinical practice guidelines and the rise of evidence-based medicine—the push for better knowledge about the effects of treatment and the use of this scientific evidence in medical decision-making (Evidence-Based Medicine Working Group 1992). Continuing evidence that many people do not receive health care most likely to give the best outcomes (McGlynn et al. 2003), or are endangered by the health care they receive (Brennan et al. 2004; de Vries et al. 2008), has provided the impetus for concerted quality improvement initiatives in a number of countries. Many of these initiatives have been characterised by clinician leadership, with government support and funding often underpinning or providing infrastructure once substantial clinical support has been gained.

In Australia, there have been sustained voluntary efforts by clinicians to improve quality and safety of care. This chapter focuses on three areas. First, individual clinicians and professional societies—particularly those concerned with more technical aspects of care delivery such as renal medicine and intensive care—have developed a variety of data registers to capture information on processes and outcomes of care and provide feedback to participating clinicians. Second, multiple health professional and specialty organisations have initiated the production of clinical practice guidelines in Australia and have highlighted the need to promote implementation of guideline recommendations and evidence-based practice. In 2000, the first national organisation with the specific aim of improving uptake of best available evidence into routine practice was formed following representations to government from medical leaders and representatives of the clinical colleges. Finally, the chapter will discuss the enthusiastic adoption of collaborative quality improvement initiatives within parts of the health sector over the last ten years. While these initiatives have been extensively funded and supported by federal and state governments and government agencies, they depend on voluntary participation by clinicians.

CLINICAL REGISTRIES

The basis for all efforts to improve quality and safety is the capacity to monitor the care being delivered. One approach to monitoring care has been the development of clinical registries or medical data registries (Drolet and Johnson 2008). Clinical registers are databases that systematically collect health-related information on individuals who are treated with a particular surgical procedure, device or drug, diagnosed with a particular illness or managed via a specific health care resource. The system or organisation governing the register is known as the registry. Information in clinical registers is captured on an ongoing basis from the defined population (Australian Commission on Safety and

Quality in Health Care 2008). Registries collect data about real-world clinical populations, not the somewhat artificial populations of clinical trials. Ideally, they encompass the entire relevant clinical population, thereby allowing monitoring of all patients by all providers and removing selection biases.

Clinical registries have been established and operated with the aim of improving patient care and outcomes through greater understanding of events, treatments and outcomes. The data collected by a registry over time are analysed and used to identify positive and negative trends, and these analyses are used—generally by clinicians—to lead to improvements in practice, and in medication and device usage. Clinical registries can identify and investigate variation in processes and clinical outcomes. Factors leading to such variability can then be investigated further, with the ultimate aim of improving patient care. Registries can drive quality improvement in many ways: indirectly through the fostering of competition, or more directly through evaluating compliance with best-practice guidelines, and through informing policy areas such as regulation and pricing policy. Where data are collected on devices and the like, registries can also play a role in post-market surveillance and notification. Where they have been introduced at a state or national level, registries have become one of the most clinically valued tools for quality improvement (Eyenet Sweden 2005).

Clinical quality registers are a particular subset of clinical registers. The primary purpose of a clinical quality register is to improve the safety or quality of health care provided to patients by collecting key clinical information from individual health care encounters, which enable risk-adjusted outcomes to be used to drive quality improvement. Clinical quality registers can be the most suitable and accurate method of providing monitoring and benchmark data and, where applicable, offer significant potential to improve health care performance across institutions and providers. Clinical quality registers should be focused on conditions and procedures where outcomes are thought to vary and where improvements in quality have the greatest capacity to improve quality of life and/or reduce costs.

Many of the clinical registries in Australia have been developed as research activities, often by committed and innovative clinicians, and frequently within particular environments—for example, teaching hospitals, academic units and professional bodies, while the voluntary nature and clinical leadership still remain vital to the success of clinical registries, the real value of registries is perhaps unappreciated and the full potential yet to be realised. More recently, there has been a recognition that these efforts have the potential to provide significant information and feedback into the quality and safety of clinical practices (Eyenet Sweden 2005; Gliklich and Dreyer 2007). Among the more prominent examples of clinical registries in Australia are the ANZDATA, ANZICS and AOA NJRR registries.

Australia and New Zealand Dialysis and Transplant Registry (ANZDATA)

This registry records the incidence, prevalence and outcome of dialysis and transplant treatment for patients with end-stage renal failure. ANZDATA collects information for the purpose of monitoring treatments and performing analyses to improve the quality of care for people with kidney failure. It collects data from renal units in Australia and New Zealand, claiming coverage of 100 per cent of patients who have received dialysis and transplantation services in the two nations. The Registry releases reports on a variety of topics, including an Annual Report examining the rates and treatment of kidney failure in Australia and New Zealand. The Registry asserts that it plays a major role in ensuring the quality of patient care and that it does this by sending to each kidney unit an annual report outlining their activity. These reports also compare the outcome of the treatment they provide with that of other units throughout the two countries. Reports are also produced at a state and national level, and analyses may also be produced for renal units, government health departments and industry concentrating on particular aspects of renal failure management (ANZDATA 2008).

Australian and New Zealand Intensive Care Society (ANZICS) Centre for Outcome and Resource Evaluation (CORE)

This bi-national peer review and quality assurance program has provided audit and analysis of the performance of Australian and New Zealand intensive care since 1992. The main adult patient database now contains data on over 800,000 patient episodes, one of the largest single datasets on intensive care in the world. The associated Australian and New Zealand Paediatric Intensive Care Registry, ANZPICR, contains over ten years of paediatric admission data. As well as benchmarking performance in intensive care, these data sets also provide an invaluable resource for the intensive care community and other health care sectors. The data has led to publications on treatment of ICU patients, including analyses of factors such as blood glucose control, kidney injury, sepsis, inter-hospital transfer of patients, after-hours discharge, and so on. (Bagshaw, Bellomo et al. 2008; Bagshaw, George et al. 2008; Flabouris et al. 2008; Moran et al. 2008; Pilcher et al. 2007; Stow et al. 2007). It enables resource planning to assist in daily activities, research and service delivery. Examples include local hospital staffing and resource planning, statewide infrastructure planning, influenza pandemic planning and biosecurity and terrorism planning (ANZICS 2008).

Australian Orthopaedic Association National Joint Replacement Registry (AOA NJRR)

In 1993, the Australian Orthopaedic Association recognised a need for a national joint replacement registry. At the time, outcomes of this type of surgery in Australia were unknown and it was not clear who was receiving joint replacements or the types of prostheses and techniques being used. The Commonwealth Department of Health and Ageing agreed to fund the Australian Orthopaedic Association to establish the Registry from 1998, and data collection started September 1999.

The purpose of the National Joint Replacement Registry is to define, improve and maintain the quality of care of individuals receiving joint replacement surgery. This is done by collecting a defined minimum data set that enables outcomes to be determined on the basis of patient characteristics, prosthesis type and features, method of prosthesis fixation and surgical technique used. The registry measures revision surgery (where a prosthesis is replaced) and mortality. Analysis of revisions, combined with a careful analysis of the timing and reasons for revision, ensures this can be used as an accurate measure of the success or otherwise of a procedure. The analyses are used to inform surgeons, other health care professionals, governments, orthopaedic companies and the wider community. The AOA NJRR has contributed directly to the quality of care, particularly to changes in clinical practice. These have included changes in the use (or non-use) of particular prostheses and techniques (de Steiger et al. 2008). The stated aims of the NJRR include providing accurate information on the use of different types of prostheses in both primary and revision joint replacements, evaluating the effectiveness of different types of joint replacement prostheses and surgical techniques at a national level, the provision of confidential data to individual surgeons and hospitals to audit their joint replacement surgery, and educating Australian orthopaedic surgeons in the most effective prostheses and surgical techniques to achieve successful outcomes (AOA NJRR).

The success of these and other registries here and abroad has led to the development of further registries, a call for the development of new registries and the increased application of analyses of the data held (e.g. see Cameron et al. 2008; Chew et al. 2008; Evans 2008; Scott 2008).

A criticism that has been levelled at clinical registries is that they can be expensive activities with unclear benefits. Certainly, registries may require considerable investment to develop and sustain. However, this cost needs to be compared with the cost savings and/or health quality improvements gained from the information and analyses. For example, the National Joint Replacement Registry has apparently influenced changes in clinical practice (de Steiger et al. 2008), and captures information on revision rates following hip and knee surgery. Over the past four years, the proportion of hip and knee procedure revisions has declined from 14.8 to 11.1 per cent and from 10.4 to 7.9 per cent respectively. These declines are in large part attributable to monitoring systems incorporated into the registry design that detect poorly performing prostheses. The annual cost saving has been estimated at $44.6 million. Given that the cost of running the Registry is approximately $1.5 million per annum, this represents a significant value (Graves 2008).

However, these examples may be the tip of the clinical registries pyramid in Australia, and much of the remainder of that pyramid consists of registries with high aspirations whose benefits have been harder to realise. The value and impact of some clinical registers has been limited by such factors as unnecessarily extensive collection of data, poor quality control, inadequate governance procedures, lack of adequate funding, or lack of linkage to an effective operator arm for gaining quality improvement in clinical practice. These limitations have curtailed their contribution to clinical quality improvement, as have the following:

- No national standard exists against which funding applications by clinical registries can be written or assessed.
- No routine processes exist to ensure that clinical registries improve safety and quality. For example, many registries take a significant period of time to collate data, reducing their ability to provide timely information to health care providers and to support clinical quality assurance and improvement.
- Registry processes, data and technology are neither uniform nor standardised, creating significant inefficiencies and hampering inter-operability with other information systems.

- Some registries collect data items that do not conform to national definitions, thereby limiting the utility and comparability of the data.
- Data quality, including completeness, is often compromised. Some registries seek information from the routine administrative collections to determine completeness or to match data with administrative collections (including hospital statistics or deaths) to extend or validate the registry information.

The potential value of clinical registries, along with the limitations of many registries, has led the Australian Commission on Safety and Quality in Health Care (ACSQHC) to develop a project aimed at enhancing the understanding, utility and application of clinical registries.

The ACSQHC, the NHMRC Centre of Research Excellence in Patient Safety at Monash University and the National E-Health Transition Authority (NEHTA) have collaborated to develop operating principles and technical standards for Australian Clinical Quality Registries (ACSQHC 2008). These are registers that are (potentially) national in coverage, and are primarily focused on supporting improvement in clinical practice, particularly clinical safety and quality.

A core function of Australian Clinical Quality Registries must be the ability to improve clinical practice and health outcomes and be capable of accurately capturing the state of health care in Australia. For registers to meet their full potential in informing the state of health care in Australia, confidence is needed in the quality and relevance of the data. The purpose of the proposed operating principles and technical standards is to:

- provide a means of improving existing clinical registers and enhancing the value of the information they provide;
- provide guidance for the establishment and maintenance of new Australian Clinical Quality Registries aiming to measure quality of care; and
- suggest a best-practice model to which both new and existing Australian Clinical Quality Registries should adhere.

An Australian Clinical Quality Registry is a registry whose purpose is to improve the safety or quality of health care provided to patients, and thus it must demonstrate potential for significant impact and relevance on quality and safety. The improvement should be commensurate with cost and effort. The data collected, and the subject-matter or 'content' of a registry, should be clearly relevant to clinical practice.

The role and position of Australian Clinical Quality Registries needs to be defined within the context of the broader safety and quality effort. We need to better understand:

- where registries fit in the context of other quality and safety activities currently used throughout the health system;
- what criteria should be used to assess whether a registry should be implemented over an alternative approach; and
- what synergies exist between registries and other safety and quality activities. For example, it may be that registry data can be used as part of national accreditation standards or national performance indicators.

In addition to understanding how registries fit into the wider quality and safety movement, the ways in which quality can be measured by registries and used to drive system improvement needs further research, and clinicians need to be integral to this work. The use of predetermined quality process and outcome indicators, soundly based on the literature or at least on consensus judgments of experts, and embedded into registries, is one approach to measuring quality. In considering what measures to use to assess performance, clinical quality registries need to ensure they adhere to their purpose and avoid 'scope creep'. While measuring outcomes is important, in some situations there are limitations in only using direct outcome measurement, such as when there are long time lapses before outcomes are measurable, or when numbers are small or there are questions about the adequacy of risk stratification, or about confounding.

Furthermore, work is also needed to identify how data can be used to drive change at the clinical interface. It may be that quality improvement is driven by the production of outputs, such as quality indicators from clinical registries and routine feedback to providers, teams within institutions, professional accreditation/auditing bodies and the public. These outputs might include warning signals that trigger when performance falls below predetermined levels. The use of these data by multidisciplinary teams should facilitate quality improvement activities by identifying areas of need and assessing performance relative to efforts to improve care. Additionally, the operating principles for Australian Clinical Quality Registries require that a registry has a documented procedure for addressing significant and unexplained variances in the quality and safety of care. Such an 'outlier' procedure needs to be sophisticated and flexible enough to address the issues and involve the various stakeholders, such as clinicians, facilities, peak bodies, consumers, funders and jurisdictions, as appropriate (ACSQHC 2008).

A characteristic of successful registries, and a very significant element of the future success of clinical quality registries, is the central role played by clinicians. The ACSQHC recognises this in the draft *Operating Principles and Technical Standards for Australian Clinical Quality Registries* which describe the various roles for clinicians, consumers, peak bodies, funders, jurisdictions and other stakeholders in the further development, operation and impact of registries (ACSQHC 2008).

Clinical registries can have a key role in monitoring and improving the quality and safety of Australian health care. They have the potential to provide a strong evidential base for determining the efficacy, safety and quality of providers, interventions, medications, devices and treatments. Many of the gaps in knowledge we have identified will be addressed over the next few years as Australian Clinical Quality Registries are further developed in the context of the wider quality and safety agenda. The structures and governance of an Australian Clinical Quality Registry form a nexus that connects clinicians, administrators, peak bodies, jurisdictions and consumers. These connections can be used to build confidence and transparency in Australian health care and help ensure that our activities are focused on the patient. In the coming e-health-enabled environment, the utility and impact of registries should flourish as both a source and destination for information and analyses.

CLINICAL PRACTICE GUIDELINES

Attempts to identify and specify what should be happening in clinical practice occurred at the same time as the moves to capture data to improve knowledge about what was actually happening.

The United States was the first country to develop clinical practice guidelines on a significant scale, starting in the 1930s when the American College of Surgeons produced guidelines on the organisation of cancer services in hospitals, and a manual on fracture care (Weisz et al. 2007). Production of guidelines soared in the 1970s, stimulated by the National Institute of Health's Consensus Development Program, and has continued to rise. PubMed, the US National Library of Medicine service that provides access to citations from biomedical literature, introduced 'practice guidelines' as a document type in 1992 and citations each year continue to increase. Outside the United States, Dutch and Swedish organisations started guideline development in the 1980s, with organisations in other countries starting production of guidelines in the 1990s (Burgers et al. 2003). Some countries, such as the United Kingdom, Germany, France and New Zealand, have national agencies with a coordinated program of guideline production. In Australia, development of clinical practice guidelines has never been centralised in this way, although the National Health and Medical Research Council (NHMRC)—a statutory authority established in 1936—has had an identified role in providing health advice from the time of its inception. The 1992 *NHMRC Act* identifies a role for the Council to issue guidelines and subsequent amendments provide for it to approve guidelines developed by other bodies. Consistent with the concerns of the times and the origins of the Council, for many decades following its establishment the focus was on public health advice, particularly infectious diseases and infant and child welfare (NHMRC 1996). The work program of the Council expanded over the years, particularly from 1993 onwards, to include provision of evidence-based advice on aspects of clinical practice. However, it does not have funding for a dedicated clinical practice guidelines program. Federal and state governments currently provide funding support for a number of clinical practice guidelines, but development of these guidelines in Australia continues to rely heavily on voluntary contributions of time by health professionals and on the efforts of professional specialty associations.

A number of factors are believed to have played a role in promoting the growth of clinical practice guidelines internationally. One reason was the increasing difficulty in meeting demand for medical services with the expansion of new medical technologies, rising public expectations and an ageing population. This cost imperative, combined with the data documenting quality problems that showed striking variations in care, prompted interest from health care purchasers, such as governments and health insurance companies. Another factor was the dramatic increase in medical knowledge and the discovery and development of new and complex interventions that required standardised techniques and elaborate protocols. The role of professional organisations in developing and promoting clinical practice guidelines has variously been portrayed as fulfilling their professional responsibility to present current knowledge and expert opinion to their members, policy-makers and the public; or alternatively, as a way to preserve professional autonomy and resist external regulation.

Clinical practice guidelines range from consensus-based documents—statements by a group of experts, with or without reference to evidence—to more explicitly evidence-based guidelines, developed after the systematic retrieval and appraisal of literature that separates opinion from evidence. A major shift from professional consensus to documents developed with more scientific rigour took place in the 1990s. There was greater investment worldwide in guidelines programs that employed methods experts, and gained input from all relevant stakeholders including consumers, rather than relying solely on the collective expertise of clinicians. Development of a clinical practice guideline can now cost several hundred thousand dollars, depending on the complexity of the issue and whether the guideline has been developed according to rigorous methods with systematic searching and appraisal of the research literature. This professionalisation of the guideline development process means that clinical groups which lack substantial funding have either moved away from auspicing guideline development, or the guidelines they produce often fail to meet current standards for guideline quality. However, even in countries with well-funded centralised guideline programs, clinical contributions to expert advisory groups are often made on a voluntary basis.

The most commonly accepted definition of clinical practice guidelines is still that developed by Field and Lohr: 'systematically developed statements to assist practitioner and patient decisions about appropriate health care for specific clinical circumstances' (Field and Lohr 1992). Recently, an alternative definition which reflects the move to make guidelines explicitly evidence based has been gaining acceptance: 'A guideline is a document with recommendations and instructions to assist health care professionals and patients in clinical decision making, based on research findings and consensus among experts, in order to make effective and efficient clinical practice explicit.' (Van Everdingen et al. 2004).

The growth in numbers of clinical practice guidelines observed in other countries has also occurred in Australia. A cross-sectional survey in 1993 (Ward and Grieco 1996) identified 34 clinical practice guidelines from 32 organisations. A later survey (Buchan et al. in preparation), aimed at identifying all clinical practice guidelines produced or endorsed for use in Australia between 2003 and 2007, identified 306 clinical practice guidelines, with over 80 groups and organisations involved in their production. A large number of these guidelines were produced by clinical colleges or specialty associations, including groups representing nursing and allied health professionals. While a considerable number of guidelines in the later survey were produced with government funding and support, many others were developed by specialty organisations or groups of health care professionals with no stated external funding support.

The 1993 survey (Ward and Grieco 1996) identified several quality problems, including no description of the processes used (if any) for retrieving and synthesising evidence. In 1995, the National Health and Medical Research Council published the first in a series of guides providing 'guidelines for guidelines', outlining the processes that should be used to develop high-quality clinical practice guidelines (NHMRC 1995). By 2007, nearly a third of the guideline documents gave some description of the processes for reviewing evidence. It is clear that substantial funding support is required to develop multi-disciplinary clinical practice guidelines where recommendations are based on a thorough review of the available scientific research evidence. The clinical area with the most sustained effort to develop a suite of evidence-based guidelines is cancer care (see Box 4.1).

Box 4.1 The Australian Cancer Network

The Australian Cancer Network (ACN) was established in 1994 by the Cancer Council Australia and the Clinical Oncological Society of Australia, with the aim of improving cancer services and cancer care. One of its key roles is to develop and disseminate evidence-based clinical practice guidelines for the prevention, diagnosis and management of cancer. The network is composed of more than 70 interest groups, including medical and nursing colleges, specialty associations, specialist cancer bodies and consumer groups. Leading clinicians voluntarily contribute their time and expertise to the guideline development process.

In 1995, a working party chaired by Professor Tom Reeve from the ACN produced the first NHMRC evidence-based guideline on management of early breast cancer—chosen because there was recognition of the large burden of disease and substantial variations in practice in Australia. The process used to gain support from the clinical community included a Breast Cancer Consensus Conference (which, despite its name, was explicitly evidence based and based on the model used by the United States National Institutes of Health), held in 1994. The early breast cancer guideline was accompanied by a version designed for consumers produced in October 1995 by the then newly formed NHMRC National Breast

Cancer Centre, which also disseminated and evaluated the guidelines. The guidelines were well accepted. A survey of Australian surgeons who managed breast cancer (Carrick et al. 1998) (150 respondents—64 per cent response rate) reported that surgeons were generally positive about the guidelines, with more than 80 per cent of respondents believing that they were useful in improving women's management. Subsequent studies of the management of breast cancer in Australia (McEvoy et al. 2004; White et al. 2004; Drummond et al. 2005) found that there had been several important changes in practice since the guidelines had been published. Surgeons treating breast carcinoma patients in two states where studies were undertaken had changed their practice patterns consistent with the national guidelines. Following development of the guidelines, a National Audit of Breast Cancer was initiated, supported by the Royal Australasian College of Surgeons. This audit now occurs on a continuing basis and provides information about the surgical treatment of early breast cancer in Australia and New Zealand. It allows surgeons to compare their practice data against a number of standards established as indicators of best practice (Royal Australasian College of Surgeons 2008).

The ACN have now produced more than ten evidence-based guidelines on all aspects of detection and management of breast cancer, skin cancer, prostate cancer, lung cancer, bowel cancer, brain cancers, lymphomas and gynaecological cancers. While funding from government helps support the development and production of these guidelines, the contribution to the guideline development process from clinical experts in cancer care continues on a voluntary basis.

Although there has been extensive involvement by clinicians in the production of clinical practice guidelines because of their potential to improve care quality and outcomes for patients, clinicians have also been concerned about possible adverse effects of clinical practice guideline production and promulgation. Issues include the loss of clinical autonomy with allegations about 'cookbook medicine', the potential for legal action if guidelines are not followed, and the potential for misuse by government authorities to impose cost-cutting and standardise medical practice. However, a systematic review of clinicians' attitudes to clinical practice guidelines, undertaken in 2000 (Farquhar et al. 2002), found that most of the clinicians surveyed were supportive of clinical practice guidelines. This study systematically reviewed surveys of clinicians' attitudes published in English between 1990 and 2000. Surveys with fewer than 100 respondents or with response rates below 60 per cent were excluded. The literature search found 153 surveys of clinicians' attitudes, of which 30 (20 per cent) met the inclusion criteria. Studies were from the United States, Canada, the United Kingdom, Italy, Israel, Denmark, the Netherlands, Ireland and Australia. Four Australian studies surveying general practitioners, cardiologists and surgeons were also included in the review (Gupta et al. 1997; Carrick et al. 1998; Girgis et al. 1999; Shah et al. 1999).

The systematic review found that most clinicians agreed that guidelines were a helpful source of advice (weighted mean 75 per cent), good educational tools (weighted mean 71 per cent) and were intended to improve quality of care (weighted mean 70 per cent). But sizeable numbers agreed that guidelines were intended to cut health care costs (weighted mean 53 per cent), and would increase litigation or disciplinary action (weighted mean 41 per cent). There were also sizeable minorities—about one-third—who agreed with the propositions that guidelines reduce physician autonomy, are over-simplified or 'cookbook' medicine, and are impractical and too rigid to apply to individual patients. Similar concerns about cookbook medicine and the potential to increase the number of malpractice suits were raised in a later survey of Australian surgeons' attitudes towards colorectal cancer guidelines (Gattellari et al. 2001).

While health care professional groups have been at the forefront of the development and evolution of clinical practice guidelines in Australia, the limits of what volunteer efforts can achieve in this area have now been reached. Developing evidence-based guidelines is an expensive activity which requires specialist methodological skills as well as specific clinical expertise in the guideline subject area. Funding development of this kind of guideline is beyond the capacity of most health professional groups and associations. Guidelines that do not have this kind of methodological rigour will not reflect the most accurate, up to date and unbiased synthesis of the scientific literature and expert opinion (Hasenfeld and Shekelle 2003). It is time to consider the value of a more coordinated approach to guideline development, and a more substantial national investment in this area, similar to that of other developed nations.

The best evidence to date on whether clinical practice guidelines improve care quality comes from a systematic review of studies of guideline dissemination and implementation strategies published between 1966 and 1998 (Grimshaw et al. 2004; Grimshaw et al. 2006). This review considered 235 studies that used controlled study designs (randomised controlled trials, controlled clinical trials, controlled before and after studies, and interrupted time series) to evaluate guideline dissemination and implementation strategies that target medically qualified health care professionals, and that reported objective measures of provider behaviour and/or patient outcome. The studies were conducted in fourteen different countries, although most (71 per cent) were conducted in the United States. They covered primary care, inpatient settings and generalist outpatient settings. The review included 309 comparisons from the 235 studies of an intervention group versus a control group. The majority of studies (73 per cent) evaluated different combinations of interventions against a 'no intervention' control group, or against a control group which also received one or more interventions. The interventions studied were dissemination of educational materials, educational meetings, reminders, audit and feedback and patient-directed interventions.

Overall, the majority of comparisons (86.6 per cent) observed modest to moderate improvements in care. Reminders were the strategy most consistently observed to be effective—the median absolute improvement in performance was 14.1 per cent in fourteen cluster randomised comparisons. Educational outreach only led to modest effects (median absolute improvement 6.0 per cent in thirteen cluster randomised comparisons of multifaceted interventions involving educational outreach), as did audit and feedback (median absolute improvement 7.0 per cent in five cluster randomised comparisons). Dissemination of educational materials—a comparatively low cost intervention— had similar effects to more intensive interventions (median absolute improvement of 8.1 per cent in four cluster randomised comparisons). Multifaceted interventions were not necessarily more effective than single interventions.

However, the overall quality of the studies was poor and the reviewers concluded that there was an imperfect evidence base to support decisions about which guideline dissemination and implementation strategies were likely to be efficient under different circumstances. Several studies of guideline implementation have been undertaken in the years since this systematic review, and an updated review examining later studies would be likely to find fewer methodological problems, and thus be able to provide greater guidance on the effectiveness and efficiency of strategies to improve guideline uptake.

There has been an increasing international focus on producing actionable guidelines and on finding ways to ensure dissemination and uptake. Australia was the first country to establish a national agency, the National Institute of Clinical Studies, formed in 2000, to improve health-care by helping close the gap between best available evidence and current clinical practice. The Institute was established following representation to the Minister of Health by leading clinical experts in evidence-based care and representatives of the medical colleges, about the need for a group to lead the continuous improvement of clinical practice and its delivery. It existed for just over six years as a Commonwealth-owned company with a board of directors, predominantly medically qualified, who were appointed by the Minister for Health. During this time, it worked with a number of clinical groups on a variety of programs to improve use of evidence in clinical care. By the end of 2005–06, the year before it joined with the NHMRC, clinical teams from over 70 per cent of all major Australian hospitals and 42 per cent of Divisions of General Practice had participated in programs run by the Institute on topics such as increasing the use of prophylaxis in patients at risk of deep vein thrombosis, improving the management of pain relief for people with cancer, and improving management of heart failure (National Institute of Clinical Studies 2006).

COLLABORATIVE QUALITY IMPROVEMENT

During the 1990s, the focus internationally on changing the knowledge, skills and habits of individual clinicians enlarged to include consideration of the context and system within which individual clinicians operate. This was stimulated by influential reports on the need to improve safety and quality of care, such as those from the US Institute of Medicine (Institute of Medicine 1998). The use of quality improvement methods, with an emphasis on clinical leadership, to improve clinical care increased. In particular, from 1995 onwards the 'Breakthrough Series' collaborative quality improvement approach developed by the United States-based Institute for Healthcare Improvement (IHI) gained popularity (Institute for Healthcare Improvement 2003).

The 'Breakthrough Series' is a short-term approach (from six to fifteen months) to collaborative quality improvement, based on the belief that much existing scientific knowledge that would help improve the processes and outcomes of care is not used in routine practice. It aims to help organisations make 'breakthrough' improvements in the care they deliver. The theoretical literature about quality improvement collaboratives identifies the following key features (Schouten et al. 2008):

- There is a specified topic with either large variations in care or with gaps between best evidence and current practice.
- Clinical experts join with experts in quality improvement to identify and share scientific knowledge, best practice and methods for improvement.
- A number of multi-professional teams from multiple sites join together in a focused time-limited effort to improve care.
- Teams use a model for improvement that involves identifying aims, setting measurable targets, testing changes on a small scale and collecting data.
- Teams participate in a series of structured meetings over a defined timescale to learn, exchange ideas and improve care.

Teams collect data to measure the impact of the changes they have made in their practice settings during 'Action Periods' between the structured meetings that function as learning sessions. This iterative process is often referred to as the 'Plan, Do, Study, Act' cycle. This model has considerable face validity, was extensively promoted by persuasive health care leaders, and has elements that appeal to policy-makers, managers and clinicians. Collaborative quality improvement initiatives spread from their US base and were adopted in a number of European countries, including the United Kingdom, Norway, Sweden and the Netherlands (Institute for Healthcare Improvement 2007).

In Australia, emergency care was one of the first clinical areas where collaborative quality improvement methods were used. During the late 1990s, there were considerable demand pressures in emergency departments, with widespread publicity about adverse effects on patient care and concerns for patient safety. The need to respond to these pressures helped drive the diffusion of collaborative continuous quality improvement (CQI) projects in major hospital emergency rooms. In 1999, an emergency care team from one major Melbourne public hospital participated in an IHI emergency care Breakthrough Collaborative Program with a number of United States hospitals. The team reported improvements in delivery of clinical treatments and some success in improving patient flow (Toncich et al. 2000). Their apparent success and enthusiasm about the benefits of the approach, combined with a high level of public and political concern about conditions in emergency departments, prompted investment the following year by the Victorian state government in a statewide emergency collaborative.

Government funding covered central administration costs, licensing fees and training with IHI, a patient satisfaction survey, and a payment to hospitals for employing additional staff so that teams from the emergency departments had time designated to undertake the quality improvement project. Staff from eighteen large public emergency departments took part in this collaborative program over an eight-month period. The collaborative teams reported significant improvements in 32 of the 47 clinical projects (e.g. reducing time to thrombolysis, and reducing time to antibiotic administration for specific clinical conditions), and in 24 of the 39 operational improvement projects (such as reducing turn around times for supporting services and reducing time to inpatient admission) (Bartlett et al. 2002). There was also substantial enthusiasm from participating teams about their involvement with the collaborative program, with half the teams describing their experience as 'excellent'.

The first national collaborative quality improvement program, with participation of emergency department staff from 47 Australian hospitals, was launched in 2002 by the National Institute of Clinical Studies (see Box 4.2).

Box 4.2 Quality collaboratives

In 2002, the National Institute of Clinical Studies wrote to all 160 Australian hospitals with emergency department attendances of greater than 20,000 per annum and invited them to participate in a quality improvement collaborative. Hospitals were expected to meet the costs associated with participation. In most cases, participation by hospital teams was voluntary, although one state government required its public metropolitan hospitals to participate and provided financial support to these hospitals to fund participants' travel to national meetings and to employ fill-in staff. Members of four state emergency nurses' associations, and the President, Chair of Quality, and Chair of Standards for the Australasian College for Emergency Medicine were part of the planning group.

Hospital teams were provided with a list of possible topic areas that could be selected for improvement. The common choice was reducing time to pain relief; 45 of the 47 hospitals included this among their project areas. Most other topics chosen by participating hospital teams involved reducing time to treatment—for example, reducing time to thrombolysis; reducing time to pathology or x-ray testing, or improving patient flow through the emergency department.

Teams met face to face three times over a six-month period and took

---

part in monthly conference calls around specific topic areas. A web-based information exchange system allowed for real-time data entry and graphing of results against targets, posting of protocols and resources and a chat forum for the teams involved. Entry to the system was password protected but all teams were able to view the data from each participating hospital. The 47 participating hospitals nominated 95 projects in total. In 63 of the 95 projects, there was self-reported improvement: 36 projects showed an improvement of 30 per cent or more in their indicator measurements. In 28 of the 95 projects, the team's nominated improvement target was met at the six-month formal end of the collaborative project.

Reducing time to analgesia was the overall focus of the collaborative, and 45 of the 47 participating hospitals focused on this area. Of 41 hospitals for which there was sufficient data, 34 hospitals reported an improvement in their time to analgesia, with nine of the hospitals achieving their identified target reduction time. In seven hospitals, time to pain relief actually worsened over the course of the collaborative period but, overall, median time to pain relief for patients reduced by 20 minutes.

Many clinical teams remained keen to continue the project after it had formally drawn to a close. Six months after the project was originally scheduled to end, 41 of the 47 original hospitals continued to participate in regular teleconferences and web-based exchange of information, and eighteen hospitals still regularly entered data tracking their performance on the originally selected indicators.

Collaborative quality improvement programs in other areas quickly followed. The Australian Council for Safety and Quality in Healthcare conducted the National Medication Safety Breakthrough Collaborative in 2003–04 with clinical teams from 100 Australian hospitals. The two key goals were to improve medication safety by reducing medication-related harm by 50 per cent among patients or clients of participating health care teams, and to develop a national network and system to sustain and transfer improvements in medication safety in health services across Australia. An evaluation in 2006 found that the collaborative had lifted the profile of medication safety in Australia, and that participating teams reported that many changes had been made to improve medication safety in their hospitals and health services (Australian Council for Safety and Quality in Health Care 2006).

The Australian Primary Care Collaboratives Program began in 2004 with funding to cover the costs of the program provided by the

Australian Government. The program focused on improving care for patients with chronic disease, specifically chronic heart disease and diabetes, and on improving access to primary care. The program was inspired by the reported dramatic success of the UK National Primary Care Development team in improving quality of care for patients. This UK program, using the IHI Breakthrough methods, was undertaken on a large scale (2000 participating practices with 11.5 million patients), and reported a fourfold reduction of mortality from existing coronary disease in participating practices compared with others, and multiple reductions in waits and delays between primary and secondary care (Knight 2004).

Initially, over 170 Australian general practices with over 950 full-time equivalent general practitioners covering 580,000 patients took part. They reported significant improvements in a number of indicators, such as blood glucose measured as glycated haemoglobin (HbA1C) levels in diabetic patients, large increases in the number of diabetes and coronary heart disease (CHD) patients meeting blood pressure targets, and an increase in the proportion of patients seen on the day of their choice from 67 per cent to 81 per cent (Farmer et al. 2005; Smith 2006). Eighteen months after the scheme began, people taking part in the program continued to report improvement in indicators of care quality (McCredie 2006). Eventually, approximately 600 practices participated in the first phase of the program. In 2007–08 the government provided funding to continue and expand the program with the aim of eventually involving 1000 general practices in collaborative quality improvement efforts (Improvement Foundation Australia 2008).

These collaborative quality improvement methods generate substantial enthusiasm and belief in their effectiveness among many participants. The use of data collection and analysis for problem diagnosis, small-scale tests of hypotheses about potential ways to improve, and revision of interventions based on data feedback are all compatible with the scientific training of health professionals. The concepts are not complex or difficult to understand. The idea of better sharing and managing knowledge so that it can be translated into practice is logical and appealing. As well as striking an intellectual chord with health care workers, there is also clearly something powerful about the collaborative process that participants find emotionally engaging and enjoyable. It applies some of the techniques that are routinely used by many other forces in society to give people rewarding experiences and so influence behaviour. There is an opportunity to network and socially engage with peers, and to share a common higher purpose that provides benefits to others and contributes to the good of society generally. Learning sessions often feature speakers with motivational messages, and many of the best-known proponents of collaboratives have charismatic, inspirational speaking styles. During learning sessions, people make public commitments about changes they will attempt to make, and testify about the success or failure of their efforts. Within the collaborative community, there is a strong ethic of sharing and providing help to others. Although several millions of dollars are spent every year on health care meetings, many of these conferences focus on the latest knowledge about what should be done for specific conditions or diseases. Other meetings aim to develop skills, knowledge and networks within a particular health care discipline. It is comparatively rare for members of multidisciplinary health care teams to meet and talk about how they could be working together to deliver care more effectively. The appeal of collaborative methods for health professionals probably lies as much in the approach taken as it does in the results achieved.

However, despite the widespread uptake of these quality improvement collaboratives, and the considerable investment in them worldwide, there is relatively little strong research evidence about their effectiveness. A systematic review of empirical studies of the effectiveness of quality improvement collaboratives identified 72 papers reporting studies of quality improvement collaboratives, which contained data on the effectiveness of care processes or outcomes, and which were published between January 1995 and June 2006 (Schouten et al. 2008). The majority of the studies were uncontrolled and over 60 per cent of these studies were based on self-report measures of participating teams. While many of the uncontrolled studies reported dramatic improvements in patient care and organisational performance, almost all of these studies had design limitations: study designs relied almost entirely on post measurement, were not able to account for secular trends, and included only anecdotal information or selected samples from self-selected sites. The reports of effectiveness from all Australian collaborative quality improvement initiatives also have these features. The review team found nine studies where controlled designs had been used to measure the effects of quality improvement collaboratives on processes of care or outcomes of care—seven of these reported on collaborative quality improvement initiatives which were explicitly based on the IHI Breakthrough Series model used in Australia. Most of the controlled studies also had significant flaws—including possible differences in baseline measurement, limited data on characteristics of control sites, no specification of blinded assessment and possible contamination.

Overall, the controlled studies showed moderate positive results, and the review team concluded that the evidence of the impact of quality improvement collaboratives was positive but limited, and stressed the importance of obtaining a deeper understanding of the relative strength of this intervention—to look into the 'black box' of the intervention and study the determinants of success or failure. It is not clear whether collaborative quality improvement methods are more or less cost-effective than other approaches to stimulating clinical care improvement (Øvretveit et al. 2002). Also, little is known about the extent to which any improvements made during the course of a collaborative quality improvement program are sustained once the intervention has ceased, or whether the methods to improve care learned by the health professionals involved are applied to other clinical topics.

CONCLUSION

As the capacity for intervention has grown, and the ways of delivering health care become more complex, the risks of compromised safety and quality of patient care have also grown. Voluntary efforts by clinicians to improve care are important, but in areas such as data registers, and clinical practice guideline development and implementation, the methods and management systems needed to support high quality efforts now require a more organised approach. While interventions to improve care by focusing on knowledge, skills and behaviour change of individual clinicians are still important, approaches that target health care teams, organisations and the system as a whole are needed to reflect the reality of current patterns of health care provision in Australia. Government has provided funding and infrastructure for collaborative quality improvement initiatives that rely on voluntary participation by health care providers and clinicians, and in many areas there has been enthusiastic participation, but strong evidence of lasting effectiveness or of cost-effectiveness is lacking. Better evidence about the effectiveness and cost-effectiveness of other approaches to guideline implementation and quality improvement efforts in health care is also needed to guide future investment. While voluntary efforts to improve safety and quality will remain a key aspect of professionalism, other approaches are needed if the challenges to safety and quality of care are to be comprehensively addressed.

REFERENCES

Australia and New Zealand Dialysis and Transplant Registry (ANZDATA) 2008, *ANZDATA Registry Report 2007*, eds S. McDonald, S. Chang and L. Excell, Australia and New Zealand Dialysis and Transplant Registry, Adelaide

Australia and New Zealand Intensive Care Society (ANZICS) 2008, *Final Report of Alpha-testing of the Draft Operating Standards and Technical Design*, ANZICS, Melbourne

Australian Commission on Safety and Quality in Health Care (ACSQHC) 2008, *Operating Principles and Technical Standards for Australian Clinical Quality Registries*, ACSQHC, Canberra

Australian Council for Safety and Quality in Health Care 2006, *Evaluation of the National Medication Safety Breakthrough Collaborative: Final Report*, Urbis Keys Young, Sydney

Australian Orthopaedic Association National Joint Replacement Registry (AOA NJRR), <www.dmac.adelaide.edu.au/aoanjrr/index.jsp>, accessed 3 April 2009

Bagshaw, S., Bellomo, R., and George, C. 2008, 'Early blood glucose control and mortality in critically ill patients in Australia', *Critical Care Medicine*, in press

Bagshaw, S., George, C. and Bellomo, R. 2008, 'Early acute kidney injury and sepsis: A multicentre evaluation', *Critical Care*, vol. 12, no. 2, p. R47

Bartlett, J., Cameron, P. and Cisera, M. 2002, 'The Victorian emergency department collaboration', *International Journal of Quality Health Care*, vol. 14, no. 6, pp. 463-70

Brennan T.A., Leape L.L., Laird N.M., Hebert, L., Localio, A.R., Lawthers, A.G., Newhouse, J.P., Weiler, P.C. and Hiatt, H.H. 2004, 'Incidence of adverse events and negligence in hospitalised patients: Results of the Harvard Medical Practice Study I. 1991', *Quality and Safety in Health Care*, vol. 13, no. 2, pp. 145-51

Buchan, H., Currie, K., Lourey, E. and Duggan, G., *Australian Clinical Practice Guidelines 2003—2007*, in preparation

Burgers, J., Grol, R., Klazinga, N., Makela, M. and Zaat, J. 2003, 'Towards evidence based clinical practice: An international survey of 18 clinical guideline programs', *International Journal of Quality Health Care*, vol. 15, no. 1, pp. 31-45

Cameron, P.A., Gabbe, B.J., Cooper, D.J., Walker, T., Judson, R. and McNeil, J. 2008, 'A statewide system of trauma care in Victoria: effect on patient survival', *Medical Journal of Australia*, vol. 189, no. 10, pp. 546-50

Carrick, S.E., Bonevski, B., Redman, S., Simpson, J., Sanson-Fisher, R.W. and Webster, F. 1998, 'Surgeons' opinions about the NHMRC clinical practice guidelines for the management of early breast cancer', *Medical Journal of Australia*, vol. 169, no. 6, pp. 300–5

Chew, D.P., Amerena, J.V., Coverdale, S.G., Rankin, J.M., Astley, C.M., Soman, A. and Brieger, D.B. 2008, 'Invasive management and late clinical outcomes in contemporary Australian management of acute coronary syndromes: Observations from the ACACIA registry', *Medical Journal of Australia*, vol. 188, no. 12, pp. 691–7

Cochrane, A.L. 1989, *Effectiveness and Efficiency: Random Reflections on a Health Service*, 2nd ed., Nuffield Provincial Hospitals Trust, Glasgow

de Steiger, R., Graves, S.E., Davidson, D.C., Tomkins, A., Miller, L., Stanford, T., Pratt, N., Ryan, P., Griffith, E. and McDermott, B. 2008, 'AOA—National Joint Replacement Registry—Does it result in a change of practice?', Registry Interest Group meeting, 14 November 2008

de Vries, E.N., Ramrattan, M.A., Smorenburg, S.M., Gouma, D.J. and Boermeester, M.A. 2008, 'The incidence and nature of in-hospital adverse events: A systematic review', *Quality and Safety in Health Care*, vol. 17, no. 3, pp. 216–23

Drolet B.C. and Johnson, K.B. 2008, 'Categorizing the world of registries' *Journal of Biomedical Informatics*, vol. 41, no. 6, pp. 1009–20

Drummond, R., Power, A., Evans, A., Luxford, K., Blakey, D., Delaney, G. and Rodger, A. 2005, 'Changes in practice of breast cancer radiotherapy 1998 –2002: An Australasian survey', *Australasian Radiology*, vol. 49, no. 1, pp. 44–52

Evans, S. 2008, 'Clinical registries and quality measurement', *Australian Patient Safety Bulletin*, no. 10, p. 8

Evidence-Based Medicine Working Group 1992, 'Evidence-based medicine: A new approach to teaching the practice of medicine', *Journal of the American Medical Association*, vol. 268, no. 17, pp. 2420–5

Eyenet Sweden 2005, *Handbook for Establishing Quality Registries*, Eyenet Sweden, Karlskrona

Farmer, L., Knight, A. and Ford, D. 2005, 'Systems change in Australian general practice: Early impact of the National Primary Care Collaboratives', *Australian Family Physician*, vol. 34, AFP Supplement, pp. 44–6

Farquhar, C., Kola, E. and Slutsky, J. 2002, 'Clinicians' attitudes to clinical practice guidelines: A systematic review', *Medical Journal of Australia*, vol. 177, no. 9, pp. 502–6

Field M.J. and Lohr K.N., eds 1992, *Guidelines for Clinical Practice: From Development to Use*, Institute of Medicine, National Academy Press, Washington, DC

Flabouris, A., Hart, G. and George, C. 2008, 'Impact of interhospital transfer on outcomes of patients admitted to Australian or New Zealand tertiary level

ICUs: Comparison with similar patients admitted from the Emergency Department using the ANZICS Adult Patient Database', *Critical Care and Resuscitation*, in press

Gattellari, M., Ward, J. and Solomon, M. 2001, 'Implementing guidelines about colorectal cancer: A national survey of target groups', *ANZ Journal of Surgery*, vol. 71, no. 3, pp. 147–53

Girgis, S., Ward, J.E. and Thomson, C.J.H. 1999, 'General practitioners' perceptions of medicolegal risk', *Medical Journal of Australia*, vol. 171, no. 7, pp. 362–66

Gliklich, R.E. and Dreyer, N.A., eds 2007, *Registries for Evaluating Patient Outcomes: A User's Guide*, prepared by Outcome DEcIDE Center [Outcome Sciences, Inc. dba Outcome] under Contract No. HHSA290200500351 TO1, AHRQ Publication No. 07-EHC001-1, Agency for Healthcare Research and Quality, Rockville, MD

Graves, S. 2008, 'Benefits and limitations of registries', *Nordic Orthopaedic Federation Conference*, Amsterdam, the Netherlands, 11–13 June 2008, <www.nof2008.com/home>, accessed 3 April 2009

Grimshaw, J., Eccles, M., Thomas, R., MacLennan, G., Ramsay, C., Fraser, C. and Vale, L. 2006, 'Towards evidence based quality improvement', *Journal of General Internal Medicine*, vol. 21, no. S2, pp. S14–20

Grimshaw, J., Thomas, R. and MacLennan, G., Fraser, C., Ramsay, C.R., Vale, L., Whitty, L., Eccles, M.P., Matowe, L., Shirran, L., Wensing, M., Dijkstra, R. and Donaldson, C. 2004, 'Effectiveness and efficiency of guideline dissemination and implementation strategies', *Health Technology Assessment*, vol. 8, no. 6, pp. 1–72

Gupta, L., Ward, J. and Hayward, R.S. 1997, 'Clinical practice guidelines in general practice: A national survey of recall, attitudes and impact', *Medical Journal of Australia*, vol. 166, no. 2, pp. 69–72

Hasenfeld, R. and Shekelle, P.G. 2003, 'Is the methodological quality of guidelines declining in the US? Comparison of the quality of US Agency for Health Care Policy and Research (AHCPR)', *Quality and Safety in Health Care*, vol. 12, no. 6, pp. 428–34

Improvement Foundation Australia 2008, *Overview of Australian Primary Care Collaboratives (APCC) Phase II*, <www.improve.org.au./APCC/apcc_phase2.html>, accessed 9 October 2008

Institute for Healthcare Improvement 2003, *The Breakthrough Series: IHI's Collaborative Model for Achieving Breakthrough Improvement*, IHI Innovation Series White Paper, Boston

——2007, *A History of IHI*, <www.ihi.org/NR/rdonlyres/E8194CFD3BB4-4B42-9317-7941F4C7C6D9/0/IHI_Timeline_2007_R4.pdf>, accessed 9 October 2008

Institute of Medicine 1998, *Statement of Quality of Care: National Round-table on Health Care Quality—The Urgent Need to Improve Health Care Quality*, <www.iom.edu/CMS/3809/18658.aspx>, accessed 9 October 2008

Knight, A. 2004, 'The collaborative method: A strategy for improving Australian general practice', *Australian Family Physician*, vol. 33, no. 4, pp. 269-74

McCredie, J., 2006, 'Collaboratives program has real world benefits', *Australian Doctor*, 27 October

McEvoy, S., Ingram, D., Byrne, M., Joseph, D.J., Dewar, J., Trotter, J., Harper, C., Haworth, C., Harvey, J.M., Sterrett, G.F., Jamrozik, K. and Fritschi, L. 2004, 'Breast cancer in Western Australia: Clinical practice and clinical guidelines', *Medical Journal of Australia*, vol. 181, no. 6, pp. 305-9

McGlynn, E.A., Asch, S.M., Adams, J., Keesey, J., Hicks, J., DeCristofaro, A. and Kerr, E.A. 2003, 'The quality of health care delivered to adults in the United States', *New England Journal of Medicine*, vol. 348, no. 26, pp. 2635-45

McPherson, K., Wennberg J.E., Hovind, O.B. and Clifford, P. 1982, 'Small area variations in the use of common surgical procedures: An international comparison of New England, England and Norway', *New England Journal of Medicine*, vol. 307, no. 21, pp. 1310-14

Moran, J., Bristow, P., Solomon, P., George, C. and Hart, G. for the Adult Database Management Committee (ADMC) of the Australian and New Zealand Intensive Care Society (ANZICS) 2008, 'Mortality and length-of-stay outcomes, 1993–2003, in the national Australian and New Zealand intensive care adult patient data base', *Critical Care Medicine*, vol. 36, no. 1, pp. 46-61

National Health and Medical Research Council 1995, *A Guide to the Development, Implementation and Evaluation of Clinical Practice Guidelines*, Commonwealth of Australia, Canberra

—— 1996, *Sixty Years of the National Health and Medical Research Council 1936-1996*, Commonwealth of Australia, Canberra

National Institute of Clinical Studies 2006, *Annual Report 2005-2006*, NICS, Melbourne

Pilcher, D., Duke, G., George, C., Bailey, M.J. and Hart, G. 2007, 'After-hours discharge from intensive care increases the risk of readmission and death', *Anaesthesia and Intensive Care*, vol. 35, no. 4, pp. 477-85

Øvretveit, J., Bare, P., Cleary, P., Cretin, S., Gustafson, D., McInnes, K., McLeod, H., Molfenter, T., Plsek, P., Robert, G., Shortell, S. and Wilson, T. 2002, 'Quality collaboratives: Lessons from research', *Quality and Safety in Health Care*, vol. 11, no. 4, pp. 345-51

Royal Australasian College of Surgeons 2008, <www.surgeons.org/Content/

NavigationMenu/Research/ASERNIPS/ASERNIPSAudits/National_Breast_Canc.htm>, accessed 19 October 2008

Schouten, L., Hulscher, M., van Everdingen, J., Huijsman, R. and Grol, R. 2008, 'Evidence for the impact of quality improvement collaboratives: Systematic review', *British Medical Journal*, vol. 336, no. 7659, pp. 1491–4

Scott, I. 2008, 'Why we need a national registry for interventional cardiology', *Medical Journal of Australia*, vol. 189, no. 4, pp. 223–7

Shah, S., Tonkin, A., Ward, J. and Harris, P. 1999, 'Implementation of nationally developed guidelines in cardiology: A survey of NSW cardiologists and cardiothoracic surgeons', *Australian and New Zealand Journal of Medicine*, vol. 29, no. 5, pp. 678–83

Smith, P. 2006, 'Collaboratives triumph: Revolutionary GP program shows dramatic results', *Australian Doctor*, 7 April, p. 1

Stow, P., Pilcher, D. et al. 2007, 'Improved outcomes from acute severe asthma in Australian intensive care units (1996–2003)', *Thorax*, vol. 62, no. 10, pp. 842–7

Toncich, G., Cameron, P.A., Virtue, E. and Bartlett, J. 2000, 'Institute for Healthcare Improvement collaborative to improve process times in an Australian emergency department', *Journal of Quality in Clinical Practice*, vol. 20, nos 2–3, pp. 79–86

Van Everdingen, J.J.E., Burgers, J.S., Assendelft, W.J.J., Swinkels, J.A., Van Barneveld, T.A., Van de Klundert, J.L.M., eds, 2004, *Evidence-based richtlijn-ontwikkeling: Een leidraad voor de praktijk [Evidence-based guideline development: A Practical Guide]*, Bohn Stafleu Van Loghum, Houton

Ward, J. and Grieco, V. 1996, 'Why we need guidelines for guidelines: A study of the quality of clinical practice guidelines in Australia', *Medical Journal of Australia*, vol. 165, no. 10, pp. 574–6

Weisz, G., Cambrioso, A., Keating, P., Knaapen, L., Schlich, T. and Tournay, V.J. 2007, 'The emergence of clinical practice guidelines', *Millbank Quarterly*, vol. 85, no. 4, pp. 691–727

Wennberg, J. and Gittelsohn, A. 1973, 'Small area variations in health care delivery', *Science*, vol. 182, no. 4117, pp. 1102–8

White, V., Pruden, M., Giles, G., Collins, J., Jamrozik, K., Inglis, G., Boyages, J. and Hill, D. 2004, 'The management of early breast carcinoma before and after the introduction of clinical practice guidelines', *Cancer*, vol. 101, no. 3, pp. 476–85

5

INTEGRATING CORPORATE AND CLINICAL GOVERNANCE

Heather Wellington and Paul Dugdale

INTRODUCTION

Governance of the health care system occurs at multiple levels and involves bureaucracies, regulatory boards, complaints commissioners, hospital managers, clinician leaders and clinicians. Although the term 'clinical governance' has special meaning in health care, governance can be viewed as a set of generic concepts, structures and processes which span sectors and domains. Good governance in an organisation arranges for the judgments that need to be made in the operation of the organisation to be properly informed, then appropriately made and implemented.

This chapter considers the clinical governance of health services as institutions. It considers what we can learn from governance concepts, knowledge and failures in non-health settings. It brings into perspective the challenges of governing safety and quality of health care at an institutional level, with a particular focus on the key role of specialist medical practitioners in clinical governance. We consider the relationship between corporate governance and clinical governance; the elements of good governance generally; some of the drivers of conduct and performance in hospitals; barriers to good governance; the structure of the public health care sector and its implications for good governance; the availability of clinical governance tools and techniques; and the future of clinical governance.

THE EVOLVING GOVERNANCE AND MANAGEMENT OF HOSPITALS

Many hospitals were established by philanthropists in the latter part of the nineteenth century as welfare-based institutions for people who were sick and impoverished. Legally, governance control rested with boards of trustees, but control for practical purposes was exercised by medical practitioners, who authorised admissions, discharges and the use of resources. These institutions gradually were transformed into organisations which provided care based on scientific principles. The discovery of sulpha drugs in the 1930s and the manufacture of penicillin in Australia from 1944 had profound impacts on the ability to provide effective health care. As care became more complex, the number of health care professions increased, hospitals' dependence on governments for funding increased and governments demanded higher levels of accountability. These changes led to hospitals developing professional administrative structures to replace medically led hierarchies.

The modern health service is a large, complex and diverse organisation, often operating over multiple sites, which continues to be challenged by the increasing complexity and diversity of care (Braithwaite and Travaglia 2008). Pharmaceuticals, devices and interventional techniques have developed over the past half-century at an astonishing pace, requiring health services to adapt and readapt to increasing professional and consumer expectations and new ways of delivering health care. During this period of profound change, governance and management systems have struggled to keep pace.

Corporate governance

The Australian Securities Exchange (ASX) (ASX Corporate Governance Council 2007) defines corporate governance as 'the framework of rules, relationships, systems and processes within and by which authority is exercised and controlled in corporations'. The ASX goes on to say that corporate governance 'encompasses the mechanisms by which companies, and those in control, are held to account'. Leadership, delegation, engagement, accountability and risk management are thus essential elements of corporate governance.

The governing entity (which, in a corporation, usually is a board of directors) is the focal point for the governance system and is responsible for ensuring that a sound system of governance is in place. It is the board's responsibility to ensure good governance of the organisation and to account to shareholders for doing this (see Cadbury report 1992). This does not mean that the board alone designs and implements the organisational governance system—successful systems of health service governance encompass all aspects of the organisation's structure and operations and depend for their success on the engagement of professionals at all levels. Ultimately, however, the board is responsible for ensuring the integrity and performance of the organisation's governance systems.

At the heart of good governance lie appropriate arrangements for making the judgments that are part of the successful operation of the organisation. In many different domains and locations, people with the appropriate capabilities obtain useful information to make informed judgments about what to do, and about what the organisation does. With good governance, mistakes will still be made and strategic errors will still occur, but they will have involved the exercise of judgment rather than occurring as a result of poor information, lack of decision-making or inadequate consideration.

Clinical governance

The phrase 'clinical governance' was defined by Scally and Donaldson in 1998 as 'a system through which NHS organisations are accountable for continuously improving the quality of their services and safeguarding high standards of care by creating an environment in which excellence in clinical care will flourish' (1998: 61). Clinical governance is viewed variously as a component of corporate governance or, alternatively, as something that is analogous to, but separate from, corporate governance.

We believe that adoption of the phrase 'clinical governance' has had a profound impact on the health care system. The phrase has fostered recognition of the need for strong clinical leadership and robust accountability for the safety and quality of clinical services. We do not believe, however, that the definition of 'clinical governance' as proposed originally by Scally and Donaldson fully conveys the key elements that contribute to the effective governance of clinical services. In particular, creating an environment in which excellence in clinical care will flourish is necessary, but not sufficient, for good clinical governance. Good governance also requires robust systems for monitoring the quality of care, engaging clinicians, managing risks and addressing poor-quality or unsafe care (see Figure 5.1).

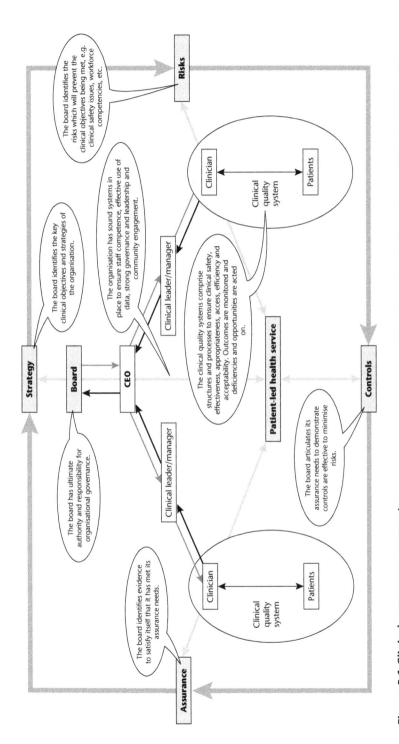

Figure 5.1 Clinical governance concepts

Source: Adapted from concepts from the Health Care Standards Unit

The governing entity of any organisation, clinical or non-clinical, is responsible for governing all organisational domains of activity, including business performance, human resources management, information technology, occupational health and safety, and product safety and quality. We believe that clinical governance should be conceptualised as a component of overall organisational governance. Clinical governance, under this paradigm, is simply the governance of clinical care—that is, the system of leadership, delegation, engagement, accountability and risk-management that applies to clinical services.

Ultimately, responsibility for ensuring the integrity and effectiveness of that system rests with the governing entity, which clearly must do more than create 'an environment in which excellence in clinical care will flourish'. In arranging the governance of the organisation, the governing entity must arrange for good clinical judgments to be made by capable people, with the right information and support. It also needs to arrange for these judgments to be subject to appropriate monitoring, review and correction, and to be appropriately aligned with the wide variety of other judgments being made throughout the organisation. Below, we describe the elements of good governance in a commercial context and then consider how these elements may apply in a health care setting.

Strategic leadership

Don Argus, a leading Australian company director, has said that a director who cannot articulate a meaningful strategy for the company should not be on the board.[1] In light of what is known about opportunities, risks and adverse events in health care, it is difficult to envisage a meaningful strategy for a health care organisation that does not comprehensively address the safety and quality of clinical services.

A meaningful strategy to improve clinical safety and quality is a critical component of all health care governance systems, and all members of the governing entity should be able to articulate the elements of that strategy.

Effective delegation

In order to fulfil its responsibilities, the governing entity of all but the smallest organisations should delegate substantial operational authority and responsibility to its appointed chief executive officer, and simultaneously implement effective mechanisms to ensure appropriate accountability for performance. Effective delegation requires that adequate resources will be available for deployment by the managers who are responsible for the delegated functions. We note, however, that in many health services responsibility for clinical quality continues to be divorced from authority to deploy the resources necessary to manage it.

Many well-publicised governance failures in health care and other settings have been characterised by a failure of delegation—in particular, there has been a lack of clarity about who is responsible and accountable for ensuring that systems for the delivery of care are properly structured and operating well. The final report of the public inquiry into children's heart surgery at the Bristol Royal Infirmary 1984–95 noted: 'There was confusion throughout the NHS as to who was responsible for monitoring the quality of care.' (Bristol Royal Infirmary Inquiry 2001). Similarly, the Inquiry into Obstetric and Gynaecological Services at King Edward Memorial Hospital highlighted responsibility and accountability for clinical care, and supervision of junior staff as key issues (Douglas et al. 2001). Many of its recommendations were aimed at ensuring clarity of responsibility for these essential functions.

Clarity about who is responsible for ensuring the adequacy of safety and quality systems is a key criterion for effective clinical governance. Our observation is that this responsibility continues to be opaque in some health services.

Accountability

Traditionally, the safety and quality of medically led care in hospitals was viewed as the responsibility of medical practitioners, their professional bodies and regulatory authorities such as medical boards. The responsibility of health services and their governing entities was considered limited to the provision of a safe environment in which medical practitioners could practise their craft. There was a heavy reliance on self-regulation and little recognition of the team-based nature of health care, and therefore of the importance of safety and quality systems. Many governing entities did not establish systems to monitor or control the safety and quality of care. Those who did often encountered resistance from medical practitioners who believed that oversight of clinical care was the sole responsibility of clinicians.

Neither the law nor public expectations support this view. While it is clear that each individual who delivers health services has a personal, professional and legal responsibility to do so with appropriate care, for many years the law has recognised that health care organisations also have both ordinary and non-delegable duties of care to patients. As employers, health services may be vicariously liable for the acts or omissions of their employees or agents. Contemporary approaches to safety and quality emphasise the need to focus on organisational systems rather than individuals (O'Leary 2003). The community also looks to government and governing entities to explain governance failures in health care safety and quality, and clearly expects that organisational systems will be in place to safeguard the safety and quality of care.

Given these legal duties, contemporary understanding and community expectations, it makes little sense to claim that health services and their governing entities have no role in the governance of clinical services that are provided utilising their staff and/or facilities, or that external bodies such as professional colleges (who are most unlikely to have any direct legal liability for the quality of care provided in an individual hospital over which they have no management control) are accountable for the safety and quality of those services.

Complementing effective systems of delegation, therefore, good governance clearly requires implementation of appropriate organisational systems to monitor, review and respond to organisational performance. These systems should be in place throughout the organisation and should include effective processes for reporting to the governing entity on organisational performance, including clinical performance. Regular comprehensive reports should be provided to the governing entity, enabling it to gain a clear picture of the organisation's operational and strategic performance. In health care, these reports should have an appropriate focus on both business and clinical performance. This monitoring and review responsibility of the board is widely recognised in contemporary governance literature—for example, the Cadbury Committee noted that 'all directors ... whether they have executive responsibilities, have a monitoring role and are responsible for ensuring that the necessary controls over the activities of the company are in place—and working' (Cadbury 1992: Recommendations).

Failure of the governing entity to question management appropriately was identified as one of the key contributors to the collapse of the HIH Insurance group, the major companies of which were placed in liquidation in March 2001 in the largest corporate failure ever seen in Australia. The subsequent royal commission noted that:

> The hand and influence of Williams [the former chief executive officer] were paramount. In itself, there is nothing inherently wrong with a

strong and forceful influence guiding the affairs of a corporation. Indeed, in Australian corporate life there have been many examples of successful businesses built in such a way. But in the modern commercial context such influence must be subject to the countervailing effect of close review, debate and questioning. This appears to have been a commodity in short supply at HIH. (Owen 2003: Volume 1)

The Commissioner, the Hon. Justice Owen, continued: 'I gained the impression that the general approach of the board and of senior management was unduly deferential. No doubt it was in most cases subconscious, and it would come as a surprise to some of those involved that an outside observer would hold such a view.' (2003).

Similarly, the PriceWaterhouseCoopers investigation into foreign exchange losses at the National Australia Bank noted that, although the Principal Board Audit Committee was not alerted directly to any issues in respect of currency options, 'After reading the supporting papers, probing of management may have revealed the seriousness of some of the control breakdowns.' (PriceWaterhouseCoopers 2004: 3).

A positive governance culture facilitates scrutiny by the governing entity of service development proposals and healthy debate between the governing entity and management about organisational performance. The governing entity is recognised by its members, management and the broader organisation as having a legitimate role in challenging assumptions and questioning recommendations. In the health care context, the governing entity's responsibility to monitor and review clinical services and question proposals for service development should be recognised by all stakeholders, including clinicians. Once the legitimacy of this role is recognised, stakeholders are more likely to react constructively rather than defensively to the important debate and questioning that are a critically important element of effective governance.

An effective risk-management system

The ASX states that: 'The board is responsible for reviewing the company's policies on risk oversight and management and satisfying itself that management has developed and implemented a sound system of risk management and internal control.' (ASX Corporate Governance Council 2007: 32). In the commercial context, five key risk oversight roles have been attributed to boards:

- Approve the firm's risk appetite as a component of its strategy;
- Understand and question the breadth of risks faced by the company;
- Ensure robust oversight of risk at the board committee and senior management levels;
- Promote a risk-focused culture and open communication across the organisation;
- Assign clear lines of accountability and encourage an effective risk-management framework. (Watson and Geny 2006)

A health care organisation's risk profile will consist of risks in a range of domains including financial, reputational, human resources and clinical. Ensuring an effective clinical risk management system is in place, especially in the context of the known high risks of health care, is a core responsibility for the governing entity. As well as a retrospective analysis of adverse events, the risk management system needs to have a prospective focus on the safe design of clinical systems and support mechanisms.

Effective cultural leadership

Responsibility for cultural leadership clearly rests with the governing entity. The National Australia Bank's experience with foreign exchange losses, which it announced to the market in January 2004, highlights the importance of leadership and culture in good governance. The report on the subsequent investigation noted:'The Board and CEO must accept responsibility for the "tone at the top" and for the environment in which management did not report openly on issues in the business.' (PriceWaterhouseCoopers 2004).

In health care organisations, the governing entity also must accept responsibility for the 'tone at the top'. This means that the governing entity must lead a culture of safety and quality—a culture that both supports and requires clinicians' involvement in safety and quality systems and does not tolerate dangerous non-compliance.

The necessity for independence in governance systems

Most contemporary governance standards identify an appropriate level of independence of directors as a key prerequisite to good governance. For example, the ASX Corporate Governance Council's Principles of Good Corporate Governance and Best Practice Recommendations (2007) suggest that a majority of the members of corporate boards, including the chairperson, should be independent directors, with independence judged according to whether the director:

- has a substantial shareholding;
- has served for a prolonged period on the board;
- has recently been employed as a senior executive of the company;
- has recently been engaged as a professional adviser to the company;
- is a material supplier or has a material contractual relationship with the company; or
- has any other relationship with the company which could compromise his or her independence.

The rationale is that the independent director is in a better position to question and exercise objective judgment about the affairs of the company, unencumbered by external interests including the interests of majority shareholders or members of the company's management team. Independence is seen as a safeguard of good governance, particularly on behalf of minority shareholders.

We comment further on the issue of independence in health service governance systems later in this chapter, but note that where health services are not governed by independent boards, other mechanisms to assure appropriate levels of governance independence may need to be instituted.

BARRIERS TO GOOD GOVERNANCE OF HEALTH CARE ORGANISATIONS

Although the concepts of good governance described above are increasingly acknowledged and are progressively being applied to the health care sector, there are many barriers to the implementation of effective governance systems, including:

- unique professional cultures and subcultures which impact on clinician engagement;
- traditional methods of employing or engaging medical practitioners;
- debilitating workforce shortages;
- a paucity of evidence-based clinical governance tools; and
- in some jurisdictions, a lack of a clearly identifiable governing entity for each health care organisation, with a resulting merging of regulatory, governance and operational responsibilities.

We explore some of these barriers in more detail below.

Engagement of medical practitioners in clinical governance

Although a degree of independence is considered essential to the effectiveness of governance systems, good governance also depends on structures and processes which are embedded in the day-to-day operations of the organisation. The most effective governance occurs when there are:

- a common organisational vision and strategy which are subscribed to by all stakeholders;
- well-designed systems for delivering services and monitoring, responding to and demonstrating accountability for their safety and quality; and
- an organisational culture of continuous improvement and an unwavering commitment to service safety and compliance with evidence-based standards.

An effective governance system cannot be imposed unilaterally. The governing entity can lead the organisational culture and invest in organisational systems, but those systems will not operate effectively without the engagement of the key professionals who work within them. The issue of engagement of medical practitioners is a particularly serious one, because they have 'plenary legal authority' and very little happens in health care without their endorsement (Reinertsen et al. 2007).

For such engagement to occur, medical practitioners need to recognise the need for and legitimacy of governance systems. There are, however, well-documented differences in management and professional subcultures in the health care sector which have made the task of engaging medical practitioners, and therefore governing health care organisations, exceedingly complex. These subcultures are deeply entrenched and to some extent are perpetuated by the system of post-graduation pre-vocational learning for medical practitioners in Australia, which continues to be based primarily on an apprenticeship model.

Tension between medical professional aspirations for clinical autonomy and the recognised need for individuals and organisations to comply with clinical systems and account for their clinical performance have been well documented over many decades and continue to pose a major clinical governance challenge in the twenty-first century.

Sir George Newman, the first chief medical officer at the Ministry of Health, said to the British Medical Association in 1920:

> The state has seen in the profession a body insistent on the privacy and individuality of its work, the sanctity of its traditions and the freedoms of its engagements. The profession has seen in the state an organisation apparently devoted to the infringement of these traditions and incapable of putting anything worthy in their place. It has feared the imposition of some cast iron system, which might in practice make the practitioner of medicine servile, dependent and fettered. (Kendall and Lissauer 2003: 4)

It was only in the mid-1980s that individual general managers replaced consensus management teams dominated by doctors in the UK National Health Service. The British Medical Association responded to that proposed reform in the following terms:

> It could be interpreted from the [Griffiths] report that a somewhat autocratic 'executive' manager would be appointed with significant delegated powers, who would—in the interests of 'good management'— be able to make major decisions against the advice of the profession ... it should be clearly understood that the profession would neither accept nor cooperate with any such arrangement—particularly where the interests of patients are concerned. (Harrison 1999: 7)

Donald Irvine, former president of the UK General Medical Council, has described the culture of medicine in the United Kingdom in the following terms:

> The profession remained 'wedded' to a 19th-century professional culture, when society was changing profoundly. In the 20th century, the profession was vigorously progressive in developing medical science and technology, while remaining deeply conservative on matters of attitude and human relationships about which patients care greatly. Attitudes to paternalism, communication and patient consent exemplified this. (Irvine 2004: 272)

Irvine concludes that unqualified professional autonomy has become demonstrably inappropriate and is incompatible with evidence-based practice. He describes 'inappropriate autonomy, manifest as divisive tribalism aggravated by the fragmentation caused by specialisation, [which] has resulted in a profession less and less able to act creatively as a coherent entity.' (Irvine 2004: 272).

Research on New Zealand health care students suggests that, even before commencing their training, medical students believe that clinical work should be the responsibility of individuals in contrast to nursing students who have a collective view and believe that work should be systematised. Pharmacy students are at a mid-point on this continuum (Horsburgh et al. 2006).

This very strong professional culture of personal accountability—in particular an entrenched belief that service quality is determined mainly by individual competence and performance—together with well-documented cynicism of the motivation, competence and/or per-formance of non-clinical managers has impeded the full engagement of the medical profession in clinical governance. Recent major health system inquiries in Victoria and New South Wales have confirmed a significant division between public health service managers and clinicians, including a significant lack of trust by clinicians in managers (see Garling 2008; Victorian Government Department of Human Services 2005).

Internationally, there have been calls for a rewriting of the 'implicit compact between the government, the medical profession and the public' and re-establishing 'responsible autonomy' as the primary organising principle for clinical work (Ham and Alberti 2002; Degeling et al. 2003). At issue here is the ethos of arranging for judgments to be made. The traditional medical ethos is that the best arrangement is for each senior clinician to make their own judgments, and be respons-ible for them to their patients. The ethos we are proposing is that, in a health care organisation, there must be a layering of arrangements for making clinical judgments. There should be joint decision-making over protocols, agreements over standard approaches for common clinical activities, peer review of clinical performance, and an alignment of the clinical activities and other activities in which the organisation is engaged, with clinicians and other senior staff understanding and taking account of the judgments that each makes.

In several jurisdictions, horizontal clinical networks are being implemented as a strategy to improve clinician engagement (Dunbar 2008), although they generally are still developmental and their effectiveness has not been evaluated in the Australian context. Clarity of roles, responsibilities and authorities is critical for the effective functioning of clinical networks. Consistent with this observation, a recent review of clinical engagement in clinical management structures in New South Wales (unpublished, referred to in the Garling report 2008) recommended clearer definition of the role of hospital and hospital network general managers in the clinical stream environment.

At a whole-of-system level, we consider that relationships between the professional colleges and health bureaucracies need to be strengthened significantly. Most of the professional colleges work primarily through their fellowship bases, and we observe that many colleges feel dis-empowered by an inability to influence operational decision-making in individual hospitals and health services, as well as at a system-wide level.

Professional colleges are in a unique position to advise health services on issues of clinical standards, credentialling, scope of clinical practice, competence and performance, all of which are critical elements of an effective clinical governance system. The establishment of sound systems for developing, receiving and valuing such advice will foster good decision-making and support good clinical governance.

It is clear that relationships between the medical profession and the health care system need significant further development to sustain the improvements in clinical governance that have been achieved in recent years. More research is required into the structures and processes that facilitate meaningful clinical engagement while ensuring continuing clarity of authority and responsibility for core health service operational and governance functions.

The influence of workforce shortages

Internationally, there are serious shortages of health care professionals (Productivity Commission 2005). In Australia, there is both a shortage and a maldistribution of doctors, and in recent years suggestions that medical practitioners in some specialties may be leaving the public sector and concentrating only on private sector work. Many public sector governing entities and managers fear that if they require medical practitioners to engage in onerous clinical governance activities, they may not be able to retain an adequate workforce. This situation is exacerbated by the overall shortage of medical practitioners, the relatively more attractive remuneration opportunities in the private sector for procedural specialists, the perceived greater value accorded by private hospitals to medical practitioners, less complex private sector working environments and the developing opportunities to engage in teaching and research in the private sector (Morey et al. 2007). In rural areas, where medical workforce shortages are most acute, the consequences of losing a medical practitioner because of a failure to resolve mutual concerns about clinical governance are potentially very serious for health care organisations.

These factors combine to increase apprehension by governing entities that, if they require participation in clinical governance systems that incorporate requirements that medical practitioners perceive to be unduly onerous, those clinicians may simply seek a less burdensome working environment elsewhere, leaving the organisation without coverage in critical clinical areas. Workforce shortages are believed to have been a significant contributing factor to the clinical governance deficits that occurred at the Bundaberg Base Hospital (Davies 2005).

Nevertheless, governing entities, particularly of public sector organisations, may be required to balance the potential consequences of a total loss of a service against the potential consequences of a poorly governed service with inadequate accountability arrangements. Clinically informed guidance that addresses whether no service is better than an unsafe service would help governing entities to make rational decisions in such circumstances.

The structure of hospital medical staff and implications for good governance

Australia has a mixed public/private health care system which has served the nation well, but which creates challenges associated with governing a specialist medical workforce with a relatively high proportion of part-time participants in both the public and private sectors. Many medical specialists in Australia work part time in both the public and private sectors. In Victoria, industrial conditions have favoured part-time employment of specialist medical practitioners in public hospitals over full-time employment, although a recent review suggests that there has been an increase in the number of specialists working only in one or other sector (Morey et al. 2007). That review noted that, as expectations regarding clinical governance increase, hospitals are identifying the need to engage more full-time staff.

Some private hospitals appoint large numbers of medical practitioners with an expectation that many of those practitioners will engage with the hospital on an infrequent basis. The focus has been on developing a large medical staff with the potential to attract large numbers of patients to the hospital, even if the frequency with which individual specialists admit patients is low. Reducing the size of the medical staff to a core group of specialists who admit patients regularly may be a preferable arrangement from an operational and clinical governance perspective, but its practicality is limited because of its potential impact on the hospital's occupancy, and therefore its commercial viability. In the private sector, engagement of full-time specialist staff remains the exception, and in both the public and private sectors, a predominantly part-time staffing structure is more usual. In some circumstances, the extent of individual professionals' regular contact with the organisation may be quite limited.

It is extremely difficult to engage individuals in team-based processes of clinical care and organisational governance processes if they are not exposed to them regularly. We have seen some of the most inspiring quality and clinical governance systems operating in health service settings where there is continuity of senior staff working well together across disciplines within a common vision and mission, highlighting the value of teamwork (Braithwaite and Travaglia 2005). The typical structure of the medical workforce in large hospitals, however, means that clinical engagement processes need to be designed specifically to influence and accommodate relatively more individuals than would be the case with a predominantly full-time workforce.

We believe that all health care organisations should review their medical staff structure to ensure its compatibility with organisational governance aspirations. This is a critical strategic issue which can be influenced by a planned and systematic appraisal of the optimal structure, the current structure and the steps necessary to close any identified gaps.

THE STRUCTURE OF THE PUBLIC SECTOR AND ITS IMPLICATIONS FOR GOOD GOVERNANCE

Victoria is the only Australian jurisdiction that has retained independent boards of governance of public health services. The Victorian system of health service governance most closely mirrors the commercial governance system. There is a clear separation between government (as the regulator, funder and owner of public hospitals) and public health service boards of governance that appoint the chief executive officer, hold him or her to account, and ultimately are accountable for the performance of their organisations. Following a 2003 independent review, the governance structure of the Victorian system was strengthened with the objective of balancing governance autonomy with account-ability to the minister (Victorian Public Hospital Governance Reform Panel 2003).

There are significant accountability safeguards in the Victorian system of public health service governance, including reporting requirements to the department and the minister, a broad statutory right for the minister to issue written directions to the board with which the board must comply, and a similarly broad right for the departmental secretary to issue directions to the health service with which it also must comply. In addition, the minister may appoint delegates to boards, may recommend to the Governor in Council that one or more directors are removed from a board, and may recommend the appointment of an administrator to exercise the powers of the board.

In other jurisdictions, there is a more direct relationship through the state or territory departments of health to government. In some jurisdictions, independent statutory authorities complement this system of direct bureaucratic governance. For example, in New South Wales, area health services are established by the *Health Services Act* 1997 as corporations which are managed and controlled by a chief executive, who in turn is subject to the control and direction of the Director-General. The Act also provides for the establishment of statutory corporations with specific governance functions—the Clinical Excellence Commission, for example, is a statutory corporation which is governed by a board and has a broad charter that includes the following areas:

- promotion and support of improvement in clinical quality and safety in public and private health services; and
- monitoring clinical quality and safety processes and performance of public health organisations and reporting to the Minister thereon. (New South Wales Clinical Excellence Commission 2004: 3)

The Final Report of the Special Commission of Inquiry into Acute Care Services in New South Wales Public Hospitals (Garling 2008) recommended the continuation of the basic system structure and specifically advised against a return to hospital-based or health service-based boards of governance.

In all Australian jurisdictions, organisational governance arrange-ments are complemented by independent statutory bodies with authority to receive and investigate complaints, such as the Health Complaints Commissions in each state and territory.

We note that there is no empirical evidence about whether well-selected, trained and supported governing boards are more effective governors of clinical services than appointed administrators and bureaucrats. Most Australian jurisdictions have experienced highly publicised clinical governance failures, including Bundaberg, Mackay, Royal North Shore, King Edward Memorial Hospital, Royal Adelaide Hospital radiotherapy errors and Adelaide Women's and Children's Hospital chemotherapy errors (see Chapter 15). Victoria, with its locally based boards, has not been immune, with publicity highlighting concerns about safety, quality, accountability and culture at the Alfred Hospital.

The issues of the role of community based boards and the benefits of locally based governance were firmly on the agenda nationally in 2007, in relation to the Mersey Campus of the North West Regional Hospital in Tasmania. The Tasmanian government had accepted the recommendation of a planning exercise (led by one of the authors, Heather Wellington) that, to ensure sustainability of safe, high-quality services, the roles of the Mersey and Burnie Campuses of that hospital should change significantly, with the Mersey Campus moving from an acute community hospital to a specialist hospital with a focus on high-throughput, short-stay elective medical and surgical care, aged care and rehabilitation.

This recommendation was made following many years of concern about the safety and sustainability of services provided at the Mersey Campus, and repeated structural changes including a period during which the hospital was governed and managed by the private sector. The recommendation was unpopular with some staff and a proportion of the community. Following a community campaign, the issue came on to the national political agenda in the lead-up to the 2007 federal election, when then Prime Minister John Howard announced the federal government would assume responsibility for the hospital from the Tasmanian government and put in place a community-led governance structure. Specifically, the Prime Minister announced that the Commonwealth would:

• support the community operating the Mersey Hospital as a community-controlled and Commonwealth-funded institution; and
• support the establishment of a Mersey Community Hospital Trust, comprising regional local government, business and health profession leaders, to run the hospital on behalf of the community.

The proposed structure had many of the features of a community-based board of governance, representing a significant departure from the way in which the remainder of the Tasmanian public health system was (and continues to be) governed.

Much of the Australian health bureaucracy and many independent policy analysts reacted very negatively to that decision (Sayer 2007; see also Doggett and Burns 2007; Richardson 2007), as did Health Ministers in other jurisdictions who were reported as saying that:

- putting local boards in charge of hospitals would simply add another level of bureaucracy to the system and drain already limited resources; and
- the system of hospital boards had been tested and was found not to work.

The Commonwealth assumed ownership of the Mersey Community Hospital on 23 November 2007. The newly elected Rudd Labor government announced shortly after its election that, rather than proceeding with the establishment of a community trust, it intended to appoint a religious, charitable or private sector organisation to operate the Mersey as a public hospital. Efforts to identify a suitable provider failed, however, and on 18 July 2008 Health Minister Nicola Roxon announced that the state of Tasmania would manage the Mersey Community Hospital on behalf of the Commonwealth. The hospital is now being managed by the Tasmanian government, in accordance with an agreement with the Commonwealth, under governance arrangements that otherwise are indistinguishable from those that apply to the entire Tasmanian public hospital sector.

Like most health planners and policy analysts, we think the Prime Minister's intervention was seriously misguided, not because it involved the establishment of a local governing entity, but because that governing entity would have been given the unmanageable task of overseeing the continuation of services that repeatedly had been demonstrated to be unsustainable. In addition, community-based boards cannot operate without support. Much of the success of the Victorian public health service governance model stems from the significant investment made by the state in board selection, training, remuneration and support— none of which was in place in Tasmania to support a local governing entity in the north-west.

Nevertheless, the Prime Minister's intervention highlighted the question of how best to structure health services in order to deliver safe services to a community. Regardless of the structural arrangements that are adopted for public health services, the elements of good governance, including leadership, delegation, engagement, accountability and risk management, need to be reproduced within a framework that enables an appropriate degree of independent scrutiny. As described above, we consider that clarity of roles and responsibilities, independent monitoring of operational performance and robust questioning of assumptions and proposals are critically important elements of clinical governance. The extent to which Australia's jurisdictional public health systems are designed to support these roles will be a key determinant of the sustainability and effectiveness of their clinical governance systems.

Noting a lack of empirical evidence, we nevertheless consider that, in the current challenging and volatile health care environment, characterised by high degrees of politicisation and intense public interest, it is arguably more difficult to achieve the appropriate structures and independence in the absence of governing boards. We are strong advocates for definitive research into this important health system design issue.

Standardising tools and techniques for good clinical governance

Governing entities can only govern on the basis of the information available to them. There is an onus on a governing entity to demand relevant and appropriate information, and the failure of various governing boards to do so has been identified as a contributing factor in some prominent governance failures (see, for example, the PriceWaterhouse-Coopers (2004) report into the NAB foreign trading problems).

Effective oversight of clinical performance depends on:

- agreed standards for the delivery of quality health care (see Chapter 9);
- reliable information systems for determining whether agreed standards have been met—encompassing structures, processes and outcomes (see Chapter 14); and
- a method of reporting the ensuing performance information in a meaningful way throughout the organisation to the governing entity.

Such standards should usually cover structures (e.g. necessary staff numbers and competencies, equipment requirements), processes (e.g. 'best-practice' policies and procedures) and outcomes (e.g. adverse event and functional improvement rates). Consistent with contemporary regulatory theory, standards should focus on outcomes rather than inputs, allowing clinicians, managers and organisations to deploy local resources innovatively for best results.

There are particular problems, however, in accessing the information needed to govern clinical services. The challenge in health care is that there is a paucity of standards for the structure, delivery or outcomes of quality care. Even if appropriate standards were readily available, reliable systems for monitoring and reporting compliance are lacking. Contrast clinical governance systems with financial governance systems, where international accounting standards are complemented by robust local compliance frameworks which clearly define the necessary structures, processes and outcomes expected of modern hospital financial systems. In an environment where standardised tools for monitoring and reporting performance in clinical safety and quality are lacking, there is a risk that efforts to develop relevant tools will be duplicated across the system.

There is also a strong desire within the sector to identify a core suite of indicators of clinical performance which can be used to assess the safety and quality performance of the organisation 'at a glance'—a 'balanced scorecard' or similar approach. While monitoring of high-level clinical performance indicators can be a useful clinical governance tool, clinical governance obligations cannot be satisfied through such an approach in isolation. We are concerned that most of the governance failures that have occurred, both within and outside the health care system, would not have been identified through high-level monitoring of key performance indicators. In health care, it remains exceedingly difficult to identify reliable performance indicators, although some are emerging in some areas and the number available will continue to expand in the future, greatly aided by the establishment of risk-adjusted clinical registries. Some of the highest risk events, however, are relatively rare and occur only when a number of risk factors align—simply monitoring usual performance will almost certainly fail to alert organisations to any fundamental flaws in the design of their clinical systems, which may align under certain circumstances to produce catastrophic results (Reason 2000).

In addition, many safety and quality problems will not be detected by clinical indicator monitoring because data collection systems are unreliable or indicators simply do not exist in many key areas of performance. Error rates reported in the peer-reviewed literature, for example, suggest that expected error rates are much higher than those that are reported in most hospitals, highlighting the inadequacy of current data collection and reporting systems (see Chapter 9). In the absence of reliable systems, such clinical indicator rates can only be used as broad indicators of local trends and a stimulus for further investigation.

We encourage governing entities to work with their management teams to agree on an organisational safety and quality framework. Many such frameworks have been published—most identify core dimensions of quality including safety, effectiveness, appropriateness, accept-ability and access. In addition, organisational characteristics including approaches to credentialling and staff competency, data and information management, leadership and governance and consumer engagement are all key determinants of service quality.

The safety and quality framework should provide an agreed foundation for the organisation's clinical governance system which, consistent with the core governance functions described in this chapter, should incorporate planning, investing, monitoring, reviewing, reporting, responding and managing risk across the range of services that the organisation provides, and across all of the relevant dimensions and determinants of service quality.

In a mature governance system, much of the activity will be proactive rather than reactive. The governance system should enable assurance that standards of care are being applied appropriately (and answer the question: If not why not?), that expected outcomes are being achieved, and that key risks are being identified and managed before they materialise. A focus on standards will move the governance process from a retrospective review of adverse events, to a prospective process of ensuring services are designed and delivered sustainably and within an appropriate risk-management framework. We consider that the mature clinical governance system of the future will be much more comprehensive, standardised and proactive than the systems that operate today.

We also believe that external accreditation processes are likely to have an increasingly important influence, similar to the influence of external audit in the corporate environment. The Australian Council on Healthcare Standards' EQuIP program has been the most commonly used program in Australian hospitals over the past several decades (see Australian Council on Healthcare Standards 2006; and Chapter 13). Based on a traditional accreditation model, it has had a strong focus on peer-based learning and evidence of improvement rather than compliance, which has been a cause for some criticism on the basis that knowledge of improvement alone is of little benefit in the absence of a clearly defined baseline. In more recent years, the accreditation model has been refined and mandatory criteria have been introduced, enhancing the meaning of accreditation and the reliance which can be placed on it. Work currently underway by the Australian Commission on Safety and Quality in Health Care to reform standards and accreditation processes across the health care system should ensure that accreditation becomes an even more valuable governance tool in the future (Australian Commission on Safety and Quality in Healthcare 2008).

CONCLUSION

The introduction of the term 'clinical governance' has had a profound impact on the delivery and monitoring of health care in Australia. Although the term is used widely, there are various interpretations of its meaning. We believe that clinical governance is an element of a broad system of organisational governance, that there is a common set of governance processes which apply, regardless of the sector or context, and that significant lessons can be learnt from the concepts, techniques and failures of governance in non-health care settings.

Governance, together with the structures through which it courses, is about ensuring the primacy of judgment over the affairs of the organisation. Good judgment should sit at the centre of the operation, enterprise, strategy and ethics of the organisation. Good governance empowers judgment throughout the organisation. It is about placing people into the kinds of roles and activities that their capacity for judgment suits; about bringing deliberations into relations with each other in arrangements that promote good, informed judgments; and about monitoring the combined effects of these judgments and the operating environment on organisational performance. Good governance depends on robust processes of questioning and debate in a continuous effort to assure and improve the quality of services. In the commercial context, independence of the governing entity from organisational owners is seen as important—but independence is difficult to achieve in the public health care system, in which government owns, operates, funds, regulates and monitors performance.

The structure of Australia's health care system means that governance is exercised in different ways in different jurisdictions. The impact of different system structures on the effectiveness of clinical governance has not been evaluated empirically. We believe that the tools and techniques of clinical governance are developing and will continue to improve. We support further research on the impact of system structure on the effectiveness of clinical governance.

ACKNOWLEDGMENT

The authors would like to thank Yin-Lan Soon for research assistance in preparation of this chapter.

REFERENCES

ASX Corporate Governance Council 2007, *ASX Corporate Governance Principles and Recommendations*, 2nd ed., ASX Corporate Governance Council, Sydney

Australian Commission on Safety and Quality in Healthcare 2008, *Final Report on the Review of National Safety and Quality Accreditation Standards*, Australian Commission on Safety and Quality in Healthcare, Sydney

Australian Council on Healthcare Standards 2006, *The ACHS EQuIP 4 Guide, Part 2—Standards*, Australian Council on Healthcare Standards, Sydney

Braithwaite, J. and Travaglia, J. 2005, 'The ACT Health inter-professional learning and clinical education project: Background discussion paper #1. The value, governance and context of inter-professional learning and practice', Braithwaite and Associates and the ACT Health Department, Canberra

——2008, 'An overview of clinical governance policies, practices and initiatives', *Australian Health Review*, vol. 32, no. 10, pp. 10–22

Bristol Royal Infirmary Inquiry 2001, 'Learning from Bristol: The report of the public inquiry into children's heart surgery at the Bristol Royal Infirmary 1984–1995', Bristol Royal Infirmary Inquiry, London

Cadbury, A. 1992, *Report of the Committee on the Financial Aspects of Corporate Governance*, The Committee on the Financial Aspects of Corporate Governance and Gee and Co, London

Davies, G. 2005, *Commissions of Inquiry Order (No. 2) 2005: Final report.* Queensland Government, Brisbane

Degeling, P., Maxwell, S., Kennedy, J. and Coyle, B. 2003, 'Medicine, management, and modernisation: A "danse macabre"?', *British Medical Journal*, vol. 326, no. 7390, pp. 649–52

Department of Health of Western Australia Office of Safety and Quality in Health Care 2003, *Introduction to Clinical Governance: A Background Paper Information Series No. 1.1*, Department of Health of Western Australia, Perth

Doggett, J. and Burns, E. 2007, *Road Test: Mersey Valley Hospital Takeover*, Centre for Policy Development, Sydney

Douglas, N., Robinson, J. and Fahy, K. 2001, *Inquiry into Obstetric and Gynae-cological Services at King Edward Memorial Hospital 1990–2000: Final Report*, Department of Health, Government of Western Australia, Perth

Dowton, S.B., Stokes, M.L., Rawstron, E.J., Pogson, P.R. and Brown, M.A. 2005, 'Postgraduate medical education: rethinking and integrating a complex landscape', *Medical Journal of Australia*, vol. 182, no. 4, pp. 177–80

Dunbar, J. 2008, 'Integration and coordination of care', *Inaugural Rural and Remote Health Scientific Symposium*, 6–8 July, Brisbane

Garling, P. 2008, *Final Report of the Special Commission of Inquiry: Acute Care Services in New South Wales Public Hospitals*, New South Wales Government, Sydney

Generational Health Review 2002, *South Australian Generational Health Review: Consultation summary*, Government of South Australia, Adelaide

Ham, C. and Alberti, K.G. 2002, 'The medical profession, the public and government', *British Medical Journal*, vol. 324, no. 7341, pp. 838–42

Harrison, S. 1999, 'Structural interests in health care: "Reforming" the UK medical profession', European Consortium for Political Research, University of Leeds, Leeds

Health Care Standards Unit, *The Standards for Better Health: Improving Board Assurance*, <www.hcsu.org.uk/index.php?option=com_docman&task=doc_view&grid=634>, accessed 10 January 2009

Horsburgh, M., Perkins, R., Coyle, B. and Degeling, P. 2006, 'The professional subcultures of students entering medicine, nursing and pharmacy programmes', *Journal of Interprofessional Care*, vol. 20, no. 4, pp. 425–31

Irvine, D. 2004, 'The profession: Time for hard decisions on patient-centralised professionalism', *The Medical Journal of Australia*, vol. 181, no. 5, p. 272

Kendall, L. and Lissauer, R. 2003, *The Future Health Worker*, Institute for Public Policy Research, London

Kuhlmann, E. and Saks, M. 2008, *Rethinking Professional Governance: International Directions in Health Care*, Policy Press, Bristol

Menadue, J. 2007, 'Obstacles to health reform', *Australian Healthcare Reform Alliance Summit*, Centre for Policy Development, Canberra

—— 2008, *Another Design Problem in Health: No-one Runs Hospital*, Centre for Policy Development, Canberra

Morey, S., Barraclough, B. and Hughes, A. 2007, *Ministerial Review of Victorian Public Health Medical Staff: Report of the Review Panel*, Victorian Government Department of Human Services, Melbourne

New South Wales Clinical Excellence Commission 2004, *Directions Statement*, New South Wales Department of Health, Sydney

O'Leary, D. 2003, *Patient Safety: Instilling Hospitals with a Culture of Continuous Improvement*, Testimony before the Senate Committee on Governmental Affairs, 11 June

Owen N., *Report of the HIH Royal Commission*, Commonwealth of Australia, Canberra, 2003

PriceWaterhouseCoopers 2004, *Investigation into Foreign Exchange Losses at the National Australia Bank*, PriceWaterhouseCoopers, Melbourne

Productivity Commission 2005, *Australia's Health Workforce Research Report*, Commonwealth of Australia, Canberra

Reason, J. 2000, 'Human error: Models and management', *British Medical Journal*, vol. 320, no. 7237, pp. 768-70

Reinertsen J.L., Gosfield, A.G., Rupp, W. and Whittington, J.W. 2007, *Engaging Physicians in a Shared Quality Agenda*, IHI Innovation Series white paper, Institute for Healthcare Improvement, Cambridge, MA

Richardson, J. 2007, 'Mersey Hospital: A potentially fatal intervention', *Australian Policy Online*, <www.apo.org.au>, accessed 3 April 2009

Sayer, L. 2007, 'Hospital grab sparks alarm', *Hobart Mercury*, 3 August 2007

Scally, G. and Donaldson, L.J. 1998, 'Clinical governance and the drive for quality improvement in the new NHS in England', *British Medical Journal*, vol. 317, no. 7150, pp. 61-5

Van Der Weyden, M. 2005, 'The Bundaberg Hospital scandal: The need for reform in Queensland and beyond', *Medical Journal of Australia*, vol. 183, no. 6, pp. 284-5

Victorian Government Department of Human Services 2005, *Leading Clinical Governance in Health Services—The Chief Executive Officer and Senior Manager Roles*, Victorian Government Department of Human Services, Melbourne

Victorian Public Hospital Governance Reform Panel 2003, *Victorian Public Hospital Governance Reform Panel Report*, Victorian Government Department of Human Services, Melbourne

Victorian Quality Council 2005, *Better Quality Better Healthcare*, Victorian Government Department of Human Services, Melbourne

Watson, M. and Geny, H. 2006, *Special Comment: Best Practices for a Board's Role in Risk Oversight*, Moody's Investor Service Inc., <www.corpgov.deloitte.com/binary/com.epicentric.contentmanagement.servlet.ContentDeliveryServlet/CanEng/Documents/Board/The%20Directors%27%20Series/Archive/2007/October/Handout/BestPracticesForBoard%27sRoleInRiskOversight.pdf>, accessed 20 December 2009

NOTE

1   This comment by Don Argus was reported in *The Weekend Australian*, 5-6 October 2002, as quoted in the report of the HIH Royal Commission (Owen 2003).

6

TRANSFORMING CLINICAL GOVERNANCE IN QUEENSLAND HEALTH

Stephen Duckett

The state of Queensland covers about one-fifth of the Australian land mass and contains one-fifth of the Australian population (around four million people). Queensland Health is the state government authority responsible for providing public hospital services to this population through 28 large public hospitals with 8256 beds, treating 740,804 admitted patients in 2007–08, and a further 145 smaller hospitals with 1937 beds treating 90,830 patients in the same period.

Queensland Health employs 66,200 staff and, in addition to responsibilities for public hospital provision, provides public health services and regulates private hospitals. Queensland is Australia's most dispersed state, with the majority of the population residing outside the capital, and with significant regional coastal cities such as Bundaberg, Rockhampton, Townsville and Cairns. Until 2005, the state had only one medical school, the University of Queensland, located in Brisbane. Commonwealth funding to Queensland for medical places has traditionally been lower than for other states, resulting in lower per capita numbers of medical graduates than the rest of the country—contrast South Australia at around fourteen new medical graduates per 100,000 population per annum with seven per 100,000 in Queensland.

Queensland has had difficulty in recruiting Australian-trained doctors to work outside the south-east corner of the state, which has meant a heavy reliance on internationally trained medical graduates to staff its rural and regional services. These recruitment difficulties provided the environment in which Dr Jayant Patel was recruited to provide surgery at Bundaberg Base Hospital and for 'Bundaberg' to become notorious, the subject of editorial critique (Van Der Weyden 2005) and journalistic exposé (Thomas 2007). Complaints about Dr Patel's work at Bundaberg eventually stimulated an independent Commission of Inquiry (Davies 2005), an independent management consulting review (Forster 2005), a shake-up of the Queensland Health organisational structure, and the replacement of the Minister for Health and the entire top echelon of the department. The author of this chapter was appointed to Queensland Health as part of that leadership transformation, with responsibilities including clinical governance reforms and, more broadly, the culture change agenda. This chapter draws on that experience as a participant observer, attempting to reflect dispassionately on the contemporary issues. However, because many of the changes described here are still new, it is not yet possible to incorporate evidence of the success or failure of the changes implemented.

It is important to note that the Davies Commission of Inquiry focused not only on Dr Patel and the Bundaberg Base Hospital, but also reviewed a 'psychiatrist' appointed to Townsville Hospital who did not have a medical degree, as well as appointments and other issues at Charters Towers, Rockhampton, Prince Charles and Hervey Bay hospitals. Dr Patel was thus a lightening rod for widespread problems in Queensland Health. He was the most politically salient and visible symptom of the underlying problems with clinical governance in the Queensland public hospital system at the time.

One of the critical issues found by Davies (2005) in his inquiry was that the problems about Dr Patel emerged early in his employment at the hospital: the first serious complaint about Dr Patel occurred within eight weeks of his commencing (2005: 171, para 3.406). There were 22 complaints against Dr Patel during the 24 months of his employment at Bundaberg. Taking into account periods of leave, there was 'about one formal patient complaint or formal staff report for each month he actually worked' (2005: 416, para 6.269). Independent investigations conducted as part of the Davies Inquiry confirmed that many of these complaints raised valid, serious questions about the competence of Dr Patel. A critical issue in Bundaberg, therefore, was not a problem of identifying aberrant practice, but rather of acting on this knowledge.

Davies went on to review the handling of complaints against Dr Patel, the appointment processes for Dr Patel and the nature of these complaints.

Queensland Health policies about complaints and appointments were, on the whole, endorsed. A second issue identified by Davies, and related to the first, was that while Queensland Health policy was appropriate, problems arose in whether and how the policies were implemented.

A third important deficiency identified by Davies was 'a culture of concealment' (2005: 473), emanating from Cabinet and the Minister's office through senior levels of the organisation to shape the culture of the whole organisation. Fourth, both Davies and the separate Forster report also identified the failure to engage clinicians in policy- and priority-setting throughout the organisation as a critical issue.

Queensland Health is a unitary organisation, in that services are delivered by employees of the organisation, and the Director-General has line management responsibility stretching to every employee in every service delivery point throughout the organisation. At the time of writing (early 2009), Queensland Health was structured into fifteen districts with district chief executive officers accountable directly to the Director-General, with no boards of directors to provide intermediate governance of services. It is not the purpose of this chapter to review the strengths and weaknesses of boards versus a unitary organisation, but the latter does have the unique potential of facilitating a statewide rollout of policy changes because of line management accountability.

QUEENSLAND HEALTH'S NEW CLINICAL GOVERNANCE FRAMEWORK

The new post-Bundaberg approaches to clinical governance use a range of regulatory instruments from multiple levels of the regulatory pyramid (see Table 6.1). The regulatory instruments themselves are part of overall system changes, and no one regulatory instrument is required to carry the whole burden of transforming clinical governance.

More fundamentally, the transformation of clinical governance in Queensland Health, set in train by the new executive, emphasises culture change and a new set of values to apply throughout the organisation. The values underpinning the changes are not unique to patient safety and clinical governance, or to Queensland, but are common in other systems of public governance (Edwards 2002; Harlow 2006; Williams and Young 1994). In this chapter I outline how these values of accountability, transparency and participation are effected in the design of clinical governance in Queensland, with attention paid to the tensions inherent in living these values.

Table 6.1 Queensland regulatory pyramid: Standard characterisation

Pyramid element	Queensland Health example
Command and control	Independent Health Quality and Complaints Commission sets standards for public and private providers, with power to review adverse events, patient complaints
Meta-regulation	Central policies specify ways in which district health services are to manage safety issues and to some extent, the intra-district clinical governance approach
Co-regulation	Queensland Audit of Surgical Mortality conducted by Royal Australasian College of Surgeons, funded by Queensland Health
Economic instruments	Statutory requirement for public reporting of quality of care Clinical practice improvement payment (Duckett, Collins et al. 2008)
Self-regulation	Within policy framework, district autonomy in internal approach to audit Requirement for district review of identified potential safety issues Performance monitoring of districts using statistical process control (Duckett et al. 2007)
Voluntarism	Development of statewide clinical guidelines involving strong clinical engagement and leadership

These process values respond directly to the issues identified in the Davies and Forster reports—issues of ensuring action is taken, policies are implemented, relevant information disclosed and clinicians engaged. Many of the instrumental changes implemented in Queensland Health are shaped by more than one of the underpinning process values.

Drawing on Tuohy's (1999) work, one can identify a number of ways in which the health care system is shaped or controlled: through culture, norms and mores; through financial incentives and markets; and through organisational structures and legal or organisational regulatory processes. Generally, policy-makers only have access to the latter two clusters of policy instruments and, even for these, the more they are orthogonal to the dominant culture of a system, the weaker will be their ability to shape and transform the care system. Shifting culture, including changing the underlying process values, is difficult and relatively slower to achieve than the other instruments. Culture is also less visible, with no landmark legislation or budget splash, and does not attract political and media attention to the same extent as the more visible economic or regulatory/structure changes. However, shifting culture is quintessentially what leadership is about—indeed, it can be argued that creating and shaping culture is the only important thing leaders do (Schein 1992). If a shift in culture is achieved and embedded, it is more profound and longer lasting than other changes. The new process values outlined in this chapter were thus seen as a key part of the major transformation of the culture of Queensland Health, with the objective of achieving the more profound shifts that are necessary to ensure long-lasting change.

As Table 6.1 shows, a range of new policies and practices have been introduced as part of the new clinical governance framework, with many of these adapted from strategies in place in other organisations. The new policies are mutually reinforcing, using a range of levers with provenance in different over-arching domains (e.g. human resource policies and finance policies as well as clinical governance). The original definition of the clinical governance framework referred to a 'web' of policies to emphasise both the multiple strands and the interacting nature of the policies, better to catch any problems (Duckett 2007).

What might make Queensland unique is implementation of such a range of strategies over the relatively short period of the three years following the external reviews. But this chapter argues that these new strategies and policies are less important than the attempt to change the culture of Queensland Health by shifting the discourse to emphasise accountability, transparency and participation (or engagement) with concomitant policy changes in line with the new discourse and values.

The change in clinical governance processes was paralleled by a major emphasis on workplace culture and leadership change. This was based on the view that, in order to achieve culture change, there needed to be changes in leadership at every level of the organisation—not necessarily changes in personnel, but rather changes in leadership behaviours. The culture change role of the leader was recognised early, as was the need to improve the skills of leaders throughout Queensland Health. This reflected an underlying theory about leadership: that leadership is not an inherent personality trait but rather that leadership behaviours can be learnt and are amenable to change (Heifetz 1994; Heifetz and Linsky 2002).

The transformation of workplace culture and leadership was managed by a distinct group within the Queensland Health Centre for Healthcare Improvement, this Centre also being responsible for the safety and quality agenda. In that way, the links between the safety and quality agenda and the organisational culture agenda were emphasised and reinforced. The workplace culture and leadership change processes employed have been described elsewhere (Crethar et al. 2009). These involved workplace culture surveys (to track staff attitudes and morale), action plans developed by districts responding to issues identified in the surveys, and a number of programs to up-skill managers at all levels of the organisation to reinforce a broader range of leadership behaviours and to encourage reflection on the implementation of these leadership behaviours. This leadership development program is one of the largest undertaken in any organisation in Australia, inside or outside the health sector. For example, about 5000 staff participated in a two-day leadership development workshop (for 500 staff this became an annual residential workshop), with a maximum of around 25 staff participating in each workshop. The workshops were generally structured around organisational units (e.g. the district leadership team would all attend a single workshop), but cross-cutting workshops also were developed— for example, programs for emerging clinical leaders. These workshops were particularly important in developing the leadership behaviours of participants, especially relating to the values of accountability and participation.

ACCOUNTABILITY

The new Queensland clinical governance approach places a strong emphasis on accountability. There are two main aspects to this: emphasising that responsibility for clinical governance is vested in line management (as is responsibility for other aspects of organisational performance), and the idea that managers should be held to account for performance relating to clinical governance issues.

An emphasis on line management responsibility signals that clinical governance is not a side issue and the preserve of clinicians (medical or non-medical), but rather that clinical governance, the safety of patients and the quality of services are the core business of Queensland Health. It recognises that adverse events, for example, might be caused because of defects in the management or communication processes of the organisation, and are not simply the result of problems within the clinical realm. It also forces clinical governance issues to be considered part of the same decision-making processes as budget and access issues.

Importantly, when things go wrong, accountability up the organisational chain is via line management, and disciplinary procedures are also the responsibility of line management. This emphasis on reinforcing the importance of line management is in response to the apparent failure of line management in Bundaberg and other locations investigated by the Davies Commission. Emphasising the role of line management increases accountability, and hopefully line management attention to quality issues.

Line management responsibility and accountability can only occur if there is clarity of roles and responsibilities, and when the place of clinical governance in these roles and responsibilities is not simply a tokenistic afterthought. New policy documents and 'implementation standards' provided this clarity, with explicit statements of the roles and responsibilities of managers, medical directors, directors of clinical units and officials in the corporate office (see Queensland Health 2008a), as well as clear policies for reporting and managing clinical incidents (see Queensland Health 2008b).

A new Clinician Performance Support Service (CliPSS) was established to support the conduct of performance appraisal of clinical staff. The aim was to ensure that, where performance issues of clinical staff are identified, organisational processes exist to work with clinicians to change their behaviours.

External accountability was strengthened through the creation of an independent Health Quality and Complaints Commission in 2006. This Commission has wide-ranging powers to investigate quality or safety events, and also to establish standards for health organisations (including public and private hospitals and non-institutional services such as general practice). The *Health Quality and Complaints Commission Act* 2006 (Qld) imposes a statutory duty on all health providers (including Queensland Health) to:

> establish, maintain and implement reasonable processes to improve the quality of health services provided by or for the provider, including processes—

(a) to monitor the quality of the health services; and

(b) to protect the health and well being of users of the health services (Section 20).

The Commission was reviewed by a Parliamentary Committee after its first two years of existence and, despite recommendations for some changes in the way the Commission approached its work, there was endorsement of the importance and need for an independent oversight body.

Internal accountability was strengthened by an emphasis on the use of statistics to monitor variation in outcomes of care (mortality, complication rates) on a monthly basis. Queensland Health monitors 30 indicators and flags to hospitals (both public and private) when their outcomes appear to be different from the state average (positive or negative). A hierarchical system of reporting was introduced with a requirement for various levels of the organisation to report on the nature of the investigations undertaken in response to the variations identified, and on the action taken as a result of those investigations (Duckett et al. 2007; Clinical Practice Improvement Centre 2008).

A statewide system of clinical incident reporting has been introduced which enables any member of staff to report a clinical incident (including near-misses), and also allows statewide reporting of patterns of incidents. There are structured reporting requirements for serious clinical incidents (sentinel events) and a requirement that a 'root cause analysis' be undertaken when a serious clinical incident occurs. Corporate tracking of the progress of root cause analyses includes monitoring action on the outcomes of the analysis.

There are, of course, tensions involved in this new emphasis on accountability. First, the significantly enhanced monitoring and reporting creates an additional local workload. There is clearly a trade-off, for example, in the statistical control processes as to what level variation from the state average is deemed to be aberrant and warrants further investigation. The broader the 'control limits' are, the fewer local investigations will be triggered, but in turn the more likely it is that real differences in clinical practice will not be identified and addressed. The converse is also true: narrower control limits will increase the number of investigations that do not reveal systematic underlying problems, but might pick up such issues earlier. Different participants will place different emphasis on the balance of false negatives and false positives in any such reporting process.

A second tension occurs in the balancing of the importance of safety and quality and other organisational imperatives. In most organisations, managers spend their time on the urgent and immediate, and find it difficult to invest time in the longer term strategic and cultural shifts necessary to reposition an organisation. Thus, investigations and reporting of clinical incidents often involve significant management time, whereas preventive action (for example, in managing fatigue risk) may be delegated or attract less management attention.

Finally, the tension between meeting budget targets, meeting activity or access targets and meeting clinical governance requirements is not easy to manage. Organisational and government processes typically place significant emphasis on both budget and access issues: budget performance can easily be measured to the last cent; waiting times are regularly reported and are also a matter of public concern. In contrast, safety and quality issues principally attract interest with individual reported events or publication of data. The sustained approach necessary to attempt to reduce the incidence of adverse events does not provide an immediate reward to managers, and hence often does not attract management attention.

All these tensions are relevant in Queensland Health's emphasis on accountability. Recognising the tensions is important and the first step in the process. The main strategies pursued in response are to affirm the importance of clinical governance issues in key performance indicators for managers as well as ensuring the safety and quality issues are kept directly on the agenda of the senior management team in Queensland Health and in meetings with chief executives.

TRANSPARENCY

Transparency has been defined as:

> a principle that allows those affected by administrative decisions, business transactions or charitable work to know not only the basic facts and figures but also the mechanisms and processes. It is the duty of civil servants, managers and trustees to act visibly, predictably and understandably. (Transparency International 2008)

This process value clearly links with the other two values of accountability and participation (Oliver 2004). Internal transparency is facilitated by the clear specification of roles and responsibilities, which also facilitates clarity of accountability. Transparency is also facilitated by an organisational culture in which staff feel safe to report clinical incidents, near-misses and poor performance by colleagues. Thus, moving from a culture of concealment to one of transparency requires changes throughout the organisation, not only in the corporate office.

External transparency, the reverse of the 'culture of concealment', is becoming part of Queensland Health's *modus operandi*. Queensland Health now reports publicly on notifications in its clinical incident reporting system (Queensland Health 2008c). These reports serve both internal and external purposes. Internally, they indicate to staff that reporting of clinical incidents is valued and that action arises from this reporting. Externally, they indicate that Queensland Health acknowledges that clinical incidents occur, and also reinforces responsiveness to these incidents and their underlying causes. The number of clinical incidents reported in the Queensland Health system is increasing: 46,990 incidents were reported in 2006–07, an increase of 30 per cent from the previous year. The increased number of incidents reported was cited as a sign of the health of the organisation in the public report: 'it demonstrates the successful implementation of policies, systems and cultural reform that encourage staff to identify and report problems' (Queensland Health 2008c: 8).

The clinical incident reporting system is designed to make it easy to report clinical incidents, and to stimulate reporting in line with the philosophy that unless problems are known they cannot be addressed or managed. Reporting is promoted with an emphasis on identifying system factors that might have led to the incident, emphasising a 'just culture' rather than a search for a single professional at fault.

A short training program, known as Human Error and Patient Safety (HEAPS), has been developed for clinical staff. It emphasises the just culture approach, and the importance of reporting clinical incidents in order to strengthen and legitimate assertiveness, and also to create room for junior staff to intervene if they identify a clinical risk.

The clinical incident reporting processes specifically identify 'blameworthy events', events that are associated with drunkenness or specific intent, in order to distinguish that minority of events from the vast majority of events that are the result of actions of well-intentioned staff.

Reporting and analysis of consumer complaints and feedback has also been strengthened by the introduction of a statewide information system (PRIME CF) that records complaints and their outcomes.

Summary reports are provided to the local consumer consultative body, the health community councils.

In addition to these internal reporting processes, external reporting of safety issues has been strengthened. The Health Quality and Complaints Commission receives extensive reports on hospital activities against its published standards, and has the power to investigate specific incidents. Surgical mortality is now voluntarily reported to the Royal Australasian College of Surgeons' Queensland Audit of Surgical Mortality, funded by Queensland Health, but run as a peer-review process under the auspices of the professional college (Royal Australasian College of Surgeons 2008).

Transparency about clinical incident reporting is part of a wider transparency agenda. Queensland Health now reports publicly on a range of performance measures—for example, waiting times for elective surgery, number of patients waiting for outpatient bookings, and ambulance bypass. This reporting occurs through an 'our performance' internet site (<www.health.qld.gov.au/performance/default.asp>), an annual public hospital performance report that incorporates reporting on clinical outcomes and a quarterly public hospital performance report. This extensive range of reporting is now a statutory obligation on Queensland Health under the *Health Services Act* 1991 (Qld) (section 38B) and goes beyond that proposed as part of Commonwealth reporting obligations. The New South Wales Independent Pricing and Regulatory Tribunal recently described the Queensland approach to public reporting as 'Australian best practice' (Independent Pricing and Regulatory Tribunal 2008). Documentation and evaluation of new safety and quality initiatives is also encouraged through publication in professional journals and at conferences.

There are clear tensions involved in an agenda of transparency. Most importantly, there are clear political costs of transparency due to the way the media responds. The immediate response of the tabloid media to identified issues in Queensland Health is to assume venality and incompetence within the organisation. This relatively unsophisticated reporting focuses on banner headlines that enshrine a 'name, shame and blame' approach to safety and quality, in direct contrast to the 'just culture' approach promoted internally within Queensland Health. The media give little latitude to Queensland Health in its treatment of public reports. In the case of reported rates of clinical outcomes (e.g. acute myocardial infarction 30-day mortality rates), any variation is automatically assumed to be variation in clinical performance rather than statistical variation, data-reporting errors or other reasons. To some extent, engaging with a quality ('broadsheet') media may assist to alleviate these problems, but it is unlikely that the tabloid media will ever ignore the opportunity for sensational headlines associated with adverse events.

Different styles of public reporting can also be used to inform debate. Queensland Health emphasises what action is taken if a hospital is identified as significantly different from the state average, rather than simply reporting a risk-adjusted mortality or complication rate (Duckett, Collins et al. 2008). This emphasis on action is consistent with the view that things can go wrong in the best hospitals, and what distinguishes good hospitals is that they use identification of an aberrant trend as an opportunity to learn and change, rather than an issue to be denied or covered up. Simple reporting of rates almost encourages the media to adopt a 'name, shame and blame' approach, rather than to identify those hospitals in denial versus those adopting a continuous improvement philosophy.

Despite the poor media reporting, the costs of transparency are not seen to outweigh the benefits, as public reporting is as much about internal constituencies as about accounting to the public. In the longer term, the public also needs to be educated to realise that adverse events are unfortunately common in hospitals and other health care settings, and that miracle cures and perfect care, as seen on TV, are not always the case when humans and human systems are involved in care processes.

PARTICIPATION

Partly in response to the criticism in the Forster review of the lack of involvement of clinical staff, participation was adopted as a third key process value. This value is conceptualised as covering both clinician and consumer participation.

A number of strategies have been implemented to strengthen participative processes within Queensland Health. An important submission to the Forster review proposed the development of 'managed clinical networks'. These cross-cutting, clinically-led groups would provide mechanisms for clinicians to be involved in key policy and quality improvement initiatives within Queensland Health.

Clinical networks were embraced as a key process to engage clinicians. These collaborative groups, among other aims, sought to improve performance of clinical interventions and clinical service delivery, to develop guidelines, plan services and guide key government initiatives in areas such as cancer and heart disease.

Clinicians generally welcomed the development of networks. Whether because of the network policy or for other reasons, clinicians' morale and sense of engagement with bureaucratic decision-making processes have significantly improved. For medical staff respondents, for example, the Queensland Health staff survey for April 2008 compared with April 2006 showed:

- Trust in immediate supervisor went from a 'middling' score to 'commendable' (these being standardised terms used in reporting the survey);
- Workplace morale went from a 'middling' to 'commendable';
- Participative decision-making showed a major improvement from close to a 'challenging' score to 'middling';
- Supervisor support went from 'middling' to 'commendable'; and
- Goal congruence (the extent to which personal goals are in agreement with workplace goals) went from 'middling' to 'commendable'.

The Patient Safety and Quality Board, the key oversight body for clinical governance across Queensland Health, was restructured to include greater participation from outside the corporate office, with participation now including clinical staff from a range of disciplines. The board and its processes achieved ISO 9001: 2008 quality management system accreditation in late 2008. A Director-General's clinical advisory group was also established to provide another opportunity for informal clinical engagement, and was subsequently replaced by a formal 'clinical senate' to provide a more structured mechanism for clinician engagement.

New mechanisms were also developed to strengthen involvement of consumers in policy and planning processes in the organisation. Although not yet as central to the departmental decision-making process as the clinician engagement forums, consumer involvement is growing in importance within Queensland Health. At the state level, an organisation known as Health Consumers Queensland was established, initially as a ministerial advisory committee on health consumer issues. In addition, 36 health community councils were established across the state, one for each of the districts as they were originally structured, with a statutory role under the *Health Services Act* 1991 (Qld) (section 28M) of:

(a) undertaking community engagement activities about the health of, or health care for, the community, including, for example—

(i) obtaining information and feedback from users of public sector health services about public sector health service issues; and

    (ii) considering planning proposals in relation to the delivery of public sector health services, and facilitating community debate and feedback on the proposals; and

    (iii) advocating for users of public sector health services, so as to influence decision-making about the delivery of the services;

(b) monitoring the quality, safety and effectiveness of public sector health services delivered in the council's district;

(c) considering and evaluating reports about the delivery of public sector health services in the council's district;

(d) enhancing community education about the delivery of public sector health services.

Independence of membership of the health community councils was strengthened by their being appointed by the minister following advice from the Health Quality and Complaints Commission.

The clinical and consumer engagement processes are at different stages of development. These could be located at different rungs on Arnstein's (1969) ladder of participation, with the rungs from bottom to top being: non-participation (manipulation and therapy); tokenism (informing, consultation, placation); and citizen power (partnership, delegated power and citizen control). For example, some clinical networks were given power to set priorities and allocate funds (towards the top of Arnstein's ladder). For most clinical networks, though, formal power remains in the formal line of accountability with the networks' influence being significant but informal, based on expert and information power. Failure to engage appropriately with clinicians risks alienating them with potential political costs, suggesting that clinician participation sits at least on the 'partnership' rung of Arnstein's ladder, connoting a degree of power.

Consumers hold less political sway and are 'repressed', to use Alford's (1975) language. Their degree of engagement sits across more rungs, from the bottom towards the middle. Anecdotal evidence suggests that some of the health community councils are used by others to lobby for additional resources for the relevant district which suggests sitting at the 'manipulation' level; others sit at different degrees of tokenism. Better health community councils and the fledging Health Consumers Queensland both aspire to partnership—a degree of power. No formal evaluation across different mechanisms of consumer engagement has yet been conducted, so it is too early to conclude where the actual balance of engagement strategies sits.

The engagement strategies for Queensland Health create certain inherent tensions. The interests of clinicians and consumers are not coincident, and to the extent that consultative structures consider similar issues, there is a potential for different emphases, and indeed different conclusions, to emerge from the different consultative processes.

In part because of the nascent nature of the clinical networks, deliberations of these groups can still be overtly influenced by the self-interest of participants advocating for their specialty, hospital or area. Some of the networks are more mature than others, and are thus able to deal with issues of greater complexity. A conceptual framework to guide considerations of clinical networks, the 'value cube' was developed; it highlights the importance of assessing value in terms of the perspectives of clinicians, consumers and funders. However, this is not yet routinely incorporated in the thinking and decision processes of either clinical or consumer groups (Duckett and Ward 2008).

Both clinical and consumer processes are still developing, and both groups need to develop skills in considering health policy issues. Clinical networks have evolved further down this path than the consumer bodies. However, most of the clinical networks have not embarked on formalised methods for considering policy tradeoffs, such as Program Budgeting and Marginal Analysis.

Initial clinical governance policy was *laissez-faire* in terms of the role, structure and function of networks, with a tightening across these dimensions in the second iteration of the policy. Overall, more than 40 clinical networks have developed at state or area levels, covering a wide range of clinical areas.

CONCLUSION

There has been significant change in the structures and processes for clinical governance across Queensland Health since 2005. New processes and policies have been promulgated, new organisational units established and new staff recruited. This superstructure is highly visible and is attracting attention across Australia, in part because of a deliberate promotion strategy, through journals and at conferences, designed to change the perception of Queensland Health from a safety and quality problem to a safety and quality leader.

Figure 6.1 shows a revised regulatory pyramid for the approach to responsive regulation adopted in Queensland Health. At the base of the pyramid is *regulation through culture*. The aim here is to embed a culture of safety and quality, so that staff and organisational units within Queensland Health are self-regulatory, with a pervasive culture promoting quality and safety throughout the organisation. These mechanisms are being implemented particularly through emphasising the values of participation and transparency. This is characterised by 'soft words' of culture change and leadership to drive improvement in safety and quality (Braithwaite et al. 2005). To some extent, a more open culture and a change of the operational norms of the organisation are conditions precedent for effective operation of some other aspects—especially those at the apex of the pyramid.

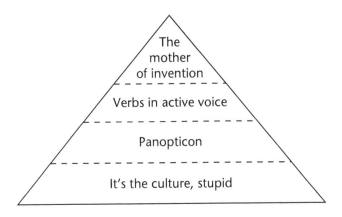

Figure 6.1 Queensland Health regulatory pyramid—alternative characterisation

The second level of the pyramid, a panopticon approach, is about *regulation through information*, emphasising the transparency value. This approach is based on the assumption that increased monitoring of activities throughout the organisation, and the use of information, will increase the likelihood that aberrant practice will be identified early, and thus reduce the risk of adverse patterns of practice. Queensland Health places a significant emphasis on statistical process control using routine data as part of this process, but new information systems have also been developed to facilitate recording and monitoring of consumer complaints and clinical incidents, the latter also including near-misses.

The third level of the revised pyramid emphasises both the importance of action (verbs or doing words) following identification of an adverse event and accountability (the active voice). Here the emphasis is on *regulation through bureaucratic processes*, and it is an essential element of converting regulation through information from 'busy work' into real service improvement. This aspect of the pyramid is underpinned by the accountability value and by the transition of 'soft words' into 'hard words' and, where necessary, sticks.

At the apex of the pyramid, 'the mother of invention' indicates an emphasis on *regulation through ideas and demonstration effects* particularly linked to the value of participation. It recognises that, because of its sorry history, Queensland Health needs to improve its performance. A range of innovative strategies have been unleashed to promote quality, such as the clinical practice improvement payment (Duckett, Daniels et al. 2008), statistical process control approaches (Duckett et al. 2007), expanding clinical simulation, and projects related to patient safety in terms of falls prevention, open disclosure, patient identification prior to procedures, and so on. The purpose is to encourage and empower innovation as part of a strategy of driving improvement in the average level of performance in the organisation (the quality agenda), rather than simply identifying and minimising the risks of poor performance or adverse events. This level of the pyramid emphasises challenging the way things are done, based on the belief that continuing to act in the same way as previously is likely to mean that the organisation ends up in the same situation as previously. Importantly, striving for improvement at the apex of the pyramid needs to be linked to culture change at the base of the pyramid. The two aspects of regulation need to be mutually reinforcing: if the culture does not accept and welcome innovation and change, it is unlikely to have an effect, and the ideas generated from pilots and the like are likely to fall on fallow ground.

The underpinning process values for the new clinical governance arrangements in Queensland Health involve fundamental shifts from the previous approaches. These values, by definition, cannot be seen but, to the extent they become embedded in the culture of Queensland Health, they will leave an enduring legacy that will be independent of organisational forms. However, it is still very early in the culture change process and the embedding of these values is still at a stage where change could easily be reversed. The values relating to participation and departmental attendance, for example, could be slowly and subtly undermined through decreasing frequency of meetings of clinicians or consumer groups. The current organisation and political leadership of Queensland Health supports and/or champions the three process values, but it is difficult to tell how long it will take for the new values to be embedded in the organisation and to develop an independent life, regardless of current participants and structures.

The three process values described in this chapter involve inherent tensions and challenges to existing internal or external players. There are costs to the organisation of adopting these values, and adherence can be undermined by external pressures, such as media reporting and the exigencies of daily political cycles. The link between development and implementation of these values and an improvement in safety and quality involves a long causal path. However, these three process values are important in terms of developing the safety and quality culture within the organisation. It is unlikely, though, that a just culture, focusing on a continuous improvement of safety and quality in the organisation, could be developed without relying either explicitly or implicitly on the three process values that have been adopted.

REFERENCES

Alford, R.R. 1975, *Health Care Politics: Ideological and Interest Group Barriers to Reform*, University of Chicago Press, Chicago

Arnstein, S. 1969, 'A ladder of citizen participation', *Journal of American Institute of Planners*, vol. 35, no. 4, pp. 216-24

Braithwaite, J., Healy, J. and Dwan, K. 2005, *The Governance of Health Safety and Quality*, Commonwealth of Australia, Canberra

Clinical Practice Improvement Centre 2008, *VLADs for Dummies*, Wiley, Brisbane

Crethar, M., Phillips, J., Stafford, P. and Duckett, S. 2009, 'Leadership transformation in Queensland Health' *Australian Health Review*, in press

Davies, G. 2005, *Commissions of Inquiry Order (No. 2) 2005*, <www.qphci.qld.gov.au/final_report/Final_Report.pdf)>, accessed 3 December 2008

Duckett, S. 2007, 'A new approach to clinical governance in Queensland', *Australian Health Review*, vol. 31, suppl. 1, pp. S16-19

Duckett, S., Collins, J., Kamp, M. and Walker, K. 2008, 'An improvement focus in public reporting', *Medical Journal of Australia*, vol. 189, nos 11/12, pp. 616-17

Duckett, S., Coory, M., Sketcher-Baker, K. 2007, 'Identifying variations in quality of care in Queensland hospitals', *Medical Journal of Australia*, vol. 187, no. 10, pp. 571-5

Duckett, S., Daniels, S., Kamp, M., Stockwell, A., Walker, G. and Ward, M. 2008, 'Pay for performance in Australia: Queensland's New Clinical Practice Improvement Payment', *Journal of Health Services Research and Policy*, vol. 13, no. 3, pp. 174-7

Duckett, S. and Ward, M. 2008, 'Developing "robust performance benchmarks" for the next Australian Health Care Agreement: The need for a new framework', *Australian and New Zealand Health Policy*, vol. 5, no. 1, <www.anzhealthpolicy.com>, accessed 3 April 2009

Edwards, M. 2002, 'Public sector governance—future issues for Australia', *Australian Journal of Public Administration*, vol. 61, no. 2, pp. 51-61

Forster, P. 2005, *Queensland Health Systems Review Final Report September 2005*, <www.health.qld.gov.au/health_sys_review/final/qhsr_final_report.pdf>, accessed 3 December 2008

Harlow, C. 2006, 'Global administrative law: The quest for principles and values', *European Journal of International Law*, vol. 17, no. 1, pp. 187-214

Heifetz, R. 1994, *Leadership without Easy Answers*, Harvard University Press, London

Heifetz, R. and Linksky, M. 2002, *Leadership on the Line*, Harvard Business School Press, Boston

Independent Pricing and Regulatory Tribunal 2008, *Framework for Performance Improvement in Health: Other Industries—Final Report*, <http://tinyurl.com/5tx7g4>, accessed 3 December 2008

Oliver, R. 2004, *What is Transparency?*, McGraw-Hill, New York

Queensland Health 2008a, *Implementation Standard 1: Roles and Responsibilities*, <www.health.qld.gov.au/quality/docs/clingovimpstand1_v3.pdf>, accessed 3 December 2008

——2008b, *Clinical Incident Management Implementation Standard (CIMIS)*, <www.health.qld.gov.au/patientsafety/documents/cimist.pdf>, accessed 3 December 2008

—— 2008c, *Patient Safety: From Learning to Action II*, <www.health.qld.gov.au/patientsafety/documents/learn2.pdf>, accessed 3 December 2008

Royal Australasian College of Surgeons 2008, 'Queensland audit of surgical mortality', <www.surgeons.org/Content/NavigationMenu/Research/Audit/QueenslandAuditofSurgicalMortality/default.htm>, accessed 17 December 2008

Schein, E.H. 1992, *Organizational Culture and Leadership*, Jossey Bass, San Francisco

Thomas, H. 2007, *Sick to Death: A Manipulative Surgeon and a Health System in Crisis—a Disaster Waiting to Happen*, Allen & Unwin, Sydney

Transparency International 2008, 'Frequently asked questions about corruption', <www.transparency.org/faqs/faq-corruption.html#faqcorr1>, accessed 3 December 2008

Tuohy, C.H. 1999, *Accidental Logics: The Dynamics of Change in the Health Care Arena in the United States, Britain, and Canada*, Oxford University Press, New York

Van Der Weyden, M.B. 2005, 'The Bundaberg Hospital Scandal: The need for reform in Queensland and beyond', *Medical Journal of Australia*, vol. 183, no. 6, pp. 284-5

Williams, D. and Young, T. 1994, 'Governance, the World Bank and liberal theory', *Political Studies*, vol. 42, no. 1, pp. 84-100

7

REGULATING HEALTH PROFESSIONALS

Kieran Walshe

INTRODUCTION

The regulation of the health professions, particularly that of doctors, is one of the longest established mechanisms for protecting patients and the public against medical errors and for assuring and improving patient safety. In the United Kingdom, regulation of the medical profession was introduced in 1858 by the *Medical Act*, which created the General Medical Council to register all qualified doctors, to oversee medical education, and to discipline doctors for infractions of their professional code of conduct. That legislation was the product not of political and public pressure to assure the quality of medical care for patients, but of professional lobbying to protect the economic interests of doctors who had completed expensive university training and found them-selves undercut by a host of less well-qualified (or unqualified) healers, some of whom were certainly 'quacks'. It can be seen as much as an act of self-interested, monopolistic professional closure as one of public-spirited, community protection (Stacey 1992; Irvine 2006). That dichotomy—between the public and the professional interest—is central to the development of health professions regulation in the past and to our understanding of current reforms and future trends.

Health professional regulation is perhaps most simply defined as the arrangements put in place to assure the quality of individual professional practice by health professionals. Those regulatory arrangements are usually placed in the hands of a statutory regulatory body or council, which manages them on behalf of government and society. The scope and nature of those arrangements often varies across professions, and between jurisdictions. However, health professions regulators generally have four main functions, discussed below.

Maintaining the register

This involves keeping a central list of all those who are members of the profession (doctors, nurses, physiotherapists, or whatever) and updating it to reflect additions, as newly trained professionals achieve registration, and removals, as some people retire, die or are removed from the register for other reasons. In some cases, that register also records additional skills or specialist qualifications achieved. The regulator may have legal powers to take action to protect the title of the profession—for example, to stop someone pretending to be a doctor who is not registered, or to stop someone doing things (like prescribing drugs, or undertaking procedures) which can only be done by a registered professional.

Setting and assuring educational standards

Usually, entry to the register is dependent wholly or in part on achieving some kind of educational qualification, often awarded by a university. Regulators often have powers of oversight of both the educational standards required for the award, and of the educational program and its management by the academic institution.

Investigating and dealing with problems

When concerns are raised about the behaviour or performance of individual practitioners, they generally fall into one of three categories. The first is *misconduct*—a practitioner acting in ways that are not generally acceptable, and which may also involve a breach of the law. Examples could include dishonesty, drink driving, falsification of records, sexual offences or other forms of personal behaviour not consistent with their professional status. The second is *poor performance*—a practitioner whose clinical knowledge, skill level or practice falls below the standards to be expected of a professional. The third is *health problems* which affect the practitioner's ability to practise, such as drug or alcohol dependency, mental illness or some forms of physical illness. The regulator usually has the responsibility for investigating complaints or concerns when they are raised, and then taking action if necessary—up to and including the removal of a practitioner from the register (see Chapter 8).

Assuring continuing competence to practise

Some, but not all regulators have a statutory responsibility to do more than just investigate problems as they occur, but to take steps to ensure that all practitioners remain competent to practise (including the great majority against whom no complaint is ever raised). This may take the form of requiring some form of continuing professional development or education, or monitoring the content of a professional portfolio or record of practice, or even requiring professionals to take tests of their knowledge and skills.

The rest of this chapter is concerned with the development of these regulatory arrangements, and explores a number of areas of particular change. However, before tackling this territory, it is worth considering how health professions regulation connects or interacts with the other systems or arrangements for regulating the quality of health care and protecting patients from the harm that exists in most health care systems, and which are discussed in other chapters. To that end, Box 7.1 sets out a brief account of an example of high-profile failure in care which occurred in a United Kingdom hospital in 2001, and which resulted in a patient's death and in an inquiry that led to a series of subsequent policy and management reforms (Toft 2001).

Box 7.1 Maladministration of vincristine at the Queen's Medical Centre, Nottingham, UK

On 4 January 2001, two doctors at QMC gave chemotherapy drugs to a daycase patient, 18-year-old Wayne Jowett, who was being treated for leukaemia. The first drug, cytosine arabinoside, was to be given intrathecally (into the spine) and was administered successfully. The second drug, vincristine, was to be given intravenously, but was erroneously given intrathecally like the first drug. When injected into the spine, vincristine is highly toxic. Although the doctors realised their error and emergency treatment was provided rapidly, Wayne Jowett died a few weeks later. A subsequent independent investigation identified many related causes of the error. The hospital's procedures for administering chemotherapy drugs were poorly defined and were not being properly followed. The two doctors concerned had only started work in the hospital two days and five weeks earlier respectively, they had limited previous experience of chemotherapy administration, and they received no formal training in

---

local procedures before being put to work. The two drugs were delivered to the ward together, were similar in appearance, and were in syringes which could be transposed or interchanged easily.

Source: Based on Miller and Capstick (2003) and Toft (2001).

This was a complex and serious adverse incident, which involved failures in three different regulatory domains. First, the organisation's processes for managing care were at fault. The systems for booking and dealing with chemotherapy appointments, and for managing its administration, were not well defined and were not followed. Second, the two doctors concerned were not competent to undertake the procedure—they had not been properly trained and did not have enough experience to recognise the error they were about to make, though their professional training should have made them aware that they were working outside their own areas of competence. Third, the way the drug itself was made and delivered was at fault. Little had been done to make it distinctive from other drugs which are given intrathecally and, crucially, it was supplied ready for use in a syringe which could be connected to either an intrathecal or intravenous needle, rather than in one which could only be connected to an intravenous needle. Since 1968, around 55 similar incidents of vincristine maladministration have been reported internationally, and most have resulted in the patient's death.

This incident highlights the need for coordinated regulatory over-sight and control in the three main loci for regulation in health care systems—oriented around institutions and the processes of care within them, people who are health care professionals, and the objects used in health care: devices, drugs and equipment. In practice, as Table 7.1 illustrates, we have separate and largely disconnected systems for regulation in these three domains, with different regulatory bodies and processes and little apparent coordination. This chapter is primarily concerned with the regulation of the health professions, but other chapters deal more directly with regulation in the other domains. In this chapter, one issue which is explored later is the interaction between institutions which employ health care professionals and which have some responsibility for ensuring they practise safely and competently, and the health professions regulators, which largely focus their work on health care professionals as individuals, and have no statutory powers of oversight of the health care organisations in which they work.

Table 7.1 Regulating the health care system

Focus for regulation	Regulatory arrangements in the United Kingdom
Institutions Organisations, structures and processes, managing the delivery of health care	Health care-specific regulators (Care Quality Commission) Health care accreditation bodies (Health Quality Service, Clinical Pathology Accreditation, etc.) Generic regulators (Health and Safety Executive, Environment Agency, etc.)
People Health care professionals	Regulatory bodies (General Medical Council, Nursing and Midwifery Council, etc.) Medical Royal Colleges Other professional societies
Inanimate objects Medical devices, pharmaceuticals, equipment	Medicines and Healthcare Products Regulatory Agency European Medicines Evaluation Agency National Institute for Health and Clinical Excellence

This chapter starts by setting the context with a brief account of the history and evolution of health professions regulation in an international context. It then proceeds to examine four major current trends or themes in health professions regulation: the relationship between society, government and the professions, the growth of health professions regulation, the internationalisation of health professions regulation, and the pressures of labour and skill-mix reform on health professions regulation. It then offers a case study of the dynamics of health professions regulatory reform, based on the recent experience of the United Kingdom. The chapter concludes by questioning how far modern systems of health professions regulation are fit for the purpose, and how they fit into the wider context of health care regulation.

SETTING THE CONTEXT: HISTORY AND EVOLUTION OF HEALTH PROFESSIONS REGULATION

The regulation of medical doctors started in most European countries in the 1800s, as the emerging allopathic movement—the precursor to modern biomedicine—sought to gain control of the diagnosis and treatment of illness and to exclude those without formal qualifications.

In the United States, the Flexner report (1910) presented a comprehensive and critical nationwide review of medical education, and led to a radical reduction and consolidation in medical schools, and to the introduction or strengthening of state-level licensing boards for doctors and, in 1912, to the formation of the Federation of State Medical Boards (Beck 2004). The development of medical regulation (and the undoubted benefits of protected title and scope of practice which it brought) stimulated calls from other group for statutory regulation. In Canada, the regulation of dentistry started in Ontario in 1868. In the United Kingdom, voluntary registration of nurses started in 1887, and a statutory scheme was created by legislation in 1919. Voluntary registration for pharmacists started with the foundation of the Royal Pharmaceutical Society in 1841, and received statutory backing in 1954. The statutory regulation of opticians and optometrists followed in 1958.

In most developed countries, there are now extensive systems of health professions regulation in place, though there are important differences in the way that health professions regulation is enacted in different countries (Kuhlmann and Saks 2008). These variations are in part a product of the structure and history of the professions themselves and of the health care system in each country, and in part a result of differences in policy direction and intent. However, they provide an opportunity for us to compare and contrast approaches and to explore the likely effects of potential changes or reforms before they are enacted. Allsop and Jones (2006) undertook an international review primarily of medical regulation which provides useful comparative data on the arrangements in the United Kingdom, the United States, Canada, Australia, New Zealand, Finland and France.

Which professions are regulated?

There is a core set of major health professions which are regulated almost everywhere—doctors, nurses, dentists, opticians and pharmacists. However, important differences continue to exist in which other health professions are recognised. For example, midwifery is recognised as a separate professional group from nursing in just over half of US states; physician assistants are not recognised as a group in most European countries while they are well established in the United States; and the regulation of psychologists, counsellors, dental technicians, operating department assistants, and complementary therapists such as acupuncturists, osteopaths and chiropractors varies widely. In most countries, there has been a continuing pressure from newer professional groups to secure statutory professional regulation, for the same reasons that doctors sought it in the nineteenth century—to establish control over their scope of practice, to limit the numbers of people practising, and to gain the status and esteem which accompany professional status.

Defining the health professions

Many countries regulate 'by title', which means they protect the name of a health profession by law, and only allow a person who has been admitted to the professional register to call themselves a doctor, nurse or whatever. However, the content or 'scope of practice' of those professions is often not explicitly defined, or it is defined mainly in terms of its inputs, like the amount and content of the education program which must be undertaken to join that profession. While competence-based approaches to training in other domains have developed rapidly, they have not been widely adopted in the health care sector. More explicit scope of practice definitions are in use in some countries, like the United States and Canada. As a result, there can be substantial differences in the way that different countries define what it means to be a health professional such as a dentist, physiotherapist or midwife. The content of the role, the skills and training required, and the way it fits into the health care process can vary so widely that moving from one jurisdiction to another is difficult, and can require retraining or the completion of a conversion qualification.

The role of the state in regulation

Almost everywhere, health professions regulation is endorsed or supported through the state by legislation which gives powers to the regulatory bodies. However, in some countries those regulatory bodies are government agencies, essentially controlled by the department of health, while in others they are quasi-autonomous bodies, with elected councils and financial independence because they are funded by registration fees charged to registrants. In broad terms, the greater the role that the state plays in funding and providing health care, the more it takes control of health professions regulation. For example, in Finland and other Scandinavian countries, medical regulation is directly undertaken by a government department; in the Netherlands it is enacted both through the government's Health Care Inspectorate and through the professional associations; while in the United States it is largely run by the medical profession itself, at both a state and federal level.

Integrated or fragmented regulation

The origins of health professions regulation—enacted one group at a time, in response to pressures from particular groups, with piecemeal and incremental development over time—have tended to produce systems of regulation which are fragmented along professional lines, with separate regulatory bodies, legislative requirements and provisions, and regulatory processes for doctors, nurses, dentists and others. In some jurisdictions, like Ontario, Canada and New Zealand, regulatory reforms have tried to reduce this fragmentation, and to create either a single regulatory body and process, or a harmonised set of arrangements across separate regulatory councils.

State, provincial or regional variations in regulation within countries

The federal structure of countries like the United States, Canada and Australia (and to some degree countries in Europe such as Germany and, since devolution, the United Kingdom) has produced systems of health professions regulation which are predominantly organised at a state or provincial level, because that is where legislative and political responsibility for the health care system is located. In these countries, while federal governments may play little or no part in health professions regulation, federated councils to deal with specialist and postgraduate registration, and to coordinate standards and organise information interchange between state or provincial boards, have developed. Nevertheless, variations in professional regulation within these countries can be substantial—for example, the number of health professions regulated varies from province to province in Canada, and until recently there has been no national medical register in Australia and doctors moving from state to state have had to register afresh (Productivity Commission 2005).

The mission and function of the regulatory body

The core function of regulatory bodies is regulation (as defined at the outset of this chapter), and their primary mission is to protect the public. However, in many countries regulatory bodies have other functions as well, such as promoting the interests of the profession, or organising and providing educational and professional development. Moreover, the nature of the regulatory territory varies. Some regulatory bodies deal with the whole process of investigating and adjudicating breaches of the professional code of conduct, while others deal only with investigation, and decisions are made by a separate and independent tribunal. Some regulatory bodies deal with all educational standard-setting while others share that responsibility with professional associations.

The governance and accountability of the regulatory body

It has already been noted that the state plays a varying, but often influential, role over health professions regulators. Some regulatory bodies are run by a council or board elected by registrants, but many have a partly or wholly appointed council or board, often with key stakeholders (such as educational institutions, hospital associations and patient groups) having some powers of nomination. Accountability to government is often secured through a requirement to report to the legislature annually. More practically, where regulatory bodies are funded by government, the executive often has considerable influence over what they do, while regulatory bodies which are mostly or wholly funded through fees charged to their registrants are more able to exercise a degree of autonomy. The challenge is to avoid regulatory capture by any one stakeholder group. Most commonly, regulatory capture is seen to occur with elected boards which end up acting in the economic or social self-interests of the registrants. However, a significant risk also exists that government, struggling with other problems like the rising costs of health care or a shortage of practitioners in key areas, will seek to use health professions regulation to tackle those problems.

The remainder of this chapter discusses four important trends in health professions regulation which, at least in part, emerge from this brief review of the international context. First, it examines societal attitudes to the health professions, and public expectations of regulation. Second, it explores the increasing intensity and scope of oversight of the health professions through regulation. Third, it discusses the internationalisation of health professions regulation which is resulting, in part at least, from increasing professional mobility and extensive economic migration. Fourth, it examines the pressures of labour and skill-mix reform, and their implications for health professions regulation.

SOCIETY AND THE HEALTH PROFESSIONS: A CHANGING RELATIONSHIP

In his preface to *The Doctor's Dilemma*, first published in 1906, George Bernard Shaw famously railed against the perversity of a health care system which gave doctors a pecuniary interest in (over)treatment, and memorably described the medical profession as a 'conspiracy against the laity'. His diatribe continued:

> Again I hear the voices indignantly muttering old phrases about the high character of a noble profession and the honor and conscience of its members. I must reply that the medical profession has not a high character: it has an infamous character. I do not know a single thoughtful and well-informed person who does not feel that the tragedy of illness at present is that it delivers you helplessly into the hands of a profession which you deeply mistrust . . . That is the character the medical profession has got just now. (Shaw 1946)

Yet the social reality was very different. For most of the twentieth century, there was an implied contract between the health professions, government and wider society (Klein 1998). The professions were granted considerable autonomy and effective self-regulation, in return for which they policed themselves effectively and helped to control the costs of the health care system (Salter 2001). Surveys of public opinion consistently showed very high levels of trust in the medical and nursing professions.

Over the last twenty years, that established relationship of trust has been eroded or even destroyed, and in its place governments have sought to put arrangements to measure and monitor the performance of health care institutions and professionals, and to make them much more explicitly accountable. In part, this reflects a wider societal trend, away from a deferential, collectivist and paternalistic society in which professionals of all kinds were revered and trusted, and towards a more equal, consumerist and individualist society in which trust, status and tradition count for much less (O'Neill 2002; Power 1997). But it has been catalysed by a number of high-profile failures in care in which many patients have been harmed by health care professionals who practised incompetently, showed arrogance and a lack of insight into their own behaviour, and were allowed to continue doing so for many years despite their deficiencies being well known to their professional and managerial colleagues (Walshe and Higgins 2002). These cases revealed the clubby, cosy, protectionist culture of some health professions, showed that standards of practice were often lax and unacceptably low, and demonstrated that the existing regulatory arrangements had failed to deal with significant quality failures (Walshe and Higgins 2002; Walshe and Shortell 2004; Faunce and Bolsin 2004).

With some notable individual exceptions, the health professions and the regulatory bodies have been slow to recognise these problems and to reform themselves. By failing to respond proactively, and to show honesty, openness and a willingness to embrace reform, the health professions regulators have tended to find themselves the unwilling subject of, rather than the initiator and author of, those reforms (Irvine 2003). George Bernard Shaw might find more public support for his caustic views of the medical profession now than he did over a century ago.

THE GROWTH OF HEALTH PROFESSIONS REGULATION

The recent history of health professions regulation in many countries has been one of expansion and growth: in the numbers of professions and professionals regulated, the range and scope of their activities which are regulated and the intensity of oversight of their performance by regulatory bodies.

The growth of health professions regulation is, of course, a product of the changing relationship between the professions and society described above. But some of the pressure for the introduction of professional regulation comes from the professions themselves, and while there is no doubt an element of philanthropic public interest in their enthusiasm, it is certainly true that regulation serves professions' economic interest by giving the monopolistic control of their work, and enabling them to control the supply of health professionals who can do that work. It can also be seen as serving their social interests, by giving them standing and respect in the eyes both of other health professions and of wider society. The growth in health professions regulation is, at least in part, a result of governments ceding to the insistent and continuing pressure for regulation from health professions and their lobby groups.

However, governments also face frequent calls to regulate a wide range of other professional and occupational groups (from plumbers and hairdressers to teachers and social workers) and the growth of health professions regulation can also be seen as part of a wider regulatory expansion in society, as more and more occupations are subject to some form of regulatory control. Regulation also results from public concerns about the quality of services and about examples of poor practice which sometimes receive extensive media attention.

To take a particularly current example, in many countries health professions regulation is now being expanded to cover a range of alternative or complementary therapies—a controversial move in the eyes of many biomedical scientists who often regard such treatments as having no basis in modern science, and no plausible theoretical explanation or demonstrated empirical effect beyond placebo (Bausell 2007; Singh and Ernst 2008). However, regulation is expanding for three reasons. First, at least some of the professional groups concerned want to be regulated—especially those (like acupuncturists and osteopaths) who often practise in collaboration with or alongside conventional medical practitioners. Second, the use of complementary therapies has expanded dramatically in recent years, which has brought more people into contact with these therapies as patients, and has made conventional medical practitioners more aware of complementary medicine. Third, there have been a number of high-profile cases of failure, in which people have been harmed by complementary therapies or have failed to access conventional therapy for curable conditions (Ernst 2001).

Only a few jurisdictions have adopted a rational and planned approach for considering the extension of regulation to new health professions, such as the province of Ontario in Canada (Allsop and Jones 2006). In 1994, Ontario introduced a system of regulation founded around a set of thirteen 'regulated acts' (such as making a diagnosis, prescribing a medication, undertaking an invasive procedure, administering an injection, and so on). It established the Health Professions Regulatory Advisory Council (HPRAC), which considers the case for regulating new groups, based on an assessment of whether the group has a distinctive body of knowledge, what risks are associated with its activities or treatments, and whether it undertakes these controlled or regulated acts.

The second area of growth in health professions regulation has been in the range and scope of those professional activities which are regulated. Traditionally, health professions regulation was mainly focused on dealing with behaviour which brought the profession into disrepute and cases of gross misconduct (Irvine 2006). The former would include criminal activity, sexual misconduct, dishonesty, and so on. The latter would involve actions or inactions which were clearly completely outside the boundaries of accepted practice—for example, refusing to visit or examine an urgent case, or making crude and inexplicable errors in diagnosis and treatment. But then regulators found themselves often having to deal with professionals whose ability to practise was impaired by their own health problems, including difficulties like depression and alcohol or drug dependency (Harrison 2008). In these cases, a more remedial approach and a continuing involvement in monitoring their return to health was often needed. As social attitudes have changed, and the number of complaints to regulatory bodies has continued to grow inexorably, regulators have also found themselves asked to deal with cases of poor performance which, while not representing gross misconduct, do seem to show that the practitioner is not competent, and cases of behaviour which, while not criminal, seem unacceptable—such as rudeness, bullying, poor communication and arrogance. Over time, and in response to these shifting expectations, health professions regulators have expanded their remit to deal with almost any aspect of the health professional's character, behaviour or performance.

The third area of growth has been in the intensity of oversight exercised by the regulatory bodies. Traditionally, health professions regulators admitted people to their register when they completed their qualifying examinations, and only reviewed their performance in response to a complaint about them. As a result, the great majority of health professionals were never subject to any review or oversight from the regulator throughout their career. But in recent years, regulators have started to require health professionals to periodically provide some form of evidence to demonstrate their continuing fitness to practise. Initially, this usually took the form of a record showing at least a certain level of participation in continuing professional development (training courses, education programs and the like). However, many regulators now require more information, such as details of current practice volumes and areas of specialisation, information on complaints or treatment outcomes, and results from appraisals by the practitioner's employer. Revalidation or recertification is made dependent on the successful completion of an assessment every few years (Pringle 2006). Moreover, some regulators now concern themselves with the conduct of people before they become health professionals, during their period of pre-qualification training (Boon and Turner 2004), and some are introducing a form of student registration.

There is little empirical evidence which would enable us to test the impact of the expansion of health professions regulation described above, or to assess its effectiveness in protecting patients and the public, though what evidence does exist is broadly, if mildly, supportive of increased regulatory scrutiny (Sutherland and Leatherman 2006). However, it probably makes more sense to see the growth of health professions regulation as a political and social response to the changing relationship between the professions and society, and a symptom of the wider shift away from trust and collegiality and towards performance measurement and accountability.

156

INTERNATIONALISATION: THE MIGRATION OF HEALTH PROFESSIONALS

It was noted earlier that health professions regulation has largely been developed at a national (or state or provincial) level and that, as a result, significant differences in regulatory arrangements exist both between countries, and even within countries between different states, provinces or regions. For most health professions and most countries, these arrangements have still worked well because the great majority of health professionals have trained and worked for their whole career in one jurisdiction.

However, there has always been a significant level of health professional migration. A World Health Organization study almost 30 years ago found that around 6 per cent of doctors and 5 per cent of nurses worked outside the country where they trained—but that about 87 per cent of these migrants were working in five countries—Australia, Canada, Germany, the United Kingdom and the United States (Mejia et al. 1979). Since then, mobility has further increased—for example, in 2001 around 29 per cent of doctors practising in the United States were migrants—mostly from India, Pakistan and the Philippines (Forcier et al. 2004). Overall, the picture is mostly one of rich, developed countries importing health professionals from much poorer, developing countries whose health care systems are already fragile and short of resources (Bach 2008). Countries which import health professionals have usually adapted their regulatory arrangements to provide conversion or qualifying processes designed to ensure that immigrant professionals match up to indigenous standards of skills, knowledge and competence (including the ability to communicate in the host language). Migrants have been willing to accept these requirements (and sometimes to make career compromises like taking less senior positions or working in shortage specialities) to secure the economic benefits of migration. Where, for geographic or social reasons, there have been significant flows of health professionals between countries (for example, between the United States and Canada), mutual recognition arrangements have tended to evolve.

The European Union has become the first international region to seek to standardise or harmonise health professions regulation across countries, so ensuring that health professionals can move freely from one country to another and still continue to practise. These changes are part of the much wider implementation of the single European market—which guarantees the free movement of goods, services, people and finance across all member states of the European Union, without tariff or trade barriers of any kind (Busse et al. 2002). Each member state must accept health professionals from other states on to its register and allow them to practise as if they were trained there. In the five largest health professional groups, where there has been harmonisation and mutual recognition of training for decades through a number of European Union directives dating back to 1975 (Jinks et al. 2000), regulatory convergence has not been too difficult, but in other professions where there are more significant differences in training, agreed competences and ways of working, regulatory harmonisation has been more difficult. Some groups—osteopaths and chiropractors, for example—are regulated professions in some European Union countries but not in others. It remains to be seen how well information about competence and fitness to practise will be shared between regulators, to prevent health professionals who are disciplined in one country simply moving somewhere else. The volume of health professional migration within Europe has always been quite limited—constrained by language differences, and by the relatively marginal economic advantages to be secured by moving between countries. But the expansion of the European Union to include ten new and economically less developed states from Eastern Europe in 2005, and the existence of surpluses of health professionals in some European countries and shortages in others, have both stimulated greater migration in recent years, just as the new single market provisions allowing mobility have come into force.

It seems likely that international migration among health professionals will continue to grow, especially in countries or regions where international agreements are reached to make movement easier (like the European Union), or in places where the economic or social incentives to move are very strong. The absolute size of migration flows does not have to be very large to present a significant challenge to professional regulators in coordinating and sharing information and maintaining professional registers. In the future, it is likely that some degree of regulatory convergence will emerge, with standards, competencies and ways of working becoming more homogenous. Indeed, the internationalisation of health professions regulation may constrain its reform at a national level, particularly in Europe.

SKILL-MIX AND LABOUR REFORM: IMPLICATIONS FOR PROFESSIONAL REGULATION

The professional self-interest which leads to pressure for regulation to secure occupational closure and monopoly, as discussed earlier, has also been a formidable barrier to redesigning professional roles and responsibilities, altering the skill-mix of the health care workforce, and introducing new roles. The history of midwifery in the United States and Canada is an illustrative case study (Spoel and James 2006). The recognition of midwives as a separate professional group has consistently been opposed by medical associations and related lobby groups, who have sought to sustain control over the birthing process by obstetricians, and to prevent the development and regulation of the midwifery profession.

It can be argued that, at its worst, professional regulation has been used to impose a host of artificial and unnecessary restrictive practices on health care organisations, constraining the way they use their staff resources and hindering innovation and improvements in efficiency and quality. An alternate view could be that professional regulation protects quality and patient safety, and provides an important defence against health care organisations cutting costs and quality by making staff work beyond or outside their level of competence. Regulation is certainly central to any labour reform, as staff costs make up about 75 per cent of the costs of providing most health care services, and making any service changes almost always involves changing the work processes or routines of health professionals (Buchan et al. 2001).

Many skill-mix reforms involve the transfer of work from one group of health professions to another, or to non-professionals, often accompanied by the routinisation of work through the greater use of clinical guidelines, protocols and decision aids. Examples include the replacement of junior doctors in the emergency department by emergency care practitioners (with a professional background as a paramedic or a nurse); the replacement of general medical practitioners with nurse practitioners; the replacement of medically trained anaesthetists by nurse anaesthetists; and the transfer of work from qualified nurses to health care assistants or personal support workers. In other areas, skill-mix reform has involved the transfer of work from dentists to dental technicians and hygienists, from pharmacists to pharmacy assistants, and from radiographers and ultrasonographers to other staff. While the empirical evidence on the cost and clinical effectiveness of these changes is sometimes limited and there is a risk that work is not transferred effectively (Richardson et al. 1998), it is still clear that health care organisations can realise significant improvements in quality and efficiency through redesigning care processes, and that usually means changing clinical roles and responsibilities (Hunter 1996).

The process of role redesign challenges existing systems of health profession regulation in a number of ways. First, it crosses the boundaries between health professions and often between regulatory bodies. New roles may combine the skills of more than one group (paramedics and nurses in emergency care practitioner roles, for example) or require an existing professional to acquire extended skills from another group (nurse anaethetists, for example). This raises questions of which regulatory body should oversee the new role, what or whose standards or expectations of competence should apply, how complaints or issues of fitness to practise will be handled, and so on. Second, the new role may run counter to well-established professional regulatory standards and expectations—for example, involving a specialist task being taken on by someone with less training and specialised knowledge. It can represent a significant challenge to the status quo, and may require amendments to existing regulatory standards. Third, the new role may require new or amended education and training programs, and regulators need to review, approve and communicate those new education requirements to academic institutions. In general terms, the more harmonised the regulatory arrangements, and the more use made of explicit scopes of practice, the easier it is to define new roles and fit them into the existing regulatory schema.

THE DYNAMICS OF REGULATORY REFORM: A CASE STUDY FROM THE UNITED KINGDOM

The arrangements for health professions regulation in the United Kingdom have been the subject of almost constant but incremental reform over the last two decades, and the broad direction of change has been much in line with the trends already outlined earlier in this chapter—extending the reach, scope and intensity of regulation; changing governance arrangements to diminish the power of the professions themselves and to give greater power to other stakeholders including employers, academic institutions, government and the public; and harmonising regulatory arrangements across the health professions. However, progress has often been painfully slow and has been made in the face of covert and sometimes overt opposition from some professional groups (Walshe and Benson 2005).

The health professions in the United Kingdom are currently regulated by nine separate councils (for doctors, dentists, nurses, opticians, pharmacists, osteopaths, chiropractors, and other health professions).

For reasons of history, there are two separate pharmaceutical regulators (one just covering Northern Ireland and the other the rest of the United Kingdom). The Health Professions Council began life regulating a range of professions allied to medicine, like therapists and medical laboratory scientists, and has become the default regulator for any new professions as government has not wanted to create any new separate councils. Each regulatory body has its own legislation, and the arrangements for undertaking the main regulatory functions set out at the start of this chapter vary to major or minor degrees from regulator to regulator. They have different terminology, fitness to practise rules, sanctions, governance arrangements, and so on.

It would be impossible to provide an account of recent changes in health professions regulation in the United Kingdom without first explaining the importance of the Bristol and Shipman inquiries—two independent investigations into major failures of care in the British National Health Service (NHS), which produced reports containing recommendations for health professions regulatory reform.

The Bristol inquiry examined poor standards of practice in paediatric cardiac surgery at the Bristol Royal Infirmary in south-west England between 1985 and 1995, which resulted in about 35 avoidable deaths (Kennedy 2001). It concluded that there was a 'club culture' among doctors which caused them to put their own professional loyalties and relationships before the safety of patients. It made almost 200 detailed recommendations, but its key recommendation in relation to regulation was that a new statutory body should be created to oversee the nine health professions regulators. The Council for Healthcare Regulatory Excellence was established in 2003 and given legal powers to monitor the performance of the regulatory bodies, to support improvement and coordination, and to review their fitness to practise decisions and appeal those which it found unduly lenient. Over the last five years, it has been an important advocate for reform, and has held the regulatory bodies to account. The then president of the General Medical Council (GMC), Donald Irvine, was a reformer who used the Bristol case to drive a series of changes aimed at making the GMC more open and accountable, and creating a system for revalidation or recertification. His reforms were opposed by much of the medical establishment, which tried to have him unseated (Irvine 2003). When his term as president finished, his successor diluted and delayed his reforms.

The Shipman inquiry examined the case of a GP in east Manchester who, over a period of two decades, deliberately killed about 215 mostly elderly, female patients with injections of morphine. The inquiry remit was broad, and it explored the workings of the General Medical Council, its fitness to practise procedures and its proposed approach to revalidation. It was highly critical of the GMC, its unwillingness to reform itself and its fitness for purpose as a regulator, and called for a whole series of reforms (Smith 2004). In response, the government commissioned two reviews—one, led by the Chief Medical Officer, of medical regulation; and one, led by the NHS director of human resources, of non-medical regulation. Those reviews and the resulting reports (Donaldson 2006; Foster 2006) resulted in turn in a White Paper which has led to the most fundamental and radical changes to health professions regulation to date (Department of Health 2007).

The current changes—still underway as the necessary legislation only passed into law in 2008—involve reform to the governance of all the health professions regulators, to move from elected and professionally dominated boards to appointed boards with representatives of a number of stakeholders. They also modernise and harmonise fitness to practise procedures and sanctions, introduce independent adjudication on those cases, and require all health professions to adopt a form of periodic revalidation. For doctors, they introduce a new local GMC adviser in each health care organisation, which should make the local handling of complaints and concerns much more effective and create better links to employers. They further strengthen the powers of oversight and intervention of the Council for Healthcare Regulatory Excellence. There are some weaknesses—the changes have been enacted using the existing mosaic of legislation (in which each regulatory body has its own Act of Parliament) when it would have been clearer and simpler to replace the existing legislative complexity with a single Health Professions Regulation Act. Moreover, government decided not to move to the use of competence-based regulation and explicit scopes of practice, which would have simplified the processes of harmonising and standardising regulatory arrangements and would have made future changes easier to introduce. Nevertheless, these reforms are more comprehensive and far reaching than any previous changes, and they have been met with little or no professional opposition and have been supported by key opinion leaders like the medical Royal Colleges.

CONCLUSION

Health professions regulation serves both the public and the professional interest, but over the last two decades there has been an international trend away from regulatory arrangements focused on the economic and social interests of doctors, nurses and other professionals and towards arrangements which give primacy to public protection and patient safety. These are not simple or straightforward reforms to enact in political terms, because the health professions have powerful vested interests and close links to the establishment and government. The progress that has been made is testament to two key forces. The first is a change in societal attitudes and expectations, in which deference to professional authority and asymmetry in knowledge and education have been replaced by the assertion of individual and collective rights for users and communities by an increasingly well-informed and confident public. The second is the accumulation of evidence from a range of sources, particularly the inquiries into high-profile failures in health care organisations, that patients were being harmed by some health care professionals who should have been stopped from practising, but were not.

The regulatory arrangements now (or soon to be) in place in the United Kingdom are intended to offer an effective modernisation of the regulatory process to make it fit for purpose in a modern health service, while retaining the strengths of the professional philosophy and altruistic motivations which have served health professionals and the public well. Today's challenge is finding a way to square that circle, and to develop a new contract between the health professions, society and government which is mutually accepted and supported.

One main area of concern remains, which was alluded to in the introduction to this chapter, and was illustrated by the example case of a patient death caused by the incorrect administration of vincristine described in Box 7.1. It is that health professions regulation, despite being perhaps the longest established mechanism for assuring patient safety and service quality in health care, remains largely disconnected from this more recent and wider movement. Indeed, the systems-focused philosophy of the advocates of safety science tends to play down the importance of individual action, motivation and contribution, and to see all or most errors as products of the system or organisation of care. But it is a mistake not to recognise the importance of individual health professionals in the system of care, or to underestimate the emphasis placed on individual responsibility and accountability in the clinical culture. More integrated approaches to assuring safety and quality are needed, which can connect the systems for measuring and assessing quality in organisations and for individual health professionals, at both the local and national levels.

REFERENCES

Allsop, J. and Jones, K. 2006, *Quality Assurance in Medical Regulation in an International Context*, University of Lincoln, Lincoln

Bach, S. 2008, 'International mobility of health professionals: Brain drain or brain exchange?', in A. Solimano, ed., *The International Mobility of Talent: Types, Causes and Development Impact*, Oxford University Press, New York

Bausell, R.B. 2007, *Snake Oil Science: The Trust About Complementary and Alternative Medicine*, Oxford University Press, Oxford

Beck, A.H. 2004, 'The Flexner Report and the standardization of American medical education', *Journal of the American Medical Association*, vol. 291, no. 17, pp. 2139-40

Boon, K. and Turner, J. 2004, 'Ethical and professional conduct of medical students: Review of current assessment measures and controversies', *Journal of Medical Ethics*, vol. 30, no. 2, pp. 221-6

Buchan, J., Ball, J. and O'May, F. 2001, 'If changing skill mix is the answer, what is the question?' *Journal of Health Research and Policy*, vol. 6, no. 4, pp. 233-8.

Busse, R., Wismar, M. and Berman, P.C. 2002, *The European Union and Health Services: The Impact of the Single European Market on Member States*, IOS Press, Amsterdam

Department of Health 2007, *Trust, Assurance and Safety: The Regulation of Health Professionals*, Department of Health, London

Donaldson, L. 2006, *Good Doctors, Safer Patients: Proposals to Strengthen the System to Assure and Improve the Performance of Doctors and to Protect the Safety of Patients*, Department of Health, London

Ernst, E. 2001, 'Intangible risks of complementary and alternative medicine', *Journal of Clinical Oncology*, vol. 19, no. 8, pp. 2365-6

Faunce, T.A. and Bolsin, S.N.C. 2004, 'Three Australian whistle blowing sagas: Lessons for internal and external regulation', *Medical Journal of Australia*, vol. 181, no. 1, pp. 44-7

Flexner, A. 1910, *Medical Education in the United States and Canada*, Carnegie Foundation for Higher Education, New York

Forcier, M.B., Simoens, S. and Giuffrida, S. 2004, 'Impact, regulation and health policy implications of physician migration in OECD countries', *Human Resources for Health*, vol. 2, no. 1, p. 12

Foster, A. 2006, *The Regulation of the Non-Medical Healthcare Professions*, Department of Health, London

Harrison, J. 2008, 'Doctors' health and fitness to practise: The need for a bespoke model of assessment', *Occupational Medicine*, vol. 58, no. 5, pp. 323-7

Hunter, D.J. 1996, 'The changing roles of health care personnel in health and health care management, *Social Science and Medicine*, vol. 43, no. 5, pp. 799–808

Irvine, D. 2003, *The Doctor's Tale: Professionalism and Public Trust*, Radcliffe Medical Press, Oxford

—— 2006, 'A short history of the General Medical Council', *Medical Education*, vol. 40, no. 3, pp. 202–11

Jinks, C., Ong, B.N. and Paton, C. 2000, 'Mobile medics? The mobility of doctors in the European Economic Area', *Health Policy*, vol. 54, no. 1, pp. 45–64

Kennedy, I. 2001, *Learning from Bristol: The Report of the Public Inquiry into Children's Heart Surgery at the Bristol Royal Infirmary 1984–1995*, The Stationery Office, London

Klein, R. 1998, 'Competence, professional self-regulation and the public interest', *British Medical Journal*, vol. 316, no. 7146, pp. 1740–2

Kuhlmann, E. and Saks, M., eds 2008, *Rethinking Professional Governance: International Directions in Healthcare*, Policy Press, Bristol

Mejia, A., Pizurki, H. and Royston, E. 1979, *Physician and Nurse Migration: Analysis and Policy Implications*, World Health Organization, Geneva

Miller, E. and Capstick, B. 2003, 'Maladministration of vincristine: clinical governance failures and recommendations for prevention', *Clinical Risk*, vol. 9, pp. 143–8

O'Neill, O. 2002, *A Question of Trust*, Cambridge University Press, Cambridge

Peck, C., McCall, M., McLaren, B. and Rotem, T. 2000, 'Continuing medical education and continuing professional development: International comparisons', *British Medical Journal*, vol. 320, no. 7232, pp. 432–5

Power, M. 1997, *The Audit Society: Rituals of Verification*, Oxford University Press, Oxford

Pringle, M. 2006, 'Regulation and revalidation of doctors', *British Medical Journal*, vol. 333, no. 7560, pp. 161–2

Productivity Commission. 2005, *Australia's Health Workforce*, Commonwealth of Australia, Melbourne

Richardson, G., Maynard, A., Cullum, N. and Kindig, D. 1998, 'Skill mix changes: substitution or service development?', *Health Policy*, vol. 45, no. 2, pp. 119–32

Salter, B. 2001, 'Who rules? The new politics of medical regulation', *Social Science and Medicine*, vol. 52, no. 6, pp. 871–83

Shaw, G.B. 1946, *The Doctor's Dilemma*, Penguin, Harmondsworth

Singh, S. and Ernst, E. 2008, *Trick or Treatment? Alternative Medicine on Trial*, Bantam Press, London

Smith, J. 2004, *The Shipman Inquiry Fifth Report. Safeguarding Patients: Lessons from the Past—Proposals for the Future*, The Stationery Office, London

Spoel, P. and James, S. 2006, 'Negotiating public and professional interests: A rhetorical analysis of the debate concerning the regulation of midwifery in Ontario, Canada', *Journal of Medical Humanities*, vol. 27, no. 3, pp. 167-86

Stacey, M. 1992, *Regulating British Medicine: The General Medical Council*, Wiley, Chichester

Sutherland, K. and Leatherman, S. 2006, 'Professional regulation: Does certification improve medical standards?', *British Medical Journal*, vol. 333, no. 7565, pp. 439-41

Toft, B. 2001, 'External inquiry into the adverse incident which occurred at Queen's Medical Centre, Nottingham, 4th January 2001', Department of Health, London, <www.dh.gov.uk/en/Publicationsandstatistics/Publications/PublicationsPolicyAndGuidance/DH_4010064>, accessed 28 January 2009

Walshe, K. and Benson, L. 2005, 'General Medical Council and the future of revalidation: Time for radical reform', *British Medical Journal*, vol. 330, no. 7506, pp. 1504-6

Walshe, K. and Higgins, J. 2002, 'The use and impact of inquiries in the NHS', *British Medical Journal*, vol. 325, no. 7369, pp. 895-900

Walshe, K. and Shortell, S.M. 2004, 'What happens when things go wrong? How healthcare organisations deal with major failures', *Health Affairs*, vol. 23, no. 3, pp. 103-11

8

NON-DISCIPLINARY PATHWAYS IN PRACTITIONER REGULATION

Ian Freckelton SC

INTRODUCTION

A number of different mechanisms exist by force of law to render health practitioners accountable and answerable for their provision of health services to the public. All have in common the pursuit of both redress for those adversely affected by unprofessional or flawed service provision and an attempt to reduce the potential for recurrence of substandard patient care. Regulation by health boards, councils and disciplinary tribunals has significant elements of the coercive, command and top-down approach because it is, for the most part, imposed in response to the expression of grievances. However, one of the features of regulation, which addresses underlying precipitants to adverse outcomes by focusing upon both performance and health, is that it is more participatory and more consonant with principles of therapeutic jurisprudence. It is less coercive and more focused upon acknowledgment and remediation.

This chapter reviews the evolving role of health practitioner bodies and external decision makers, identifying the roles, advantages and limitations of conduct, performance, health and character pathways of investigation by regulators. It identifies an international trend toward regulators' focus upon fitness for practice and validation for practice, and therefore a trend away from a preoccupation with determining whether a particular allegation of misfeasance or non-feasance is proven.

The chapter also explores the contribution made by fair trading/ trade practices enforcement litigation, malpractice litigation, health ombudsmen investigations and coronial inquiries. It analyses and contrasts the respective focuses of each of these mechanisms that are directed towards enhancing public safety, and reflects upon the complementarity of the various accountability mechanisms that exist under contemporary but evolving legislation.

THE ROLE OF PROFESSIONAL REGULATORS

The traditional focus of disciplinary regulators, such as health boards and councils, was archetypally top down (see Braithwaite et al. 2005)— to make findings about, and impose sanctions arising from, allegations of impropriety, variously termed 'unprofessional conduct', 'professional misconduct', 'infamous conduct in a professional respect' and 'unsatisfactory professional conduct'. This meant receipt of 'complaints' or, more latterly, 'notifications' from persons aggrieved by nominated conduct. Usually the aggrievements emanated from patients or their relatives, but sometimes they came from concerned professionals, competitors or other investigators to whose notice the conduct had come (such as coroners, occupational health and safety investigators, insurers, etc.). Occasionally, even third parties with an ideological agenda, which somehow touched upon the behaviour in question, initiated a complaint. An example in this regard was Senator Julian McGauran's complaint on behalf of the Right to Life lobby group to the Medical Practitioners Board of Victoria about a late-term termination of pregnancy (see *Royal Women's Hospital v Medical Practitioners Board of Victoria* 2006).

Traditionally, regulators would investigate conduct the subject of notification and themselves rule upon it. However, in many countries— including in Australia and New Zealand—the trend over the past decade has been both to increase lay participation on regulatory bodies and tribunals, and to remove final adjudication over serious complaints about professional behaviour from professional boards and councils. This has entailed disaggregation of the investigative, prosecutorial and adjudicative functions of such entities, and externalising the adjudicative and in some instances the investigative functions. The diminished professional role of regulators and the bestowal of the decision-making role in serious matters on external tribunals (whether dedicated bodies or specialist divisions of administrative tribunals) has resulted from mistrust of, and disillusionment with, what has been described as fraternalism and excessive leniency towards health practitioners in the disciplinary context by boards and councils (e.g. see Hancock 1997; Thomas 2004, 2006). The balance between endeavouring to rehabilitate practitioners whose conduct, performance or character has proved unacceptable, and taking a strong stand against practitioners who have not proved worthy of community trust, has been a difficult ongoing issue for the health professions.

THE CONDUCT PATHWAY

The essence of regulation by conduct is the determination of whether a particular impropriety, however it is formally termed, has been engaged in by a practitioner. It may have been an impropriety drawn explicitly to the attention of a regulator by a notifier, or one which the regulator has encountered by chance in the course of another investigation and which it has investigated of its own motion. It may be conduct that has caused identifiable or potential harm to a patient, or it may be conduct that has brought the profession into undeserved disrepute. For the sake of fairness, the conduct has to be identified with specificity, and there must be reasonable clarity about the timing and circumstances of its alleged commission so that the practitioner is enabled to answer the accusation. It is important to recognise in respect of both practitioners and notifiers that the stakes can be very high in conduct investigations—a career and reputation on the one hand, and serious injury or death on the other. Proof is on the balance of probabilities, in Australia on the Briginshaw standard (*Briginshaw v Briginshaw* 1938), which means that the more serious the allegation, and the potential consequences of an adverse finding for the practitioner, the more the proof must be precise and avoid surmise, suspicion or guesswork.

Decision-making tribunals determine whether the technical criteria for an adverse finding are made out—namely whether the conduct alleged has been proved and whether, as a matter of law, the conduct, as found, satisfies the definition of the misconduct alleged against the practitioner. Then there is a second phase in which the tribunal determines what consequences should follow to protect the public—the overall objective of health practitioner regulation. Such consequences cannot be punitive (*Health Care Complaints Commission v Litchfield* 1997; *Purnell v Medical Board of Queensland* 1999). Their overarching purpose is protective in two senses: minimising ongoing risk for patients; and protecting and upholding the standing of the profession (e.g. see *Ha v Pharmacy Board of Victoria* 2002). However, to that end deterrence both of the practitioner and of others who may be minded to behave similarly is a relevant consideration (*Craig v Medical Board of South Australia* 2001). So too is denunciation of conduct that transgresses ethical norms of the health professions—for instance, by reference to codes of ethics and conduct, as well as clinical guidelines. Options in terms of dispositions that can be imposed are broad. They can be tailored to the individual and the particular circumstances to most effectively accomplish the objective of protecting the public. They include deregistration, suspension of registration, imposition of conditions on registration, auditing and monitoring, mandated further education or supervision, fines, reprimands and cautions. However, there is little data on the effectiveness of such sanctions in achieving the desired aims, either in respect of the individuals concerned or others who might contemplate comparably unethical conduct.

Advantages and disadvantages of the conduct pathway

The principal benefit of a regulator's placing adverse behaviour on a conduct pathway for investigation (and potentially for determination) is that an independent decision will be made that is responsive to the aggrievements of notifiers, who are often the persons who have been adversely affected by the conduct. Resolution of allegations may establish that seriously inappropriate behaviour took place or that a significant error, without justification, was made. Thereby the notifier receives vindication for their allegation, albeit that disciplinary regulators are not able to compensate for pecuniary or non-pecuniary losses—that is the role of the civil courts. However, where unprofessional conduct is established on the evidence, the notifier has the comfort of both a formal recognition of the deficits in the practitioner's conduct, and knowledge that he or she has made a contribution to protection of other members of the public from suffering the same experience as the patient/client concerned. This is particularly so if a high-end sanction is imposed—for instance, one which affects the practitioner's registered status.

Where the matters are serious and dealt with by independent tribunals (i.e. not heard and determined by Professional Standards Panels in a closed hearing), there is a resolution to allegations that is public and transparent. Decisions by many such bodies are now published on the internet, thereby enabling community and practitioner debate about the professional issues involved, and providing a focus for ethical education of trainee practitioners. In short, a fillip is given to ethical awareness and discourse at different levels within the profession.

However, the problematic aspects of the traditional approach of the 'conduct pathway', in terms of disciplinary regulation, are that generally unprofessional conduct is not a 'once off', and that it has multifactorial aetiologies and explanations. It is usually indicative of an underlying problem in terms of competence, arising from the practitioner undertaking work beyond their skills or knowledge, being out of date or unrepresentative of the community of views in their profession, having an unacceptable style in their service provision, being mentally or physically unwell or being substance-dependent. Alternatively, a systemic problem in the workplace (inadequate staffing or resources, demands to work excessive hours, etc.) may have contributed to the individual instance of substandard health service delivery.

An adjudication limited to a specific instance may provide 'justice' so far as an individual notifier, or even the practitioner, is concerned, but it may do little to enable interventions to optimise patient safety because its focus is restricted to the subject matter of the particular material raised by the notification. The decision-making body may discern broader issues from its exploration of the particular scenario forming the subject of the allegations in the notice of hearing, but its capacity to inquire into or rule upon matters beyond the notice and to fashion sanctions that arise more generally from such matters is very limited. There is often little by way of a feedback loop from the disciplinary decision-maker to the investigative body and the practitioner concerned. This can result in an artificially limited response to what is identified as a broader problem endangering patient safety by reasons of deficits in the practitioner's capacity to provide health services. It suffers from a number of the vices of 'between parties' litigation, legalism and adversarialism, failing to address wider issues and being confined by artificially constrained factual matrices. In addition, the authoritarian approach of such imposed decision making does little to involve and enlist the cooperation of the practitioner involved. In fact, the coercive aspect of the process can be alienating, distressing and damaging for health practitioners. The process of cross-examination can be difficult for complainants and practitioners alike.

THE PERFORMANCE PATHWAY

Recognising these limitations, in the 1990s, many jurisdictions created a 'performance pathway' by which investigations inquire into whether an underlying cause exists for a particular instance of unsatisfactory conduct and what needs to be done to remediate it, thereby reclaiming a reclaimable practitioner's competence and thus providing for consumer safety. This has been described as a therapeutic jurisprudence approach (Freckelton and Flynn 2004; Freckelton and List 2004; Freckelton 2007), but it can also be characterised in a range of other ways. Most importantly, it constitutes an attempt to manage risk by identifying it, understanding it and, where possible, enabling remedial measures to be instituted in cooperation with the practitioner to guard against its recurrence. Fundamentally, it stems from the proposition that competence is not guaranteed by the mere receipt of threshold tertiary qualifications and continuing vocational practice, even if ongoing professional education is engaged in. It recognises that ongoing entitlement to registered practice needs to be earned by continuing demonstration of competency, evaluated on a number of axes. One of these is maintenance of competency for the duration of health practitioners' registered practice and demonstration of such competency as required—for instance, by revalidation requirements as are coming into force from 2009 in the United Kingdom for medical practitioners (General Medical Council 2008b). As the College of Registered Nurses of Nova Scotia puts it, a competent registered practitioner is one who is 'able to integrate and apply the knowledge, skills and judgment required to practice safely and ethically in a designated role and practice setting' (Vandewater 2004). The performance pathway acknowledges and addresses the reality that a variety of different circumstances can result in an attenuation or impairment of competency.

A significant change of orientation is commencing among regulatory bodies in Australia and New Zealand (as well as in Canada, the United Kingdom and parts of the United States) by this reconceptualisation of concerns about practitioner service delivery away from 'conduct' to professional 'performance'. However, as yet the measures are halting and somewhat patchy (see Chapter 7).

Internationally, there are various definitions of unsatisfactory or unprofessional performance, but their essence is much the same. For instance, in Victoria under section 3 of the *Health Professions Registration Act* 2005 (Vic), 'professional performance' is defined as 'the knowledge, skill or care possessed and applied by a registered health practitioner in the provision of regulated health services'. In New South Wales, section 86A of the *Medical Practice Act* 1992 (NSW) similarly defines 'professional performance' as 'a reference to the knowledge, skill or care possessed and applied by the practitioner in the practice of medicine'. There is the potential for incorporation also of the notion of 'judgment' within performance definitions.

In New Zealand, the Medical Council may assess a doctor's performance at any time in response to a concern raised by, for example, a patient, a colleague or the Health and Disability Commissioner (HDC). In conducting a performance assessment, the Council considers whether 'the health practitioner's practice of the profession meets the required standard of competence' (*Health Practitioners Competence Assurance Act* 2003 (NZ), s 36(5)).

In the United Kingdom, the General Medical Council (2008a) has constructed a performance assessment process triggered by factors such as:

- a tendency to use inappropriate or outdated techniques;
- a basic lack of knowledge/poor judgment;
- a lack of familiarity with basic clinical/administrative procedures;
- poor record-keeping or failure to keep up-to-date records;
- inadequate practice arrangements;
- concerns over referral rates;
- inadequate hygiene arrangements; and
- poor prescribing.

Its processes are typical of performance investigations conducted in many jurisdictions. The practitioner is written to by the Council and asked to submit to a 'performance assessment' where the focus of the assessment is performance rather than conduct or health. When a practitioner refuses to undergo an assessment or fails to cooperate with the process, the case is referred to a Fitness to Practise Panel to consider whether the practitioner's fitness to practise is impaired and whether action is required in relation to his or her registration.

When there is a performance assessment, it is undertaken by a 'team leader', who is a doctor, along with two or more other doctors and one or more non-doctors. The assessment procedure is flexible, with the assessors adopting such procedures and seeking such advice or information as they consider necessary in order to assess the standard of the practitioner's performance. However, almost invariably assessments involve a peer review by reference to:

- a visit to the practitioner's place of work;
- interviews with the practitioner;
- interviews with third parties, including the complainant or complainants in the case; and

- a review of a sample of the practitioner's records and practice documents.

In addition, it is standard practice in the United Kingdom for a test of competence to be undertaken, comprising formal scrutiny of the basic knowledge and skills required for the particular area of practice in which the practitioner is engaged. The assessors disclose any information they receive to the practitioner (meaning there is very little by way of confidentiality in the process from the point of view of colleagues), and allow a reasonable opportunity for him or her to comment. At the end of the assessment process, the team reports on the standard of the practitioner's professional performance.

The New Zealand, New South Wales, Victorian and Northern Territory Medical Boards have been the Australasian pioneers of a reframing of notifications away from 'conduct' to 'performance' (see Reid 2006). However, as yet, uptake of performance investigations (and assessments) is limited and a number of challenges remain. In its 2007 annual report, for instance, the Victorian Medical Practitioners Board identified that it had only undertaken fourteen performance investigations in its previous year and had determined to take no further action in half of the cases. Similarly, the New South Wales Medical Board (2007: 23) undertook only twelve performance assessments and concluded only eight of them during the same period. This was in spite of the fact that the Health Care Complaints Commission referred 163 complaints during the same period which it designated as 'performance matters'. As from 1 July 2007, the Victorian Psychologists Registration Board (2007) was enabled to undertake 'performance investigations'. However, although it had employed a 'Manager of Performance' as of 17 September 2008, it had not commenced a performance assessment.'[1]

The Victorian Medical Practitioners Board in its 2007 Annual Report (Medical Practitioners Board of Victoria 2007: 19) identified a number of challenges in relation to performance investigations:

- They tend to be prolonged, often taking over six months.
- The performance pathway is intensive and requires cooperation from the practitioner being assessed, assistance from the relevant area of expertise (e.g. a College), and considerable coordination.
- They are stressful for the practitioners who are assessed.

To these, five other considerations might be added. First, such investigations are expensive, generally requiring senior practitioners to devote between one and three days to the assessment and reporting process. In addition, they require significant involvement from regulatory board staff. Second, selection of suitable assessors, sufficiently skilled to undertake the task and prepared to do so, is far from straightforward. Third, identification of criteria by reference to which performance should be evaluated is also far from straightforward, other than in procedural clinical work. In respect of psychiatry and psychology, the challenges are particularly demanding to identify standardised and fair assessment criteria without unduly intruding into clinician–patient relationships. Fourth, performance investigations are not always welcomed by notifiers, who may be more concerned to receive vindication (or a process which facilitates a civil claim) for their specific grievances rather than precipitating a diffuse investigation into a practitioner's performance that may not involve any determination about their particular complaint. Finally, the effectiveness of performance investigations, assessments and resolutions has yet to be longitudinally evaluated.

While there is much to be said in favour of identifying and addressing root causes of individual instances of unprofessional conduct, as of 2009 the shift in regulatory focus from conduct to performance is only in its early stages. Only modest numbers of performance investigations have been undertaken in Australia and New Zealand, and there remains a level of resistance at a regulator level to invoking the 'performance pathway' rather than the 'conduct pathway'. Lawyers representing health practitioners are commencing to identify strategic advantages in the less adversarial/accusatory approach of the performance pathway and in its less public aspect. This may play a role in changing practitioners' attitudes towards it as an alternative to the conduct pathway. However, it remains to be seen whether the option which exists in the overwhelming majority of health practitioner notifications to conceptualise them as 'performance' matters, becomes the norm in investigations in the years ahead. In relation to investigations into the performance of a variety of non-procedural practitioners, particular challenges exist to formulate criteria and methodologies for performance assessments that are both fair and effective in evaluating potential practitioner deficits in competency.

THE HEALTH PATHWAY

Another explanation and context for both unsatisfactory conduct and performance is impaired health on the part of health practitioners.

Our knowledge of the health profiles of the various health professions remains limited, although it is somewhat better in relation to doctors and nurses than in relation to other professionals (see Freckelton and Molloy 2007; Psychologists Registration Board of Victoria 2008). Arguably, there is a legal duty in tort, an implied duty in contract and an ethical responsibility (see *Re Bainbridge* 2007) for health practitioners to take reasonable care to avoid their health deteriorating to a point where, if they continue to work or if they provide a particular service, they could cause foreseeable harm to the recipients of their services (see generally Freckelton and Molloy 2007). Many professional regulatory bodies have health programs which facilitate the obtaining of needed treatment for unwell health practitioners—ranging from psychiatric disorders, cognitive decline and psychological difficulties to physical ailments and substance dependencies. A function of such programs is to negotiate a respite from practice or conditions upon practice until practitioners are well enough to continue. For those with cognitive decline, the focus is upon practitioners ceasing registered practice and transferring to a non-practising category where one exists (see Adler and Constantinou 2008). The role of personality disorders, as against psychiatric disorders, remains a difficult demarcation point in relation to the health pathway.

A limitation of the health pathway is that historically it has only been activated when a notification is made by a patient or colleague that the practitioner's fitness to practise is impaired. However, such notifications are rare, since peers and employing institutions experience inhibitions about 'informing' against colleagues, in spite of the manifest risk posed by practitioners whose skills and judgment are less than required for practice. This has led to the commencement of the imposition of legislative obligations to report. For instance, in New Zealand, section 45 of the *Health Practitioners' Competence Assurance Act* 2003 (NZ) provides that:

> if a person . . . has reason to believe that a health practitioner is unable to perform the functions required for the practice of his or her professions because of some mental or physical condition, the person must promptly give the Registrar of the responsible authority written notice of all the circumstances.

In New South Wales, the Medical Board must not register a person as a medical practitioner unless satisfied that the person 'is competent to practise medicine (that is, the person has sufficient physical capacity, mental capacity and skill to practise medicine and has sufficient communication skills for the practice of medicine)' (*Medical Practice Act* 1992 (NSW), s 13(a)). As a result of a controversial amendment coming into force in 2008 (see Arnold 2008), section 71A of the New South Wales Act has gone further and now provides that a doctor commits 'reportable misconduct' if he or she practises medicine while intoxicated by drugs or alcohol (an issue highly relevant to the operation of the health pathway), or practises medicine 'in a manner that constitutes a flagrant departure from accepted standards of professional practice or competence and risks harm to some other person'. Importantly, if a doctor believes, or ought reasonably to believe, that another doctor has committed 'reportable misconduct', they must, as soon as practicable, report the conduct to the board (s 79(2)). Failure to do so will itself constitute either 'unsatisfactory professional conduct' or 'professional misconduct'.

In Victoria, a medical practitioner who concludes that another registered health practitioner is suffering from an illness or condition which has seriously impaired or may seriously impair that person's ability to practise, and may result in the public being put at risk, is obliged to notify the relevant board (*Health Professions Registration Act* 2005 (Vic), s 32).

It is likely that such obligations will become more prevalent and in due course extend to imposition of comparable requirements to employers, including hospitals and practice owners. This is part of a growing recognition that ill-health, in any of its forms, has the potential to impact adversely on professional performance and, in some circumstances, contribute to unprofessional conduct. Thus it poses a threat to patient/client safety that needs to be addressed in a responsive and prompt way. Health issues, therefore, are likely in due course to escalate in their coercive component, in terms of mandated reporting, but to continue in their negotiated, participatory style in order to endeavour to return practitioners to a condition in which they are able to continue or resume practice safely.

THE CHARACTER/FITNESS AND PROPER PERSON PATHWAY

In most jurisdictions, there is a prerequisite for ongoing registration of health practitioners that they either be 'of good character' or be 'fit and proper persons' to practise their profession (see generally Freckelton

2008a). In some circumstances this enables an inquiry into whether conduct, either engaged in within the professional environment or in a personal capacity, detracts from the appropriateness of the practitioner remaining registered: the good character pathway. However, the distinction between 'good character' and 'bad character' is simplistic and psychologically problematic (see, for example, *Melbourne v The Queen* 1999).

An example of legislation in this regard is section 3 of the Victorian *Health Professions Registration Act* 2005, which includes within the definition of 'professional misconduct' conduct of a health practitioner, whether occurring in connection with the practice of their profession or occurring otherwise, that would, if established, justify a finding that 'the practitioner is not of good character or otherwise not a fit and proper person to engage in the practice' of their profession.

Such requirements mandate adherence to high standards of conduct by health practitioners in all facets of their lives, or at least desistance from conduct that might reflect problematically upon the standing of their profession. The requirements are premised on an expectation of trustworthiness, integrity and 'worthiness' on the part of health practitioners. They also postulate that conduct in any aspect of life by a health practitioner will inevitably impact to some degree upon their reputation as a health professional, and thus the reputation of their profession—there cannot be a complete divide between professional and private life. However, as Justice Kirby has pointed out (*McBride v Walton* 1994), it is important that regulators not intrude excessively into the non-professional activities of registrants and that they not assume the mantle of 'moral policemen'. The boundaries of regulation by reference to character are still evolving.

LIMITATIONS OF REGULATION BY HEALTH REGULATORS

It can therefore be seen that the capacity of health regulatory bodies to investigate, address and, on occasion, refer to external tribunals for further action issues concerning the practice safety of health practitioners has limitations and continues to shift with changing values and attitudes, both within the professions and within the general community. While some attempts are being made by such bodies to re-route classification of notifications from the traditional focus upon 'conduct' and 'character', with all of the pejorative terminology and consequences—including adverse publicity—that accompany such designations, this has not proved substantially effective. Performance and health investigations are less adversarial and depend upon external assessment and sensitive negotiations with practitioners to adjust practice approaches and areas of fitness to practise. They are expensive, they take time, and they require sophisticated and calibrated evaluation processes. They do not always satisfy notifiers who may seek an authoritative adjudication upon whether the wrong that they have alleged has been established by available evidence. Performance and health investigations can give the impression of prob-lematically sympathetic and fraternal responses to adverse instances of health practitioner conduct, which have either caused harm or had the potential to do so. In an era of increasingly assertive con-sumerist responses, and a market-driven health care environment (see, for example, Hancock 1999), such approaches are not always acceptable to the media or welcomed by the community. On occasion, too, prac-titioners want to be vindicated and exonerated by a formal investigation of allegations against them. In a 2006 performance investigation of a Victorian medical practitioner, which found no performance deficits, neither the notifier nor the practitioner was satisfied by the performance pathway.

The combination of the four regulators' pathways leaves a need for other accountability mechanisms through the legal system. Four other responses within the legal system exist, addressing a number of regulatory lacunae:

- bringing of civil litigation;
- oversight by health services complaints commissioners;
- consumer protection actions; and
- coroner's oversight.

CIVIL LITIGATION AGAINST HEALTH PRACTITIONERS

The general topic of negligence and malpractice litigation against health practitioners is beyond the scope of this chapter (see Bennett and Freckelton 2006) (and also see Chapter 12). However, in terms of the potential for such actions to protect the safety of the community, it is pertinent that the focus of every such action (save the extremely rare phenomenon of class actions) is upon asserting the rights of an individual litigant who has been adversely affected in terms of pain and suffering or pecuniary loss by specific and identified substandard health service provision. In other words, such legal action is very much confined to particular factual scenarios (Kirby 2001), and has a limited capacity to address broader issues of community safety (see, for example, Studdert and Brennan 2001; Studdert et al. 2004).

Further, actions in tort and contract—the latter of which are rare—are compensatory. Exemplary damages (also known as punitive or vindictive damages), which hold up tortfeasors as examples and involve enhanced sums of damages, are very rarely awarded (Mendelson 1996) and in a number of places have now been abolished (see, for example, *Civil Liability Act* 2002 (NSW), s 21). The terms of settlement of malpractice litigation (only a tiny percentage of which go to judgment) are generally confidential, precluding public understanding of any de facto assumption of responsibility for adverse outcomes by insurers acting for health service providers. In addition, the overwhelming majority of cases of health practitioner negligence do not prompt the institution of litigation, meaning that it is only a small and probably unrepresentative sample of injured persons who seek and obtain pecuniary redress. This precludes broad extrapolation from decisions. It also means that such litigation has only a very modest educative impact upon health practitioners.

However, these considerations acknowledged, the awarding of significant damages to litigants has an outcome more generally for the provision of health services in a risk-aversive and cost-conscious health service environment. This can be both positive, in terms of encouraging better adherence to professional standards, and negative, in terms of conducing to the practice of defensive health care (see Studdert et al. 2005). The limitations of malpractice litigation as an inhibitant upon unprofessional conduct by health service providers have become even more pronounced since Australia's statutory tort reforms at the early part of the twenty-first century (see Bennett and Freckelton 2006).

HEALTH SERVICES COMPLAINTS COMMISSIONERS

In those jurisdictions with health services commissioners or health ombudsmen, there is the potential for both conciliation of a variety of complaints about health practitioners and also investigation of complex matters and reports to government (see Wilson 1999). However, it is comparatively rarely for these broader issues and systemic matters to be their principal focus. An example of such an exercise was the report of the Victorian Health Services Commissioner into the conduct of a former dentist, Noel Campbell, who provided health services to those with cancer (Health Services Commissioner of Victoria 2008). She found him to have misrepresented himself to patients, to have failed to secure informed consent, and to have exploited patients with the impunity of being an unregistered health services provider. Amongst her recommendations, she proposed that his case be referred for consideration for action under Victoria's fair trading legislation and that the Minister for Health consider implementation of the New South Wales scheme for regulating unregistered health practitioners (see Freckelton 2008c). Other Victorian inquiries of a similar kind were conducted into recovered memory therapy practice (Health Services Commissioner of Victoria 2005), and into a number of incidents involving registered nurses at the Royal Melbourne Hospital (Health Services Commissioner of Victoria 2002).

In New South Wales, the Health Care Complaints Commission has also reported specifically on impotency treatment services (Health Care Complaints Commission of New South Wales 1998), adverse outcomes following cataract surgery at Dubbo Base Hospital (Health Care Complaints Commission of New South Wales 1999a), incidents in the operating theatre at Canterbury Hospital (Health Care Complaints Commission of New South Wales 1999b), and into cosmetic surgery (Health Care Complaints Commission of New South Wales 1999c).

However, although the quality of these reports is of a high standard, it is apparent that such reporting and formal systemic investigation has constituted only a modest focus of the two largest health ombudsmen in Australia. By far the greatest component of their work lies within the day-to-day investigation and conciliation of complaints. This highlights both the substantial potential but also the limitations in practice of broad oversight from health services commissioners.

CONSUMER PROTECTION ACTIONS

Provision of health services is regulated in some respects by the involvement of those bodies which administer fair trading obligations. As already noted, in 2008 the Health Services Commissioner in Victoria recommended such action in relation to the cancer treatments offered by the unregistered dentist, Mr Campbell.

Illustrative of this form of accountability was a successful action brought by the Australian Consumer and Competition Commission (ACCC): in *Australian Competition and Consumer Commission v Nuera Health Pty Ltd (In Liquidation)*, an action was taken by the ACCC seeking declaratory orders in relation to various representations (described in the ACCC's statement of claim as the 'cure cancer representations', the 'prolong life representations', the 'scientific representations', the 'cure cancer future representations', the 'prolong life future representations', the 'Rana representations' and the 'Rana future representations'). These were said to contravene provisions in the *Trade Practices Act* 1974 (Cth), and that the individual respondents, Paul Rana and his sons, Christopher Rana and Micheal Rana, aided and abetted the conduct of one or more of the relevant corporate respondents. The ACCC also sought injunctive orders restraining the respondents from making or continuing to make representations to the effect of any of the impugned representations, and requiring the publication of a prescribed notice on various websites that had been maintained by one or other of the respondents. Justice Ryan stated that the evidence adduced before him:

> uniformly exemplifies conduct of the most reprehensible kind [which] reveals a consistently cynical and heartless exploitation of cancer victims and their relatives when they were at their most vulnerable. This conduct was not like that which is sometimes encountered in this context of a well-meaning but misguided administration of a single cure or treatment which the promoter genuinely believes, in the face of a body of opposing scientific opinion, to offer a prospect of arresting or delaying the progression of the disease. In this case, the evidence reveals that Mr Paul Rana, who has been the controlling mind and will of the corporate respondents, has personally taken the leading role in promoting and administering the so called 'treatments' and extorting from the patients, or their relatives, substantial upfront fees amounting to as much as $25,000 to $35,000. (2007: [7])

He found Paul Rana to have 'indiscriminately thrown together, under the aegis of the Rana System, a package of discredited or entirely unproven theories, procedures and nostrums which he has gleaned from populist literature and a range of other sources of widely varying scientific or medical credibility' (2007: [8]). He found Mr Rana to have cynically made a variety of representations to various victims that were untrue or, insofar as they went to future matters, without having any reasonable grounds for making them. Justice Ryan inferred from the uncontested affidavit evidence that the Ranas knew that each of the representations in those categories was unsupported by generally accepted science.

Justice Ryan was also satisfied that the conduct alleged against the corporate respondents and the members of the Rana family, which was uncontested, was conduct which was unconscionable within the meaning of section 51AB(1) of the *Trade Practices Act* 1974 (Cth). He commented that 'it is difficult in many respects to envisage conduct which is more deserving of that description' (2007: [10]) He made the orders sought by the ACCC and ordered the respondents, jointly and severally, to pay the ACCC's costs fixed in the sum of $150,000.

Another example of such actions is that brought by the Victorian Department of Consumer Affairs in that state's Supreme Court in 2007–08 against a national provider of optometry services, Merringtons (*Cousins v Merringtons Pty Ltd*, 2007, 2008; see generally Freckelton 2009b). The action arose from complaints by seventeen different clients of Merringtons who claimed, amongst other things, that Merringtons:

- did not provide spectacles or contact lenses in a specified or reasonable time;
- provided spectacles or contact lenses not in accordance with prescription and unfit for the purpose;
- required that prescription spectacles be tried for a period of time to allow the customer to adjust to them, when the spectacles were not fit for their purpose and without first checking the spectacles;
- did not refund amounts paid by customers despite failing to supply or supplying faulty prescription spectacles or contact lenses; and
- required that customers produce and surrender to Merringtons their original receipts for their purchase as a condition of considering whether to give the customers a refund (*Cousins v Merringtons Pty Ltd* [2007]).

The relief sought was a series of declarations and injunctions, as well as a public notice order pursuant to section 149A and 153(1) of the *Fair Trading Act* 1999 (Vic). Ultimately, Hansen J found many of the alleged contraventions proved (*Cousins v Merringtons Pty Ltd* 2007), and then was required to consider whether he should grant the relief sought by the department. He made declarations that Merringtons had engaged in a number of forms of misleading and deceptive conduct. He injuncted Merringtons from making such misleading and deceptive representations, and failing to pay refunds when reasonably requested to do so. He also ordered them to institute a compliance program, using professional assistance to the extent necessary, observing that 'the conduct of the defendants, which conduct includes their attitude of careless regard for the interests of and arrogance to the complainants, their pre-litigation conduct and continuing refusal to enter a compliance program, their "trust me" attitude, and the disregard for the interests of their customers, warrant the imposition of a compliance program' (*Cousins v Merringtons Pty Ltd* 2008: [68]). He ordered Merringtons to pay compensation to a number of the clients whom they had inconvenienced and also, and perhaps most importantly from a commercial point of view, Hansen J ordered them to take out an advertisement in the *Herald Sun* and to be displayed in its stores advising of the result of the Supreme Court proceedings.

The *Rana* and *Merringtons* decisions are examples of the potency of consumer protection actions against health service providers, and the potential that they have to unmask unacceptable conduct by health professionals and employer institutions. The orders made were a potent cocktail of provisions directed towards providing solace to adversely affected clients, and a series of deterrents with real marketplace impact to guard against repetition of the unprofessional conduct engaged in, not just by individual practitioners but in the case of Merringtons by administrative staff and those responsible for unethical policies, requiring them to implement corrections.

CORONERS' OVERSIGHT

The institution of the coroner is one of the oldest known to our legal system (Hunnisett 1961). From the earliest phases of coronership, coroners and their juries made findings (in what was termed their inquisition) about a variety of matters, including incidents involving fatalities, and added 'riders' to the inquisition designed to reduce the potential for further avoidable deaths (see Law Reform Committee of the Victorian Parliament 2006; Freckelton and Ranson 2006; Johnstone 1992; Dorries 1999; Levine and Pyke 1999). The formulation of riders has long had a particular relevance to deaths that may have been caused, or contributed to, by health service providers such as doctors, nurses and pharmacists.

Modern debates about the role of the coroner have centred upon the extent to which coroners' inquests should function as a means of inquiring publicly into the circumstances surrounding deaths, to enable coroners to make comments or recommendations designed to improve public safety (see Thomas et al. 2008; Freckelton 2008b; Hand and

Fife-Yeomans 2004). The controversies relate both to the permitted parameters of coroners' inquests—in particular, the parameters of inquiries and findings about causation and circumstances of death—and the contemporary role of riders.

In all jurisdictions in Australia and New Zealand, coroners are empowered to make such recommendations. The most recent versions of coronial legislation are those of New Zealand (coming into force in 2007) and Victoria (coming into force in 2009). Both are overtly prophylactic in their language. Thus, section 3 of the *Coroners Act* 2006 (NZ) provides that the purpose of the Act:

> is to help to prevent deaths and to promote justice through—
> (a) investigations, and the identification of the causes and circumstances, of sudden or unexplained deaths, or deaths in special circumstances; and
> (b) the making of specified recommendations or comments ... that, if drawn to public attention, may reduce the chances of the occurrence of other deaths in circumstances similar to those in which those deaths occurred.

Similarly, the preamble to the *Coroners Act* 2008 (Vic) provides that:

> The coronial system of Victoria plays an important role in Victorian society. That role involves the independent investigation of deaths and fires for the purpose of finding the causes of those deaths and fires and to contribute to the reduction of the number of preventable deaths and fires and the promotion of public health and safety and the administration of justice.

Section 1(c) of the Victorian Act explicitly stipulates that a purpose of the legislation is:

> to contribute to the reduction of the number of preventable deaths and fires through the findings of the investigation of deaths and fires, and the making of recommendations, by coroners.

The effectiveness of coroners in effectively investigating medical deaths, and in particular health deaths, has come under question in recent years (e.g. see Law Reform Committee of the Victorian Parliament 2006; Freckelton and Ranson 2006). Many deaths are not reported to coroners, thereby precluding coronial investigations. In addition, the sophistication of coroners' investigations and inquest findings and recommendations in relation to such deaths is questionable. This has raised the issue of the qualifications and experience of those appointed as coroners, together with the investigative assistance provided by bodies such as institutes of forensic medicine, and whether coroners' investigations are adding sufficient value to the ground covered by mortality and morbidity/quality assurance committees within hospitals. Their advantage is that they probe through the process of cross-examination and public hearings in a way that internal investigations cannot.

In many countries where the institution of the coroner survives, the coroner plays a de facto role as a public health official in order to identify circumstances and causes of death and make recommendations to reduce the potential for further unnecessary deaths. The coroner's jurisdiction as a death investigator is unusual in many ways, including that it is inquisitorial rather than adversarial, and because inquests are not 'between parties' litigation like civil disputes or criminal prosecutions. In addition (aside from in very limited circumstances in the Australian Capital Territory and the Northern Territory, and most recently in Victoria), coroners do not determine legal rights or entitlements—they just make findings and, if they choose, comments and recommendations. Those who are the subject of coroners' comments and recommendations, such as hospitals, need not respond in any way to them or implement them. The way to the future, though, has probably been shown by Victoria in Australasia's most recent coronial legislation, which has made it mandatory for coroners' findings and recommendations to be published on the internet, making them accessible and accountable in a way that has never previously occurred (Freckelton 2009b). Importantly, too, the ability of those subject to coroners' recommendations to 'sweep them under the carpet' has to a significant degree ended in Victoria. Under section 72(2) of the *Coroners Act* 2008 (Vic), coroners are enabled to make recommendations to any minister, public statutory authority or entity on any matter connected with a death or fire that the coroner has investigated, including recommendations relating to public health and safety or the administration of justice. If a public statutory authority or entity (such as a hospital) receives such recommendations, it is obliged to provide a written response, not later than three months after the date of receipt of the recommendations, specifying a statement of action (if any) that has, is or will be taken in relation to the recommendations. In turn, the coroner must publish the response of a public authority or entity on the internet.

The institution of coroner has evolved very considerably since medieval times. The modern coroner does not commit for trial, sit with a jury (save occasionally in New South Wales), go to scenes of death or make orders for compensation to the relatives of the deceased. But coronership plays an important ongoing role in holding those with responsibility for vulnerable members of the community, including the frail and ill, publicly accountable for the discharge of their functions. Historically, this has particularly been so in relation to poor houses, lunatic asylums and prisons. It remains so in relation to the care and treatment provided to patients by health practitioners when patients have died in the aftermath of such care. There are many circumstances in which neither criminal nor civil litigation is likely to ensue, and in which no one makes a complaint to a regulatory body, but the investigation of the coroner can expose either specific instances of substandard care or systemic defects that have led to a death which should not have happened. In such scenarios, the findings and recommendations of coroners have the potential to constitute an important check and balance, filling, in an important way, an accountability hole. The institution of coronership is in the midst of significant change, with one of its new objectives becoming an overt embracing of a prophylactic and public health role. With increasing powers to convene inquests to facilitate the making of recommendations to avoid comparably avoidable deaths in the future, and with an obligation for institutions to respond to coroners' recommendations, coronership is reinventing itself as an important participant in enhancing public safety in the health care area.

CONCLUSION

Regulation and accountability of health practitioners through legally constituted mechanisms has many different faces. Regulatory bodies such as health boards, decision-making tribunals, health ombudsmen, coroners and courts deciding fair trading actions and malpractice cases all have different focuses, all of them responsive, some of them coercive, others participatory and negotiated. However, all have in common that they constitute part of an evolving and complex fabric of accountability applicable to health practitioners. They have changed in significant ways over the past two decades, and no doubt will continue to do so in a quest for a balance between fairness and effective imposition of adherence by practitioners to high-quality practice and ethical service provision.

ACKNOWLEDGMENT

The author acknowledges with gratitude the helpful suggestions and comments of Dr Patricia Molloy, Director of Clinical Governance at Box Hill Hospital, Melbourne, Australia.

REFERENCES

Adler, R. and Constantinou, C. 2008, 'Knowing—or not knowing—when to stop: Cognitive decline in ageing doctors', *Medical Journal of* Australia, vol. 189, nos 11/12, pp. 622-4

Arnold, P.C. 2008, 'The mandatory reporting of professional incompetence', *Medical Journal of Australia*, vol. 189, no. 3, pp. 132-3

Bennett, B. and Freckelton, I. 2006, 'Life after the Ipp reforms: Medical negligence law' in *Disputes and Dilemmas in Health Law*, eds I. Freckelton and K. Petersen, Federation Press, Sydney, pp. 381-405

Braithwaite, J., Healy, J. and Dwan, K. 2005, *The Governance of Health Care Safety and Quality*, Commonwealth of Australia, Canberra

Dorries, C. 1999 , *Coroners' Courts: A Guide to Law and Practice*, Wiley, Chichester

Freckelton, I. 2007, 'Disciplinary investigations and hearings: A therapeutic jurisprudence perspective', in *Transforming Legal Processes in Court and Beyond*, eds G. Reinhardt and A. Cannon, Australasian Institute of Judicial Administration, Melbourne

—— 2008a, 'Trends in health practitioner regulation', *Psychiatry, Psychology and Law*, vol. 15, no. 3, pp. 425-34

—— 2008b, 'Good character and regulation of medical practitioners', *Journal of Law and Medicine*, vol. 16, no. 3, pp. 488-511

—— 2008c, 'Regulating the unregistered', *Journal of Law and Medicine*, vol. 16, no. 3, pp. 413-18

—— 2008d, 'Reforming coronership: International perspectives and contemporary developments', *Journal of Law and Medicine*, vol. 16, no. 3, pp. 379-92

—— 2009a , 'Regulation of health practitioners by fair trading actions', *Journal of Law and Medicine*, in press

—— 2009b, 'Rethinking the role of the coroner', *Law Institute Journal*, in press

Freckelton, I. and Flynn, J. 2004, 'Paths toward reclamation: Therapeutic jurisprudence and the regulation of medical practitioners', *Journal of Law and Medicine*, vol. 12, no. 1, pp. 91–102

Freckelton, I. and List, D. 2004, 'The transformation of regulation of psychologists by therapeutic jurisprudence', *Psychiatry, Psychology and Law*, vol. 11, no. 3, pp. 296–307

Freckelton, I. and Molloy, P. 2007, 'The health of health practitioners: Remedial programs, regulation and the spectre of the law', *Journal of Law and Medicine*, vol. 15, no. 3, pp. 366-93

Freckelton, I. and Ranson, D. 2006, *Death Investigation and the Coroner's Inquest*, Oxford University Press, Melbourne

General Medical Council 2008a, 'Doctors under investigation—performance assessments', <www.gmc-uk.org/concerns/doctors_under_investigation/performance_assessments.asp>, accessed 20 December 2008

—— 2008b, 'Licensing and revalidation', <www.gmc-uk.org/about/reform/index.asp>, accessed 23 December 2008

Hancock, L. 1997, 'Professional misconduct and avenues of complaint in Australia', in *Problem Doctors: A Conspiracy of Silence*, eds. P. Lens and G. van der Wal, IOS Press, Omsha

—— 1999, *Health Policy in the Market State*, Allen & Unwin, Sydney

Hand, D. and Fife-Yeomans, J. 2004, *The Coroner: Investigating Sudden Death*, AC Books, Sydney

Health Care Complaints Commission of New South Wales 1998, *Report into Impotency Treatment Services in New South Wales*, <www.hccc.nsw.gov.au/downloads/impo_rep.pdf>, accessed 22 December 2008

—— 1999a, *Report on an Investigation into Adverse Outcomes Following Cataract Surgery at Dubbo Base Hospital*, <www.hccc.nsw.gov.au/downloads/dubbo.pdf>, accessed 22 December 2008

—— 1999b, *Report on an Investigation of Incidents in the Operating Theatre at Canterbury Hospital*, <www.hccc.nsw.gov.au/downloads/canterbu.pdf>, accessed 22 December 2008

—— 1999c, *Cosmetic Surgery Report*, <www.hccc.nsw.gov.au/downloads/Cosmrep.pdf>, accessed 22 December 2008

Health Services Commissioner of Victoria 2002, *Royal Melbourne Hospital Report*, <www.health.vic.gov.au/hsc/downloads/rmh_report0802.pdf>, accessed 22 December 2008

—— 2005, *Inquiry into the Practice of Recovered Memory Therapy*, <www.health.vic.gov.au/hsc/downloads/final_rmt_inquiry.pdf>, accessed 22 December 2008

—— 2008, *Noel Campbell Inquiry Report*, <www.health.vic.gov.au/hsc/downloads/report_noel_campbell_1.pdf>, accessed 22 December 2008

Hunnisett, R.F. 1961, *The Medieval Coroner*, Cambridge University Press, Cambridge

Johnstone, G. 1992, 'An avenue for death and injury prevention', in *The Aftermath of Death*, ed. H. Selby, Federation Press, Sydney

Kirby, M.D. 2001, 'Tort system reforms: Causes, options, outcomes', *Journal of Law and Medicine*, vol. 8, no. 4, pp. 380–8

Law Reform Committee of the Victorian Parliament 2006, *Report on the Coroners Act 1985*, Government Printer, Melbourne

Levine, M. and Pyke, J. 1999, *Levine on Coroners' Courts*, Sweet and Maxwell, London

Medical Board of New South Wales 2007, *Annual Report 2007*, <www.nswmb.org.au>, accessed 28 October 2008

Medical Practitioners' Board of Victoria 2007, *Annual Report 2007* <http://medicalboardvic.org.au/pdf/AR_2007.pdf>, accessed 28 October 2008

Mendelson, D. 1996, 'The case of *Backwell v AAA. Negligence*—a compensatory remedy or an instrument of vengeance?', *Journal of Law and Medicine*, vol. 4, no. 4, pp. 114–30

Psychologists Registration Board of Victoria 2007, *Annual Report 2007*, <www.psychreg.vic.gov.au/images/annualreports/prbv_ar2007.pdf>, accessed 28 October 2008

—— 2008, *Health Matters for Psychologists*, <www.psychreg.vic.gov.au/images/general/health_manual.pdf>, accessed 10 January 2009

Reid, A. 2006, 'Managing poorly performing doctors', *Law in Context*, vol. 23, no. 2, pp. 91–112

Studdert, D.M. and Brennan, T. 2001, 'No fault compensation for medical injuries', *Journal of the American Medical Association*, vol. 286, no. 2, pp. 217–23

Studdert, D.M., Mello, M.M. and Brennan, T.E. 2004, 'Medical malpractice', *New England Journal of Medicine*, vol. 350, no. 3, pp. 283–92

Studdert, D.M., Mello, M.M., Sage, W.M., DesRoches, C.M., Peugh, J., Zapert, K. and Brennan, T.A. 2005, 'Defensive medicine among high-risk specialist physicians in a volatile malpractice environment', *Obstetrical and Gynecological Survey*, vol. 60, no. 11, pp. 718–20

Thomas, D. 2004, 'The co-regulation of medical discipline: Challenging medical peer review', *Journal of Law and Medicine*, vol. 11, no. 3, pp. 382–9

——2006, 'Peer review as an outmoded model for health practitioner regulation', *Law in Context*, vol. 23, no. 2, pp. 52–72

Thomas, L., Straw, A. and Friedman, D. 2008, *Inquests: A Practitioner's Guide*, Legal Action Group, London

Tracey, J., Simpson, J. and St John, I. 2001, 'The competence and performance of medical practitioners', *New Zealand Medical Journal*, vol. 114, no. 1129, pp. 167–70

Vandewater, D. 2004, *Best Practice in Performance of Health Professionals*, Background Paper for the College of Registered Nurses of Nova Scotia, <www.crnns.ca/documents/competenceassessmentpaper2004.pdf>, accessed 5 December 2008

Wilson, B. 1999, 'Health disputes: A "window of opportunity" to improve health services', in *Controversies in Health Law*, eds I. Freckelton and K. Petersen, Federation Press, Sydney, pp. 179–92

CASES

Australian Competition and Consumer Commission v Nuera Health Pty Ltd (In Liquidation) [2007] FCA 695

Briginshaw v Briginshaw [1938] HCA 34; (1938) 60 CLR 336

Cousins v Merringtons Pty Ltd [2007] VSC 542

Cousins v Merringtons Pty Ltd (No. 2) [2008] VSC 340

Craig v Medical Board of South Australia [2001] SASC 169

Ha v Pharmacy Board of Victoria [2002] VSC 322

Health Care Complaints Commission v Litchfield (1997) 41 NSWLR 630

McBride v Walton, unreported, NSW Court of Appeal, 15 July 1994

Melbourne v The Queen [1999] HCA 32; (1999) 198 CLR 1

Purnell v Medical Board of Queensland [1999] 1 Qd R 362

Re Bainbridge [2007] PRBD (Vic) 4

Royal Women's Hospital v Medical Practitioners Board of Victoria [2006] VSCA 85

NOTE

1   Personal communication, Anoushka Bondar, Notifications Manager, Psychologists Registration Board of Victoria, 16 September 2008.

9

REGULATING CLINICAL PRACTICE

William B. Runciman and Judy Lumby

CLINICAL PRACTICE: THE GAP BETWEEN WHAT IS NEEDED AND WHAT IS DELIVERED

At the heart of clinical practice lie millions of interactions between individual patients and health care professionals. What really matters during these interactions is to do, or plan to do, the right thing in the right way, and for the patients to understand what the risks, benefits and options are and be happy to accept what is done or planned (Runciman et al. 2007: 221–46). Thus, there are three phases to getting it right: first, it is necessary to make the right plan; next, to ensure that the patient has accepted the plan whilst understanding the risks and options; and third, to carry out the plan correctly.

The medical profession has traditionally 'self-regulated'. This minimal amount of regulation has largely been around codes of conduct for practitioners. Some specialist colleges have mandated that certain facilities and basic equipment be available in teaching hospitals. But how equipment is to be used, and how the practice of medicine is to be conducted, has largely been *laissez-faire*, with great latitude being afforded as to what care may be offered and how it may be provided. Compliance with evidence-based care is often resisted on the basis of a desire for 'clinical freedom' over what is disparagingly called 'cookbook medicine'. However, within the last decade there has been escalating public unease about the variability of care, the frequency with which patients are harmed by the health care process, and the fact that there appear to be no systems in place to determine when a 'rogue' practitioner is consistently well outside the bounds of what might be considered reasonable practice (Van Der Weyden 2005).

It is becoming evident that the time has come for something to be done about improving clinical practice—which, after all, consumes some 9 per cent of gross domestic product in most Western countries, and over 16 per cent in the United States alone (Organisation for Economic Cooperation and Development 2008). The resources wasted on poor quality and unsafe health care represent resources which are not spent on cost- and risk-effective health care. Some of the problems perceived with self-regulation are listed in Table 9.1.

Table 9.1 Perceived problems with self-regulation by health professionals

Principle	Problem
Autonomy	Health professionals demand and are given unreasonable levels of professional autonomy, and resist adherence to checklists and protocols.
Accountability	Health professionals are reluctant to demonstrate accountability and resist monitoring of performance, practice and outcomes.
Supervision	Health professionals discourage trainees, with varying degrees of subtlety, from seeking assistance after hours.
Transparency	Health professionals lack transparency in their own practices, accept sub-optimal performance by colleagues, and fail to report inadequacies in the system and adverse events within their practices.
Patient-centredness	Health professionals covertly or overtly impose their views, practices and plans on their patients.

Source: Runciman et al. (2007: Ch. 7).

Making the right plan

Many patients assume, when they receive health care from a professional, that what should be done for most common problems is known, and that the care they receive would be the same or very similar, irrespective of the practitioner or context. If they have high blood pressure or an abnormal blood lipid profile, they expect a standard set of tests to be done, and to be treated according to a well-established regime, ideally based on evidence, but at least based on agreed best practice, just as they would expect a standard accepted approach to getting their car serviced. However, it has been known (and published in the lay press) for over a quarter of a century that there are enormous variations in the health care received by patients in different regions of the same country, and even within the same region between different institutions and different practitioners (Wennberg and Gittelsohn 1982). The size of these variations greatly exceeds anything that could be explained by the type of disease, the type of care, or demographic or economic differences. Even common procedures, such as cardiac angioplasty and stenting, may vary eighteen-fold, and for less common procedures, such as vena cava filter placement, the variation may be as great as 26-fold (Dartmouth Institute for Health Policy and Clinical Practice 2008).

One might imagine that such variability would be limited to less common procedures, those which are difficult to diagnose or those which require complex interventions. However, work done by the RAND corporation in the United States shows that adults receive only about 55 per cent of recommended care (McGlynn et al. 2003) and children only 46 per cent (Mangione-Smith et al. 2007) (see Figures 9.1 and 9.2). The adult findings are based on rates of compliance with indicators for 30 common conditions and aspects of preventive care, and the findings for children for 21 conditions. These indicators have content, construct and face validity, and are measures of fairly basic aspects of care (McGlynn et al. 2003). For example, two of thirteen indicators for diabetes are whether the patients received diet and exercise counselling, and whether they had been prescribed ACE inhibitors if they had proteinuria. Three of 27 indicators for high blood pressure are lifestyle modification for patients with mild hypertension, drug treatment for uncontrolled mild hypertension, and changing treatment when blood pressure is consistently uncontrolled. Even a common condition like headache was associated with only 45 per cent of recommended care being carried out; two of 21 indicators are use of appropriate first-line drugs for patients with acute migraine, and a brain scan for patients with new-onset headaches with abnormal neurological signs.

It might be argued, as subjects for the RAND survey were chosen between 1998 and 2000, that the bulk of the care examined preceded the *To Err is Human* report of the Institute of Medicine of the American Academy of Science (Kohn et al. 2000), and that things have improved greatly since. However, as is evident from Figure 9.3, the average rate of change for a wide range of indicators in health care is extremely slow (Agency for Healthcare Research and Quality 2008).

Condition

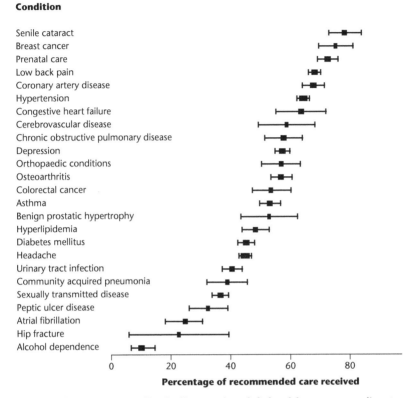

Figure 9.1 Adherence to quality indicators in adult health care according to condition

Note: The areas of the boxes reflect the number of times eligibility for a quality indicator was met for a particular condition, and the bars show the 95 per cent confidence intervals (diagram based on McGlynn, et al., 2003:2643).

Clearly, the objective stated in the Institute of Medicine (IOM) report, of halving the adverse event rate within five years, was extremely optimistic. It is clear that self-regulation, as it is currently practised, is failing patients and is eroding the credibility and standing of the medical profession.

Patient involvement

Most people have trouble assimilating complex, new verbal information in a short space of time, particularly if the information has direct implications for their personal lives. The body of medical literature is

Condition

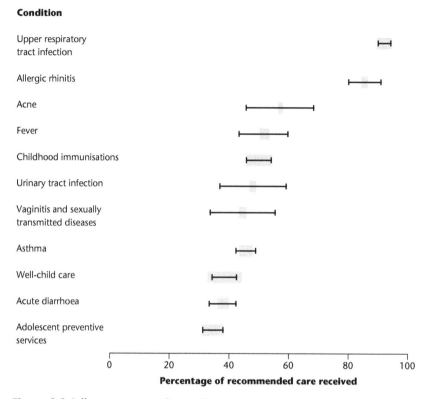

Figure 9.2 Adherence to quality indicators in child health care for according to condition

Note: The areas of the boxes reflect the number of times eligibility for a quality indicator was met for a particular condition, and the bars show the 95 per cent confidence intervals (diagram based on Mangione-Smith et al., 2007:1521).

expanding by more than 1500 articles every day, and making sense of this vast mass of information is a job for experts (Arndt 1992). There are some pamphlets and websites that practitioners may recommend to patients, but there is an ongoing problem with these not necessarily being up to date, not endorsed by relevant expert bodies, and not available in a suitable form for patients to understand. There is an urgent need for the necessary information to be presented in an authoritative, coherent form which is readily available, easy to assimilate and up to date, with pointers to where the underlying evidence may be found. Credible registers for appropriate sources of such information need to be developed and made widely available.

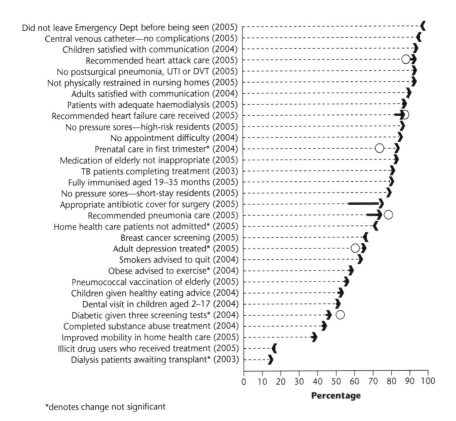

*denotes change not significant

Figure 9.3 Percentage of eligible patients who received recommended or expected care

Note: Arrowheads indicate the AHRQ estimated percentage and the direction of change from the previous year. Tails of arrows indicate average annual change. Circles are projected values estimated by adjusting McGlynn et al. (2003) indicators using the AHRQ average annual change for each comparable indicator. The McGlynn values are based on reviews of medical records from the year 2000 and the AHRQ (2008:131–5) values from administrative data up to the year shown on the x axis.

Carrying out plans correctly

To carry out plans correctly, it is necessary for the correct orders to be given and followed, and procedures or interventions to be undertaken correctly. This requires the right equipment, protocols and staff to be assembled, and the right actions to be carried out in the right sequence. Again, many patients assume that people in medical teams are trained for their roles. Further, they assume that the sorts of safety checks they see every time they fly on a commercial airline would be carried out routinely and documented by health professionals. While some of these processes are in place for some procedures in some units, there are few generally accepted standards, and emergency equipment and procedures differ widely between institutions, and usually between different parts of the same institution. Reviews of randomly selected medical records (in Australia, the United States, England, New Zealand, Denmark, France and Canada) have shown that health care-associated harm is associated with about 10 per cent of all admissions to acute-care hospitals, that 2 per cent of admissions are associated with permanent or severe harm, and that one in 300 patients dies as a result (Andrés et al. 2006). Harm is associated with over half a million admissions in Australia each year, and adverse events are managed at over a million primary care consultations annually (Britt et al. 2003).

Why should this be so?

One has to ask why highly paid health care professionals, who have undergone a prolonged induction process, should so often make plans at variance with evidence-based practice, and why so many plans are imperfectly carried out, resulting in so much harm to patients. A number of overlapping and interacting reasons why this may be so are listed (although not a comprehensive list) in Table 9.2.

Table 9.2 Factors that contribute to sub-optimal treatment of patients

Level	Problems
Individual behaviour	Errors
	Violations
	Use of mindlines not guidelines
Organisational performance	Poor work practices:
	• Inappropriate tasking
	• Poor supervision and teamwork
	• Bad rostering
	• Unstructured handovers
	Poor organisation and unavailability of protocols and guidelines
	Little or no surveillance of practice
	Equipment unavailable or unsuitable
	Perverse incentives and competing sources of income

Level	Problems
External influences	Resource constraints
	'Micromanagement' from outside

It is important to note that virtually all health care professionals are well motivated and do their best to provide safe, effective care, and that most succeed on most occasions. However, the factors in Table 9.2, singularly or in any number of combinations, frequently result in situations, events or sequences of events which may harm and occasionally hasten or cause the death of a patient. Health care is inherently risky, as many patients are frail and vulnerable and many interventions are complex. In view of this, it would seem desirable at least to reduce the variability and uncertainty of practice where this can be done.

Errors and violations

Errors are simply the 'downside of having a brain', and are by definition unintentional (Reason 1990). Most people can reduce the rates of certain types of error for short periods of time by focusing and concentrating on a particular task (Gawande 2002), but it is not possible to sustain this sort of vigilance throughout a professional life when exposure to risky situations occurs frequently and for long periods of time. Errors are ubiquitous, normal and necessary for learning (Reason 1990), but in the context of frail, unwell patients with complex, invasive interventions, even quite mundane errors can have catastrophic consequences. What is needed is a redesign of as many processes or techniques as possible so that certain errors cannot be made (see Box 9.1). These should be picked up early so that they do not have a harmful effect on patients (see Box 9.2). Means for the early detection of errors are important, as is standardisation of equipment and processes, so that everyone involved knows what should be happening and can monitor what is going on and draw attention to problems as they arise (see Box 9.3). Another step is vital here: individuals must be listened to when they draw attention to a problem, and must be respected for raising an issue; there is a lamentable history of not only ignoring warnings, but of persecuting 'whistleblowers'.

Violations are, by definition, intentional, and usually involve a trade-off such as convenience, saving time or increasing throughput or income (Reason 1990). They may become routine and manifest as bad habits, especially when it is not easy to comply with a protocol or rule in the context of a particular workplace. It is important to identify why violations are occurring and take the necessary steps to address the contributing factors (see Box 9.4). Again, having standard operating procedures allows anyone present to play a role in preventing violations from taking place and to draw attention to those that do.

Box 9.1

Brain damage or death from patients breathing mixtures of artificial gases with an insufficient percentage of oxygen occurred regularly in the past. A major cause was the juxtaposition of the control knobs for the flow of oxygen and nitrous oxide on anaesthetic machines (Barker et al. 1993). Fitting mechanical devices which prevented oxygen concentrations of less than 21 per cent eliminated this problem. The error of turning the wrong knob is still made, but this does not result in a hypoxic gas mixture, merely one with the same oxygen concentration as room air.

Box 9.2

Anaesthetists will inevitably, if occasionally, fail when they have to listen continuously for breathing circuit disconnections; such failures are a well-recognised cause of brain damage and death in paralysed patients. Audible circuit disconnection alarms (low-pressure alarms and capnographs, backed up by pulse oximeters) have virtually eliminated this problem (Runciman 2005). When they sound, the anaesthetist can reconnect the circuit and re-establish ventilation of the patient's lungs before any harm is done.

Box 9.3

An enormous amount of harm to patients has arisen from wrong concentrations or rates of drugs being infused. The use of agreed standardised instructions for how to make up solutions of drugs of the appropriate concentration and composition, and what syringes and infusion rates to use, combined with structured checklists to ensure that all is going according to plan, can greatly reduce this common, dangerous problem.

Box 9.4

It is now accepted that cross-infection, particularly with resistant organisms, is one of the major causes of morbidity and mortality in acute care hospitals. It is difficult to wash one's hands before seeing every patient if there is only one basin available in a large area, with many patients to be seen. Thus, a failure to wash hands became routine—and still is in many places. It is expensive to install basins at every bedside, but the problem has been overcome by making available an alcohol gel at each patient's bedside; this has been shown to be an effective alternative to hand washing. This does not force everyone to use the gel, but at least it makes compliance easy and practical.

Use of mindlines rather than guidelines

The term 'mindlines' refers to a phenomenon by which well-motivated people collectively devise and sanction patterns of behaviour or treatment that are at variance with evidence (Gabbay and le May 2004). Mindlines constitute collective 'rule-based' errors which institutionalise inappropriate care in certain communities of practice. Many inappropriate investigations and interventions are perpetuated by mindlines in the face of new information that renders the practices outdated and/or less risk- or cost-effective. Perverse incentives may underlie some mindlines (see Box 9.5).

Box 9.5

An example of a mindline is to routinely proceed to organise upper and lower gastrointestinal tract endoscopies as the first-line investigation for an iron deficiency anaemia. The fact that this is associated with much greater remuneration than less invasive, less costly and more appropriate initial investigations may be one factor underlying the widespread use of this approach.

Poor work practices

Many work practices set the stage for patients to be harmed, even though it is no one's intention that this should be the outcome.

Inappropriate tasking

It is a widespread practice to expect junior doctors to perform tasks for which they have had little or no training ('see one, do one, teach one'). These are often done with inadequate supervision, out-of-hours, and sometimes with assistants who are also unfamiliar with the task (see Box 9.6). People might expect that a medical emergency team would be composed of people who each have a particular role for which they have been trained, and who work to set plans and routines. This is often the case outside hospitals—for example, with ambulance and emergency workers—but is rarely the case within hospitals, in which there is a culture of 'working from first principles' rather than adhering to pre-compiled responses. Such poor teamwork often results in delays and less than ideal processes and outcomes.

***

Box 9.6

Placing an underwater seal drain for a pneumothorax is often regarded as a job for a junior doctor. Trochars (sharp metal spears) are still supplied with underwater seal drains, and these may be left in place to pierce the chest wall, at variance with prudent modern practice. The trochar may lacerate the liver, spleen, lungs or occasionally the heart. This task is often left to a junior who has only had a cursory verbal description of what to do, or may only have seen one drain inserted, sometimes by a person who themselves may have not been taught systematically.

***

Bad rostering

Rostering of staff for out-of-hours work can be very demanding if appropriate skill mixes and levels of experience are to be ensured. In some facilities, rostering is done by administrative staff who have no idea of the experience and abilities of each staff member, resulting in 'cover' being provided by people who are not up to handling many of the situations they are highly likely to encounter.

Structured handovers being ignored

This is becoming recognised as a major source of harm to patients. What has happened during a shift and what is planned are not properly documented, and are subject simply to an unstructured, cursory verbal communication, or are not passed on at all.

Little or no surveillance of practice

In many units, audits may be held to discuss things that have gone wrong, such as post-operative infections, but there is no attempt to determine objectively whether routine practices are in line with the latest evidence or for example, whether out-of-hours supervision at night is adequate.

Poor organisation and unavailability of relevant protocols and guidelines

These are also common problems. Indeed, there are some institutions where such protocols and guidelines are shown to surveyors at the time of accreditation but are, for practical purposes, rarely used during routine clinical work.

Box 9.7

It was found at a teaching hospital that there were no fewer than fourteen different types of infusion pumps and syringe drivers for administering intravenous fluids and drugs, with no provision for training or credentialling staff on any of the devices. Not surprisingly, a large number of incidents were being reported which turned out to have their origins in appropriate use of infusion devices.

Perverse incentives and competing sources of income

These are major problems in Australia (Runciman et al. 2007: 59–82). Some visiting medical officers have busy private practices, and the attention they can give to complex public hospital patients may be compromised, with a lot of reliance placed on trainees—some of whom may not yet have encountered some of the complex problems they have to deal with, with little prospect of immediate support.

Resource constraints

It is very difficult for those who are responsible for the distribution of funds to decide how they should be allocated amongst competing interests. Some of the problems outlined above have their roots in insufficient funds in the face of continuing demand.

Micromanagement from outside

This is also a major problem in some jurisdictions. For example, some hospitals are required to see all patients who present at their Emergency

Department and admit them within four hours if they require admission, whilst a major fraction of the hospital budget is contingent on waiting lists being reduced. Coupled with resource constraints, this can lead to the hospital becoming gridlocked with no patient movements possible; this has been shown to be associated with a 15 per cent increase in mortality (as well as very stressful working conditions), and may be a situation over which the local hospital administrators and clinicians have no control (Sprivulis et al. 2006).

WHAT CAN WE DO ABOUT THE PROBLEM?

In the aftermath of major reports on patient safety in 2000 and 2001 (Kohn et al. 2000; Department of Health 2000; Runciman and Moller 2001), a number of national patient safety organisations were launched, such as the National Patient Safety Foundation in the United States (<www.npsf.org>) and National Patient Safety Agency in the United Kingdom (<www.npsa.nhs.uk>). A substantial portion of their early work comprised reviews of aspects of patient safety and 'top-down' initiatives, such as the development of standards for medication charts and 'open disclosure' after adverse events. While necessary and appropriate, these initiatives have proven to be insufficient to produce widespread change. There were also some initiatives for addressing a number of rare but egregious events, such as removing concentrated potassium chloride solutions from ward stock (National Patient Safety Agency 2002), and taking steps to prevent procedures being performed on the wrong side or wrong patient (Joint Commission on Accreditation of Healthcare Organizations 2004). In parallel, and dating to before the national patient safety organisations, a large number of clinical guidelines had been produced by various organisations such as the ECRI Institute (<www.ecri.org/Pages/default.aspx>) and the National Guidelines Clearinghouse (<www.guideline.gov>). However, the pedigrees of some of these are suspect, as support had been provided by drug companies, and uptake has been limited (Grol et al. 2005). It has become apparent that the baseline compliance with basic safety and quality indicators is low (10–80 per cent) and that even intensive interventions lead only to modest changes (10–20 per cent) that are often poorly sustained (Grimshaw and Eccles 2004).

It seems that one of the problems is that mandating change from above, via the classical administrative hierarchies, has limited impact on work practices at the 'coalface'. Clinicians continue to practise in their own ways in informal but robust networks, seemingly relatively oblivious to or unconcerned about official directives (Braithwaite et al. 2009). It is apparent that both this inertia and the great variability in clinical practice may be tolerated and perpetuated by a *laissez-faire* approach to clinical practice in a climate in which 'clinical freedom' is valued over systematic self-regulation.

Responsive regulation and clinical practice

Figure 9.4 is a representation of the five levels of regulation proposed by Braithwaite et al. (2005), together with estimates of the relative contributions to each level of some of the types of organisation that are involved in the regulation of clinical practice (Runciman et al. 2007: 157-78). It is evident that the organisations involved in education, clinical practice, certification and professional behaviour have little power, and that those with the powers of command and control have little involvement in initiatives to improve clinical practice. Moreover, the financial levers in use in Australia are all associated with perverse incentives of one kind or another, and there is almost no prospect of any kind of sanction for practising in a way that may be quite idiosyncratic and markedly at variance with the available evidence. For example, registered medical practitioners can and do practise 'alternative medicine', and may actively represent that they do not provide conventional or evidence-based care.

A major problem underlying the failure of regulation of clinical practice is that, although many clinical guidelines exist, there are few clinical standards; as a result, regulatory mechanisms that do exist can gain no traction. There is no real expectation that the clinical guidelines or pathways that do exist should form the basis for routine clinical practice. Thus, although potential regulatory mechanisms exist—and how they may be brought to bear will be discussed below—until selected guidelines are elevated to clinical standards endorsed by the relevant professional organisations, there appears to be no prospect of significant sustained change. If all available levers could be used to counter the robust homeostatic mechanisms that maintain the current unsatisfactory situation, it is possible that better alignment of clinical practice with the available evidence may progressively occur.

Health care is too complex for information to be carried 'in the mind'. Information 'in the world' needs to be presented and made available in a form in which it can be accessed and used immediately without impeding workflow. This is not possible in a practical sense

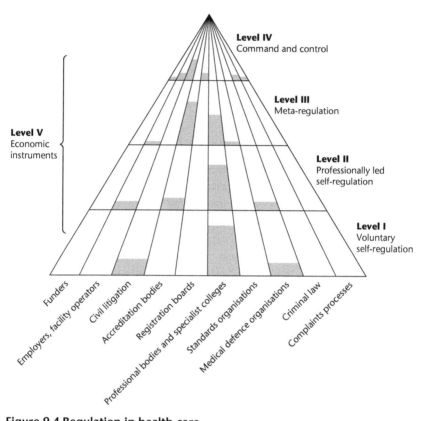

Figure 9.4 Regulation in health care

Note: The five levels of regulation proposed by Braithwaite et al. (2005), with ten types of organisation involved in regulation in health care. The shaded areas represent an estimate of the extent of involvement of each of these types of organisation at regulatory levels I–IV.

Source: Runciman et al. (2007: Ch. 7).

unless the information needed is up to date and based on evidence, wherever possible, or based on consensus by experts where there is no evidence. Also, much work is needed to determine how information should be presented so as to provide the greatest chance of correct decisions being made and carried out as intended.

Standard operating procedures, likewise, need to be available in a structured form. There is much merit in agreeing on standard ways of doing things. Such agreement does not have to wait for evidence that a particular way of doing things is better than another. The advantages of standardising processes include the fact that all health care professionals become familiar with how things are done, and that everyone involved has the opportunity to play a role in ensuring that the right equipment, staff and procedures are brought to bear on a problem. The merits of 'standardisation for standardisation's sake' are well recognised in aviation, and have contributed to the high levels of safety in this potentially high-risk industry.

There have been some successes by clinicians via 'grass roots' movements in setting standards and then seeking endorsement by the relevant professional bodies. Examples are the national and international safety standards for monitoring during anaesthesia. Widespread uptake of these de facto standards has meant that brain damage and death from certain airway and breathing problems, once regular occurrences, have become virtually 'never' events (Runciman 2005).

A proposal

If clinical standards were to be generated by groups of expert clinicians with 'street cred', they could be embodied in tools, and could then be disseminated (Runciman, Day et al. 2009). If a number of regulatory levers are then brought to bear via requirements for the use of such standards in key core clinical areas, then progress might be made. However, for this to occur the problems with patient safety and quality need to be broken down into clinically meaningful entities so that the relevant clinical standards can be brought to bear on the everyday practical clinical problems that are dealt with during interactions between clinicians and patients. The stages of such a process are listed in Box 9.8.

Box 9.8: Proposed stages of development of clinical standards

1 Determine the priorities.
2 Set clinical standards for each priority:
 • Review the literature.
 • Recruit volunteer experts.
 • Convene a national meeting.
 • Establish or plan the establishment of the standards in question.
3 Develop tools for each standard which would:
 • implicitly or explicitly incorporate the standard;
 • comprise the mechanism for guiding and documenting compliance with the standard;
 • be easy to audit at a glance.

---

4   Evaluate and improve each tool at pilot sites.
5   Obtain endorsement of the standards and tools by the relevant professional and consumer organisations:
   • Disseminate the standards for evaluation at key sites.
   • Establish mechanisms for routine surveillance and audit.
6   Use the standards for:
   • the credentialling of individual clinicians;
   • the accreditation of services and facilities.

Source: Runciman, Day et al. (2009).

Determine the priorities

What matters to patients is getting the interactions described at the beginning of this chapter right. Given the complexity of health care, it would be an overwhelming task to try to influence the behaviour of practitioners and patients across all of health care. Many of the national patient safety organisations formed around the year 2000 concentrated on 'top-down' initiatives, such as open disclosure and root cause analyses for rare, egregious problems. However, as explained below, the vast majority of the burden of disease may be addressed by setting up mechanisms for 'getting it right' in the common problem areas (Runciman, Westbrook et al. 2009). What is needed, in essence, are transparent, explicit, evidence- or consensus-based clinical standards so that the right plans are made and are then carried out correctly for the common, mundane conditions that make up the bulk of health care (Runciman et al. 2002). It is important to take a 'one hill at a time' approach (Berwick 1996).

A re-analysis of the data from the Quality in Australian Healthcare Study identified the twenty most costly adverse events (Runciman et al. 2002); the RAND Organisation identified quality indicators for 30 conditions in adults (McGlynn et al. 2003) and 21 in children (McGlynn et al. 2000; Mangione-Smith et al. 2007); the National Institute of Clinical Studies in Australia identified 23 gaps in practice (National Institute of Clinical Studies 2003, 2005); the National Institute for Health and Clinical Excellence in the United Kingdom has published over 80 guidelines (<www.nice.org.uk>); the Institute for Healthcare Improvement developed twenty interventions for five clinical conditions (Adams and Corrigan 2003); the Agency for Healthcare Research and Quality (2008) produced 27 guidelines of clinical relevance to safety; and the Stanford Evidence-Based Practice

Centre identified 25 safety practices with very strong or strong evidence of efficacy (Shojania et al. 2001).

Collating this information (see Table 9.3), produces 52 clinical problem areas that were identified by more than one of these organisations, which together embrace 744 indicators, guidelines or areas for attention. This set covers more than 90 per cent of the areas which cause the vast majority of disability-adjusted life years in Australia (Begg et al. 2008).

Set clinical standards for each priority

Having identified a clinical problem to tackle, it is important to understand what care should be recommended for that problem, and why practice may deviate from this. In order to do this, the first thing to do is to review the literature and collate other sources of information about that problem. Increasingly, these reviews should include qualitative sets of information that offer insights into what the nature of the problem is and why things do not go right. These sources include incident reports, root cause analyses, medico-legal files, complaints and coroners' recommendations.

The steps listed in Box 9.8 should then systematically be undertaken. A process by which safety standards were developed for implementation in clinical anaesthesia over two decades ago provides an example, and has been described elsewhere (Runciman et al. 2006). This involved seeking volunteer experts to review the literature and come up with 35 discussion documents, which were published in the peer-reviewed journal *Anaesthesia and Intensive Care*. These were subsequently endorsed by the relevant expert bodies, which produced formal, ratified guidelines, and this information was then disseminated to teaching hospitals. Accreditation for teaching was dependent on these and other guidelines being met. The guidelines rapidly became de facto standards and were adopted across both the public and private sectors. Subsequently, international patient safety standards were developed and endorsed by the World Federation of Societies of Anaesthesiologists, which by then had over a hundred member countries.

Promote adherence to standards

As outlined above, the problem is not that there are no good guidelines, but simply that these are not routinely followed by practitioners. In line with suggestions elsewhere in this book, all available mechanisms should be engaged to try to ensure that clinical standards are developed, disseminated and not only used, but shown to be used on a routine

Table 9.3 Clinical problem areas and clinical guidelines

	Institutes*	Sford	QAHCS	IOM	NICS	RAND	AHRQ	NICE
Basic maternal and child health	5			1	3	61	2	2
Colorectal cancer assessment and treatment	5		1		2	13	3	1
Diabetes management	5			1	1	18	2	4
Ischemic heart disease—prevention, management	5		1	1		37	2	1
Tobacco dependence treatment	5			1	1	6	1	1
Prenatal care	5			1	1	38	2	1
Heart failure management	4				2	36	1	1
Immunisation	4			2	1	57	2	
Prevention of pressure ulcers	4	1	1				2	1
Prevention of venous thrombo-embolism	4	1	1	1	1			1
Cancer pain and palliation	4		1	1				1
Depression	4			1		3	2	5
Asthma	4			1	2	27	1	
Obesity	4			1		53	1	2
Hypertension management	4			1	1	2		1
Atrial fibrillation management	3				1	27	1	1
Cerebrovascular disease	3		1	1	1	10		
Osteoporosis fractures	3	1			1	10		
Renal failure	3				1	9	2	1

	Institutes*	Sford	QAHCS	IOM	NICS	RAND	AHRQ	NICE
Prevention of medication errors and over-use of antibiotics	3	1	1	1				
Prevention of targeted classes of adverse drug events**	3	2	1				1	
Prevention of nosocomial infections	3	1	1	1				
Prevention of surgical-site infections	3	2	2				3	
Prevention of morbidity due to central venous catheter insertion	2	3						1
Prevention of morbidity and mortality in post-surgical and critically ill patients	2	2						1
Contraception and sexual health	2					9		2
Injury	2			1		1		
Diarrhoea and gastroenteritis of presumed infectious origin	2					15	1	
Tuberculosis	2						1	1
Cancer screening	2			1				1
Lung cancer	2				1			1
Breast cancer	2					10		2
Prostate cancer	2					6		1
Hyperlipidaemia	2					7		1
Drug dependence	2						2	3

Table 9.3 Clinical problem areas and clinical guidelines (*continued*)

	Institutes*	Sford	QAHCS	IOM	NICS	RAND	AHRQ	NICE
Schizophrenia	2			1				1
Neurotic, stress-related and somatoform disorders (anxiety, obsessive-compulsive disorder, post-traumatic disorder) treatment	2				1			3
Otitis media	2					7		1
Community-acquired pneumonia	2					5	1	
Influenza	2				1		1	
Chronic obstructive pulmonary disease	2					20		1
Dyspepsia and peptic ulcer disease	2					8		1
Osteoarthritis	2					3		1
Urinary tract infection	2					31		1
Sexually transmitted diseases or vaginitis	2					55	1	
Abnormal uterine bleeding	2					1		1
Caesarean delivery	2					9		1
Fever	2					32		1
Adequate staffing	2	1					1	
Prevention of falls	2		1					1

	Institutes*	Sford	QAHCS	IOM	NICS	RAND	AHRQ	NICE
Quality cancer care	2		1					1
Reducing inadequate post-operative pain management	2	1			1			

* Number of institutes that have issued guidelines in this area

** Such as analgesics, KCL, antibiotics and heparin

Note: The number of indicators, guidelines or areas for attention identified by the Stanford Evidence Based Practice Centre (Sford), the Quality in Australian Healthcare Study (QAHCS), the Institute of Medicine (IOM), the National Institute of Clinical Studies (NICS), the RAND Organisation (RAND), the Agency for Healthcare Research and Quality (AHRQ), and the National Institute for Health and Clinical Excellence (NICE).

Source: Adapted from Runciman, Westbrook et al. 2009b.

213

basis. Much groundwork is needed to go through the processes outlined in Box 9.8 for each of the problems, but the potential improvements in health care, transparency and accountability are enormous. Suggestions follow for how each of the types of organisation identified in Figure 9.4 could play a role.

Funders

At least in the United Kingdom, parts of the United States and the Netherlands, there have been trials of 'pay for performance', in which practitioners have been paid extra if certain clinical protocols are followed. Problems arose in the Netherlands when extra payments for particular services were withdrawn, and in the United Kingdom extra payments led to a large increase in the remuneration of general practitioners.

Non-payment for non-compliance would seem to be an important and, in the long term, a more appropriate potential lever. The health benefits payment agency Medicare Australia already has mechanisms by which remuneration for certain services may be limited unless certain conditions are met, or if services are provided more than a decreed number of times in a year. It is quite possible that this mechanism could be extended to payment being withheld in instances in which clinical standards were consistently not adhered to without reasons being provided. However, this would require that clinical standards and easy-to-use tools be refined, developed and accepted by the profession before such a mechanism could be put into place.

Employers and facility operators

Departments of health and many members of the public assume that employers (such as public hospitals) and facility operators (as in the private sector) can and will ensure that standards deemed desirable or necessary are adhered to. However, the experience of trying to remove concentrated potassium chloride from ward stock, or trying to ensure that the '3 Cs' (correct side, correct patient, correct procedure) protocol is followed, has demonstrated that this may, in many instances, be an optimistic expectation. Some clinicians simply refuse to comply with recommendations and memoranda, and the employers and facility operators effectively appear to be powerless. This is particularly the case in the private sector. Visiting private medical officers can choose the hospitals at which they will work, and facility operators seldom try to influence how individual practitioners carry out their work in case they take their services elsewhere (see Wellington and Dugdale, this volume, Chapter 5). It is clear that additional levers are needed if standards are to be adhered to.

Civil litigation

Tort may be used to obtain compensation if patients are harmed and it is deemed that practitioners have not exercised due care or met reasonable standards. There is no doubt that the fear of litigation under the tort system can be a powerful motivator (see Hirsch, this volume, Chapter 12). Rapid uptake of oximetry and capnography in the late 1980s and early 1990s was given impetus by the fact that practitioners would have been deemed negligent had the patient suffered serious injury or death that could have been prevented by the use of these devices. Although many professional bodies have initiatives to bring aspects of patient safety onto their agenda, a more proactive approach with respect to the development, endorsement, dissemination and enforcement of clinical standards would have a powerful effect.

Accreditation bodies

These bodies (see Berrill and Healy, this volume, Chapter 13) constitute a mechanism for improvement by providing only provisional accreditation in certain areas if facilities or health care services fail to meet standards or indicators set by relevant professional organisations. This is a regulatory mechanism which could be greatly strengthened. Accreditation organisations could also check that appropriate credentialling of clinicians has taken place. Credentialling at the moment is rudimentary in most institutions in Australia, with paperwork being completed but little actual attention being paid to whether the practitioners remain competent in their areas of clinical activity.

Registration boards

Boards have the requisite command and control powers. However, to date many have not played an active role in ensuring that minimum clinical standards are met, not least because there are few clinical standards. There is no doubt that they could act as a 'measure of last resort' for dealing with health care professionals who consistently fail to comply with standards. However, the standards have to be developed and tools to enact them disseminated before this could become a realistic proposition.

215

Professional bodies and specialist colleges

For some disciplines, such as anaesthesia, these organisations have played an active role in developing and disseminating standards for both clinical processes (such as checking an anaesthetic machine) and equipment requirements (such as ensuring the availability of suitable oximeters and capnographs). However, many professional bodies take a *laissez-faire* approach to how their members conduct their practice, and a more active approach with respect to clinical standards should be promoted.

Standards organisations

These bodies have developed a number of standards for equipment and some for clinical processes, but are generally not involved in developing clinical standards for everyday practice, although they could be. Compliance with standards is voluntary, but if clinical standards were to be developed and endorsed, the fact that they had been through the structured processes employed by these organisations would add weight to their being used for credentialling, accreditation and in civil litigation.

Medical defence organisations (MDOs)

MDOs have recently become involved in risk-management and practitioners who avail themselves of courses in risk-management and improved communication may benefit from reduced premiums. These organisations could impose increased premiums, refuse the payment of excesses, or even refuse cover if accepted formally promulgated clinical standards were wilfully violated. However, as there are virtually no clinical standards, these options are currently not realistic prospects.

Complaints processes

Patients can complain to patient advocates at the health facility level and state ombudsmen level, and to the medical registration boards. It is possible that complaints forwarded to the medical registration board may result in steps being taken by the board to make ongoing registration contingent on certain requirements being met (e.g. a review of the clinician's performance, an investigation by a public health organisation or ongoing registration with conditions). Practitioners may also be deregistered. However, registration boards generally only get involved when there are misconducts or grave misgivings about clinical practice.

CONCLUSION

The vast majority of health care is delivered during, or as a result of, interactions between patients and health care practitioners. The actions taken, or decisions made, at these interactions are less than optimal about half the time, and patients are frequently harmed by the health care process itself. Although many guidelines have been produced and a number of potential regulatory mechanisms exist, activity has been piecemeal, and there has been no coordination of effort amongst the organisations that could play a role in regulation. The health care system consumes 10 per cent of gross domestic product in Australia, and the current state of affairs and slow rate of change are unacceptable. It is time for the health care professions to be proactive in adopting techniques used in industry. Developing, disseminating and ensuring the use of clinical standards in only 50 clinical areas would lead to greatly improved care and less variation for more than 90 per cent of the conditions or circumstances that are responsible for the burden of disease in Australia. In parallel with the development of standards and tools, at least as much attention should be given to how they should be made available at the 'point of care'. It is vital that they enhance and not impede workflow, and do not intrude on contact or communication between health care professionals and patients. It is essential that mechanisms be established for standards to be undated regularly and as necessary via standing expert groups disseminating new online versions nationally. Ideally, tools could be called up and integrated into the patient's medical records, which would allow automatic audit of the performance of individuals and services with respect to standards as more sophisticated record and information systems are developed.

REFERENCES

Adams, K. and Corrigan, J.M. eds 2003, *Priority Areas for National Action: Transforming Health Care Quality*, The National Academies Press, Washington DC, <www.nap.edu/openbook.php?isbn=0309085438>, accessed 1 February 2009

Agency for Healthcare Research and Quality 2008, *National Healthcare Quality Report 2007*, Agency for Healthcare Research and Quality, Rockville, MD

Andrés, J.M.A., Remón, C.A., Burillo, J.V. and Lopez, P.R. 2006, *National Study on Hospitalisation-related Adverse Events ENEAS 2005*, Ministry of Health and Consumer Affairs, Madrid

Arndt, K.A. 1992, 'Information excess in medicine', *Archives of Dermatology*, vol. 128, no. 9, pp. 1249–56

Barker, L., Webb, R.K., Runciman, W.B. and Van der Walt, J.H. 1993, 'The Australian Incident Monitoring Study. The oxygen analyser: applications and limitations: An analysis of 200 incident reports', *Anaesthesia and Intensive Care*, vol. 21, no. 5, pp. 570–4

Begg, S.J., Vos, T., Barker, B., Stanley, L. and Lopez, A.D. 2008, 'Burden of disease and injury in Australia in the new millennium: Measuring health loss from diseases, injuries and risk factors', *Medical Journal of Australia*, vol. 188, no. 1, pp. 36–40

Berwick, D.M. 1996, 'A primer on leading the improvement of systems', *British Medical Journal*, vol. 312, no. 7031, pp. 619–22

Braithwaite, J., Healy, J. and Dwan, K. 2005, *The Governance of Health Care Safety and Quality*, Commonwealth of Australia, Canberra

Braithwaite, J., Runciman, W.B. and Merry, A.F. 2009, 'Towards safer, better healthcare: Harnessing the natural properties of complex socio technical systems', *Quality and Safety in Healthcare*, in press

Britt, H., Miller, G.C., Knox, S., Charles, J., Valenti, L., Henderson, J., Pan, Y., Bayram, C. and Harrison, C. 2003, *General Practice Activity in Australia, 2002-3*, Australian Institute for Health and Welfare, Canberra

Dartmouth Institute for Health Policy and Clinical Practice 2008, *The Dartmouth Atlas of Health Care*, The Dartmouth Institute for Health Policy and Clinical Practice, Lebanon, NH, <www.dartmouthatlas.org>, accessed 17 December 2008

Department of Health 2000, *An Organisation with a Memory—Report of an Expert Group on Learning from Adverse Events in the NHS chaired by the Chief Medical Officer*, The Stationery Office, London

Gabbay, J. and le May, A. 2004, 'Evidence based guidelines or collectively constructed "mindlines?" Ethnographic study of knowledge management in primary care', *British Medical Journal*, vol. 329, no. 7473, p. 1013

Gawande, A.A. 2002, *Complications: A Surgeon's Notes on an Imperfect Science*, Metropolitan Books, New York

Grimshaw, J.M. and Eccles, M.P. 2004, 'Is evidence-based implementation of evidence-based care possible?', *Medical Journal of Australia*, vol. 180, suppl. 6, pp. 50–1

Grol, R., Wensing, M. and Eccles, M. 2005, *Improving Patient Care: The Implementation of Change in Clinical Practice*, Elsevier, Oxford

Joint Commission on Accreditation of Healthcare Organizations 2004, *Universal Protocol for Preventing Wrong Site, Wrong Procedure, Wrong Person Surgery™ 2003*, Joint Commission on Accreditation of Healthcare Organizations, <www.jcaho.org/NR/rdonlyres/E3C600EB-043B-4E86-B04E-CA4A89AD5433/0/universal_protocol.pdf>, accessed 17 Dec 2008

Kohn, L.T., Corrigan, J.M. and Donaldson, M.S. eds 2000, *To Err is Human: Building a Safer Health System*, National Academies Press, Washington

Mangione-Smith, R., DeCristofaro, A.H., Setodji, C.M., Keesey, J., Klein, D.J., Adams, J.L., Schuster, M.A. and McGlynn, E.A. 2007, 'The quality of ambulatory care delivered to children in the United States', *New England Journal of Medicine*, vol. 357, no. 15, pp.1515–23

McGlynn, E.A., Asch, S.M., Adams, J., Keesey, J., Hicks, J., DeChristofaro, A. and Kerr, E.A. 2003, 'The quality of health care delivered to adults in the United States', *New England Journal of Medicine*, vol. 348, no. 26, pp. 2635–45

McGlynn, E.A., Damberg, C.L., Kerr, E.A. and Schuster, M.A. eds 2000, *Quality of Care for Children and Adolescents*, RAND, Santa Monica, CA, <www.rand.org/pubs/monograph_reports/MR1283/>, accessed 17 December 2008

National Institute of Clinical Studies 2003, *Evidence-Practice Gaps Report, Volume 1*, National Institute of Clinical Studies, Melbourne

—— 2005, *Evidence-Practice Gaps Report, Volume 2*, National Institute of Clinical Studies, Melbourne

National Patient Safety Agency 2002, *Patient Safety Alert*, National Patient Safety Agency, London, <www.npsa.nhs.uk/nrls/alerts-and-directives/alerts/potassium-chloride-concentrate>, accessed 1 February 2009

Organisation for Economic Cooperation and Development 2008, *Growth in Health Spending Slows in Many OECD Countries, According to OECD Health Data 2008, Chart 2: Health Expenditure as a Share of GDP 2006*, Directorate for Employment, Labour and Social Affairs, Organisation for Economic Cooperation and Development, Paris, <www.oecd.org/document/27/0,3343,en_2649_34631_40902299_1_1_1_1,00.html>, accessed 1 February 2009

Reason, J. 1990, *Human Error*, Cambridge University Press, New York

Runciman, W.B. 2005, 'Iatrogenic harm and anaesthesia in Australia', *Anaesthesia and Intensive Care*, vol. 33, no. 3, pp. 297–300

Runciman, W.B., Edmonds, M.J. and Pradhan, M. 2002, 'Setting priorities for patient safety', *Quality and Safety in Health Care*, vol. 11, no. 3, pp. 224–9

Runciman, B., Merry, A. and Walton, M. 2007, *Safety and Ethics in Healthcare: A Guide to Getting it Right*, Ashgate, Aldershot

Runciman, W.B. and Moller, J. 2001, *Iatrogenic Injury in Australia*, Australian Patient Safety Foundation, Adelaide

Runciman, W.B., Westbrook, J., Benveniste, K.A. and Day, R. 2009, 'Setting priorities and developing clinical standards', *Medical Journal of Australia*, for submission

Runciman, W.B., Williamson, J.A.H., Deakin, A., Benveniste, K.A., Bannon, K. and Hibbert, P.D. 2006, 'An integrated framework for safety, quality and risk management: An information and incident management system based on a universal patient safety classification', *Quality and Safety in Healthcare*, vol. 15, suppl. 1, pp. 82–90

Shojania, K.G., Duncan, B.W., McDonald, K.M. and Wachter, R.M. 2001, *Making Health Care Safer: A Critical Analysis of Patient Safety Practices. Evidence Report/Technology Assessment No. 43*, Agency for Healthcare Research and Quality, Rockville, MD, <www.ahrq.gov/CLINIC/PTSAFETY/pdf/ptsafety. pdf>, accessed 1 February 2009

Sprivulis, P.C., Da Silva, J.A., Jacobs, I.G., Frazer, A.R. and Jelinek, G.A. 2006, 'The association between hospital overcrowding and mortality among patients admitted via Western Australian emergency departments', *Medical Journal of Australia*, vol. 184, no. 5, pp. 208–12

Symposium 1993, 'The Australian Incident Monitoring System', *Anaesthesia and Intensive Care*, vol. 21, no. 5, pp. 501–695

Van Der Weyden, M.B. 2005, 'The Bundaberg Hospital scandal: The need for reform in Queensland and beyond', *Medical Journal of Australia*, vol. 183, no. 6, pp. 284–5

Wennberg, J. and Gittelsohn, A. 1982, 'Variations in medical care among small areas', *Scientific American*, vol. 246, no. 4, pp. 120–34

10

SURGEON REPORT CARDS

Justin Oakley and Steve Clarke

INTRODUCTION

Surgeon report cards are aggregations of comparative information about the performance of individual surgeons and surgical units. In recent years, such information has been made available to the public, particularly in the field of cardiac surgery. New York State has been publishing comparative performance data on individual cardiac surgeons' mortality rates for coronary artery bypass grafts (CABG) on the internet since 1991, and has published individual cardiologists' mortality rates for angioplasty since 2001. New Jersey and Pennsylvania have followed New York's lead and have also made performance information on cardiac surgery available. In the United Kingdom, survival rates for CABG and aortic valve replacement surgery for individual surgeons have been made available on the internet by the Healthcare Commission since 2006. This replaced a 'three-star' rating system in operation from 2004 until 2006, under which surgeons were rated as having met, failed to meet or exceeded the standards of the Society of Cardiothoracic Surgeons (Neil et al. 2004). Other countries may soon follow suit. There have been recent calls to publish surgeon performance data in the Netherlands (Lanier et al. 2003) and in New Zealand (*Otago Daily Times*, 6 February 2008).

There have been gradual moves in Australia to publish certain kinds of health care performance information, such as details about the performance of hospitals and units with various procedures, and de-identified clinician audit data (see Hughes and Mackay 2006).[1] However, unlike the United States and the United Kingdom, comparative clinician-specific performance information has not so far been published in Australia. Nevertheless, the movement to publish health care performance information has recently been gathering momentum. There have been calls to introduce clinician report cards in Australia, prompted by well-known scandals in surgery at Bundaberg Base Hospital in Queensland,[2] Canberra Hospital, and Camden and Campbelltown Hospitals in New South Wales (Clarke et al. 2005; see also Chapter 15), along with investigations into unsatisfactory outcomes of procedures by doctors such as Dr Graham Reeves.[3] Divergent complication rates between different New South Wales surgeons and hospitals for pacemaker insertion procedures have also led to calls for the public to be better informed about such variations (*Sydney Morning Herald*, 28 June 2008). The Rudd government, elected in late 2007, has demanded that public and private hospitals publish data on mortality and infection rates, and has linked public hospital funding increases to greater transparency and accountability by hospitals about their health care performance (*The Age*, 22 July 2008, 26 August 2008).[4] Some Australian surgeons see the advent of surgeon report cards as inevitable, given the increasing use of such report cards overseas.[5]

So far, the only comparative performance information on named individual surgeons that has been published is cardiac surgeon performance data, especially CABG performance data. CABG is a very useful test case for public reporting of surgeon performance data. This is because CABG is one of the most common operations conducted in the Western world, because it is conducted in much the same way throughout the world, and because there is a clear indicator of success or failure that we can use to assess performance—namely, mortality (Marasco and Ibrahim 2007). Other reasons for the focus on the CABG operation are that cardiac surgery is a major event in people's lives and that cardiac surgery is very costly. As mentioned above, lessons learned from the experience of publishing cardiac surgeon performance information have been applied in the public reporting of individual cardiologists' angioplasty mortality rates. These lessons are also being applied in the development of public reporting schemes in the United Kingdom for other surgical specialties (UK Healthcare Commission 2007), though there are challenges in developing performance indicators for specialties within which indications of success or failure are less clear than the mortality or survival statistics used to measure success in cardiac surgery. Further down the track, surgery may be a test case for other professions. Just as surgeons' performance information is now being made public, so too may performance information for nurses, lawyers, teachers, and so on.

At least three different sorts of ethical arguments can be used to support public reporting of surgeon performance information. The first type of argument is that making such information available enables patients to make better-informed decisions about surgery. The risks involved in having surgery vary according to how capable a particular surgeon is at performing a particular operation. A prospective patient who is aware of the performance ability of available surgeons is able to make a better informed decision than a patient who is not aware of the performance ability of available surgeons. So it is arguable that, on standard interpretations of the ethical doctrine of informed consent— understood primarily as being intended to uphold the value of patient autonomy—patients are entitled to surgeons' performance information, as they will be able to exercise a greater degree of autonomy if they are in possession of such information than they would be otherwise (Clarke and Oakley 2004).

The second sort of ethical argument is that, by publishing such information, the surgical profession helps fulfil a duty it has to be account- able to the community. The surgical profession is typically granted a monopoly on provision of surgical procedures in particular countries, and it is plausible to think that, in exchange for this monopoly control, the surgical profession has a reciprocal obligation to demonstrate to the community that its services are of an acceptable standard. Furthermore, the surgical profession often has a considerable degree of control over the training of surgeons, and in many countries the costs of training surgeons are borne entirely by the community or are heavily subsidised by the community. When the community has paid for the training of surgeons, the community is entitled to ensure that its investment in that training has been effective.

The third sort of ethical argument for publishing surgeon per- formance information is a consequentialist argument that stresses the overall benefits of publishing surgeon performance information. If there are such benefits overall, then consequentialist philosophers such as utilitarians will, other things being equal, be in favour of publication. This sort of argument is often presented as an economic argument for surgeon report cards, stressing the benefits in terms of increased safety and improved quality of services that result from the publishing surgeon performance information. Advocates of this consequentialist style of argument can point to evidence from studies of long-standing public reporting schemes in the United States, which suggest that publishing surgeon performance information leads to long-term increases in the quality of surgical care (Peterson et al. 1998; Chassin 2002; Marshall and Brook 2002; Hannan et al. 2003; Fung et al. 2008; Swan 2008). For example, in New York State, risk-adjusted mortality following CABG dropped 41 per cent in the first four years of public reporting and it has continued to drop. A recent study suggests that similar safely improvements are taking place in the United Kingdom as a result of public reporting, where observed mortality amongst 25,730 patients undergoing CABG surgery in north-west England dropped from 2.4 to 1.8 per cent over an eight-year period (Bridgewater et al. 2007).

These three sorts of ethical arguments can be used to support public reporting of different types of performance data. The argument of informed consent emphasises the importance of patients having access to relatively fine-grained risk information, and so can support methods of presentation such as league tables which, *inter alia*, contain mortality or survival rates for individual surgeons in a certain specialty and in a given region. The professional accountability argument is well suited to underpin more coarse-grained reporting methods, which employ thresholds to identify outliers in performance without necessarily specifying mortality rates for all surgeons above this threshhold. The publication methods supported by the consequentialist quality and safety argument will depend upon empirical research into whether health care safety and quality are more likely to be improved by publishing only hospital performance information or also clinician performance information and, if the latter, then by publishing fine-grained or only coarse-grained clinician performance data.

In this chapter, we consider the strengths and weaknesses of this quality and safety argument for surgeon report cards. We set out the argument in greater detail and then examine several objections that have been levelled against it. Despite the strong ethical arguments for publishing surgeon performance information, a variety of objections have been raised and we will consider the most important of these. First, there are those who take issue with the evidence in favour of improvements in quality and safety, and question whether the mechanisms that seem to underlie such improvements are themselves ethically justifiable overall. Second, there is the 'defensive surgery objection'. Third, there is the complaint that patients do not use performance information. And fourth, there is a moral objection to the very idea of asking patients to make choices on the basis of safety at all.

EVIDENCE AND MECHANISMS OF PATIENT SAFETY IMPROVEMENTS

A number of different mechanisms exist through which cardiac surgeon report cards have been thought to improve patient safety. It has been suggested that report cards improve the safety and quality of cardiac care because: (i) patients are less likely to choose surgeons with poorer outcomes; (ii) underperforming surgeons become more strongly motivated to improve their skills; (iii) surgeons become more risk-averse and so turn away some high-risk patients they would previously have operated on; (iv) conversely, surgeons become more risk-taking, operating on some high-risk patients they would previously have been reluctant to take on; (v) hospitals use surgeon report cards as tools to help identify problems with their surgical procedures; and (vi) hospitals restrict the operating privileges of surgeons with consistently poor performance. While various patient safety improvements have been observed after the introduction of cardiac surgeon report cards, the evidence does not conclusively show which mechanisms have led to improvements in patient safety.[6]

When public reporting of surgeon performance information was first introduced in the United States, with its market-based health care system, it was thought that better informed prospective patients would demand higher quality services and that poor performers would be disciplined by the market (Marshall et al. 2000). But while the introduction of cardiac surgeon report cards in the United States may have led to the shunning of a few poorly performing surgeons, and to patients flocking to very high performing surgeons, it is difficult to find systematic evidence of widespread 'surgeon-shopping' by patients, and so it is not clear that the cardiac care improvements that have occurred in the United States with report card schemes are attributable to such patient behaviour. In any case, surgeon report cards can facilitate informed surgeon-shopping only if patients are aware of the reports and find them comprehensible. However, public awareness and understanding of cardiac surgeon report cards, in those American states where these exist, seems to be rather limited.

In the United Kingdom, with its dominant public health care system, the argument that market mechanisms might drive quality improvements through market discipline has not been prominent. Instead, the main rationales for publishing surgeon performance information have been to enable regulators to better assess where and how performance can be improved, and to ensure the accountability of hospitals and their personnel to the general public. Likewise, the argument that surgeon report cards will improve health care quality through encouraging patients to 'vote with their feet' is less relevant to Australia, with its public health care system, than this argument is to the market-based approaches to health care in the United States.[7]

Surgeon report cards have also been thought to improve patient care quality and safety by providing stronger incentives for surgeons to improve their skills. Many surgical specialties have been developing sophisticated surgical audit processes as part of peer review of performance. Publishing identified surgeon performance information, such as the mortality or survival rates of patients operated on by named individual cardiac surgeons, clearly serves as an additional spur to improve surgical performance. There have been suggestions that cardiac surgical outcomes have improved overall since the introduction of report cards because cardiac surgeons have become more reluctant to operate on high-risk patients (such as those over 65 suffering from acute myocardial infarction), due to concerns about how the outcomes of such surgery will impact on the surgeon's overall mortality rate. The possibility of such a 'defensive surgery' reaction has led some commentators to conclude that safety and quality improvements produced by public reporting of surgeon-specific performance information come at too high a price (Vass 2002; Swan 2004). This is a very common objection to surgeon report cards, so we examine this concern in more detail below. Interestingly, the contrary suggestion has also been made: that the overall quality of surgical care in a report cards environment is enhanced because some surgeons are more prepared to operate on high-risk patients than they had been previously. Indeed, there is evidence in both the United States and the United Kingdom that high-risk patients are more likely to receive cardiac surgery after the introduction of report cards (Peterson et al. 1998; Bridgewater et al. 2007). To some extent, this will be influenced by a surgeon's level of understanding of, and confidence in, the risk-adjustment process.

Cardiac care quality and safety improvements following the introduction of surgeon report cards have been attributed not only to responses by patients and surgeons themselves, but also to reactions by health care managers and hospitals. In some cases, hospitals with cardiac surgeons who received poor report cards used these as tools to identify ways to improve cardiac care outcomes—for example, by providing better facilities and training to surgeons and surgical support staff. In other cases, where a hospital found that their relatively poor cardiac surgery outcomes were clearly due to consistently poor performance and skill on the part of particular surgeons, those surgeons were no longer permitted to undertake certain procedures, such as CABG operations. In several cases, the surgeons involved left the profession altogether (Chassin 2002).

DEFENSIVE SURGERY

One of the most common ethical objections to surgeon report cards is the defensive surgery objection. This is the concern that public reporting leads surgeons to avoid operating on high-risk patients because these patients are more likely to have unsuccessful outcomes, which would have a negative impact on a surgeon's report card. As mentioned above, some of those who raise this objection are prepared to concede that report cards have improved the overall safety and quality of patient care, but argue that high-risk patients' increased difficulty in finding a surgeon willing to operate on them is too high a moral price to pay for the various benefits of public reporting.

Sometimes the defensive surgery objection is made by people who are simply unaware that the information published in New York State and the United Kingdom is risk-adjusted; sometimes it is made by those who believe current efforts to risk-adjust such statistics are inadequate; and sometimes it is made by those who suspect that surgeons will continue to practise defensive surgery no matter how accurate risk-adjustment is. The appropriate response to those who are unaware that surgeons' report cards are routinely risk-adjusted is to point this out to them. The appropriate response to those who argue that current efforts to risk-adjust surgeons' performance information are inadequate is to ask them to help identify actual shortcomings in risk-adjustment techniques and see how these may be improved. It is not clear how to deal with the challenge from those who hold that surgeons will practise defensive surgery no matter how accurate risk-adjustment is. If figures are accurately risk-adjusted, then there can be no disadvantages to surgeons that result from taking on high-risk patients. Surgeons who choose to take on high-risk patients, and are successful, will maintain low scores. Surgeons who have been taking on high-risk patients and cease to do so under a regime of proper risk-adjustment will end up with inferior scores (Oakley 2007a: 247), so they should be motivated to adjust their attitudes to match the reality of the system under which they work. Perhaps some surgeons may believe that risk-adjustment cannot succeed because they fail to understand the system under which they are being assessed. The solution to this problem is to attempt to educate them. Perhaps some surgeons are the victim of cognitive biases which reduce their ability to understand how risk-adjustment works. If so, this is a difficult problem to solve. A possible solution would be to over-adjust for high-risk operations, so that such surgeons are rewarded so heavily for conducting high-risk operations that their biases against conducting high-risk surgery might be overcome. However, this would involve running the risk of encouraging 'offensive surgery', in which surgeons who did not exhibit such a bias sought to avoid conducting operations on low-risk patients in order to protect or enhance their reputations, and so we are reluctant to recommend it.

Two influential US surveys of cardiac surgeons' attitudes suggest that some surgeons may be engaging in defensive surgery, at least in some parts of the United States (Burack et al. 1999; Schneider and Epstein 1996). Also, some commentators argue that there is reason to suspect that New York surgeons have artificially improved their published performance figures by encouraging some high-risk patients to seek operations interstate. An oft-cited study by Omoigui et al. (1996) of such 'outmigration' provides some evidence to substantiate this suggestion. The average number of high-risk cardiac patients from New York attending the Cleveland Clinic in Ohio increased from an average of 61 per year for 1981–1988, to 96 per year for 1989–1993, the first four years in which New York State operated a report cards system. Omoigui et al. (1996) and other commentators suggest that this is a direct result of the introduction of a report card system in New York State. However, there are several reasons to doubt that these figures explain away all, or even much, of the decrease in risk-adjusted mortality that was found. A comprehensive study of outmigration from New York for 1987–1992 found no increase in outmigration from New York State for CABG referrals for the whole of this period (Peterson et al. 1998). It seems that Omoigui et al.'s (1996) findings of outmigration may be a local phenomenon, reflecting long-term patterns of referral from the western edge of New York State, which is close to the Cleveland area. Outmigration did increase from this area, but the actual increase identified by Omoigui et al. (1996) does not correlate very well with the introduction of report cards in New York State, as it commenced two years before report cards were introduced there (Chassin et al. 1996; see also Oakley 2007a). In any case, it would seem to be implausible to appeal to outmigration to explain away the results of

Bridgewater et al.'s (2007) study of CABG surgery in north-west England. In addition to finding that mortality rates had decreased significantly, the researchers also found that there was no evidence of fewer high-risk patients undergoing surgery in north-west England as a result of the publication of cardiac surgeon performance data.

Surgeons who report practising defensive surgery are typically concerned about their reputation. From an ethical point of view, however, the possible effects on patients of defensive surgery are far more important than concerns about the reputations of surgeons. Suppose that we were able to find evidence of defensive surgery—would this be ethically unacceptable? If it were to lead to the situation where high-risk patients were unable to find a surgeon at all, then this would be difficult to justify ethically. However, studies of the distribution of high-risk patients indicate that such patients are not generally being avoided by hospitals and surgeons (Peterson et al. 1998; Chassin 2004; Bridgewater et al. 2007). If anything, the anecdotal evidence of defensive surgery reactions to public reporting suggests that such responses are more likely to be made by the least proficient surgeons (Burack 1999; Hannan et al. 1995; Chassin 2002). If defensive surgery predominantly involves less capable surgeons avoiding high-risk patients, and if high-risk patients are still able to find a surgeon to operate on them, then defensive surgery may actually be beneficial for high-risk patients. So even if we were to find evidence of defensive surgery, we do not believe that this would be a knock-down objection to the publicising of surgeons' performance information. More information would be required regarding the patterns of defensive surgery that were being caused.

PATIENTS' USE OF INFORMATION

A third line of objection to publishing surgeon performance data is that patients do not, in any case, make use of the information presented in report cards (whether or not they go 'surgeon-shopping'). Werner and Asch (2007: 213–14) set up the objection like this:

> Although the idea that patients will use public report cards to select the best clinical providers is plausible, this process requires several intermediate steps that are not so assured: (1) report cards must exist; (2) patients must know about the report cards and have access to them; (3) patients must be able to understand the quality rankings and believe them; and (4) patients must act on the report card information.

There is good reason to think that the current level of understanding of report cards, particularly the complicated New York State report cards, is low (Jewett and Hibbard 1996), and that it may be difficult to easily improve people's understanding of such information, given that this would require some education in statistical methods (Clarke 2007). For this reason, there is much to be said in favour of the earlier British three-star system of rating surgeons, which had the benefit of being easy to comprehend. Furthermore, there are reasons to believe that patients do not place a high degree of trust in published report cards, and that they may often be more reliant on the opinion of friends and relatives when it comes to choosing a surgeon (Gibbs et al. 1996). In short, there are good reasons to think that most patients do not currently make much use of report cards, and they may be unlikely to do so to any great extent in the short term.

We agree that these are important considerations. However, their importance can easily be overstated and they do not add up to a case against report cards. There are several reasons that lead us to reach this conclusion. First, even if many patients do not use report cards, some do, and it is plausible to think that their choices will be improved by the use of report cards. Second, it is also plausible to think that the number of patients who do make use of report cards will slowly increase as awareness increases and trust in the system is established (see Henderson and Henderson 2007). Third, even if relatively few patients use report cards to choose between surgeons (or if choice of surgeon is not available in a public health care system), report cards help patients to autonomously *authorise* operations upon themselves in the first place. The idea that information *material* to a patient ought to be made available to them means that they ought to be provided with information that they consider *relevant* to their decision (whether information about possible side-effects or about surgeon-specific risks), even if the information is not such as to make them change their mind about having the procedure (see Oakley 2007b). Fourth, some physicians use report cards in making referrals, and it is plausible to think that the quality of their referrals is improved by the use of report cards (Schneider and Epstein 1996; Hannan et al. 1997). Fifth, it seems that, although many patients do not make use of report cards themselves, the majority are in favour of a public report card system being in place, as they see it as a means of ensuring the accountability of the medical system to the public (Kaiser Family Foundation and Agency for Health Care Research and Quality 2004).

CHOICES MADE ON THE BASIS OF SAFETY

A final objection is to the very idea of patient choice being made on the basis of considerations of safety. This objection is made by Margaret Schwarze (2007), who reasons by analogy to airline travel. According to her:

> passengers choose to fly different airlines because of the basis of the price of the ticket, the size of the seats on the plane, the number of stops the schedule of arrivals, or the luxury of the services provided. All of these choices are legitimate and valuable. We don't let passengers choose their airline based on the safety performance of the airline. It is not a legitimate choice for passengers to choose an unsafe pilot or airline; furthermore there is no value for the passenger to have the opportunity to choose between safe and unsafe pilots and airlines. (2007: 515)

One might respond to Schwarze by resisting the analogy between medicine and airline travel, but we will not pursue this path because we think that she is wrong in the case of airline travel and that the errors in reasoning here are instructive. Her basic error is factual. Airline safety information is freely available on the internet. For example, <www.airsafe.com> lists fatalities per million flights for a range of airlines, enabling a direct comparison between airlines on safety grounds. If passengers want to make choices to fly on the basis of information about safety, it is easy for them to do so. But even before the rise of the internet and the easy availability of comparative data, passengers made such choices on the basis of anecdotal evidence. Raymond, the autistic character from the 1988 film *Rain Man,* was not alone in insisting on flying Qantas rather than any other airline because of its (then) accident-free record. The fact is that some passengers do make choices of airlines on the basis of safety considerations. These are rational choices and they are legally acceptable ones.

However, we suspect that Schwarze means to express a normative, rather than a straightforwardly factual, claim. We suspect that she supposes that airlines ought to respond to evidence of lapses in safety by taking steps to make their flights safer, rather than by, say, accepting a poor safety record and competing on other grounds. We agree with Schwarze that all airlines should be required to meet a threshold standard of safely before being allowed to fly. However, if they are able to exceed this threshold then we see nothing wrong with allowing passengers to choose airlines, or even pilots, on the basis of safety considerations. The same reasoning holds for surgeons. If surgeons fail to meet a threshold of competence, then the community is entitled to refuse to allow them to practise. It is reckless to do otherwise. However, it remains rational for patients to choose surgeons on the basis of their ability to exceed this standard of competence by a greater or lesser degree.

CONCLUSION

The argument that surgeon report cards improve the quality and safety of surgical care has figured prominently in debates about public reporting of surgeon performance information. We have examined four important objections to this argument, and found that none of them provides a decisive reason against the quality and safety argument for surgeon report cards.[8]

REFERENCES

Bridgewater, B., Grayson, A.D., Brooks, N., Grotte, G., Fabri, B.M., Au, J., Hooper, T., Jones, M. and Keogh, B. 2007, 'Has the publication of cardiac surgery outcome data been associated with changes in practice in northwest England? An analysis of 25,730 patients undergoing CABG surgery under 30 surgeons over eight years', *Heart*, vol. 93, pp. 744-8

Burack, J. H., Impellizzeri, P., Homel, P. and Cunningham J.N. 1999, 'Public reporting of surgical mortality: A survey of New York State cardiothoracic surgeons', *Annals of Thoracic Surgery*, vol. 68, pp. 1195-1200

Chassin, M.R. 2002, 'Achieving and sustaining improved quality: Lessons from New York State and cardiac surgery', *Health Affairs*, vol. 21, pp. 40-51

—— 2004, 'Interview with Justin Oakley and David Neil', 13 February 2004

Chassin, M.R., Hannan, E.L. and DeBuono, B.A. 1996, 'Benefits and hazards of reporting medical outcomes publicly', *New England Journal of Medicine*, vol. 334, pp. 394-8

Clarke, S. 2007, 'Surgeons' report cards: Heuristics, biases and informed consent', in *Informed Consent and Clinician Accountability: The Ethics of Report Cards on Surgeon Performance*, eds S. Clarke and J. Oakley, Cambridge University Press, Cambridge, pp. 167-79

Clarke, S. and Oakley, J. 2004, 'Informed consent and surgeons' performance', *The Journal of Medicine and Philosophy*, vol. 29, pp. 11-35

Clarke, S., Oakley, J., Neil D.A. and Ibrahim, J. 2005, 'Public reporting on individual surgeon performance', *Medical Journal of Australia*, vol. 183, no. 10, p. 543

Duckett, S.J., Collins, J., Kamp, M. and Walker, K. 2008, 'An improvement focus in public reporting: The Queensland approach', *Medical Journal of Australia*, vol. 189, nos 11/12, pp. 616-17

Fung, C.H., Lim, Y-W., Mattke, S., Damberg, C. and Shekelle, P.G. 2008, 'Systematic review: The evidence that publishing patient care performance data improves quality of care', *Annals of Internal Medicine*, vol. 148, no. 2, pp. 111-23

Gibbs, D.A., Sangl, J.A. and Burrus, B. 1996, 'Consumer perspectives on information needs for health plan choice', *Health Care Financing Review*, vol. 18, no. 1, pp. 55-73

Hannan, E.L., Siu, A.L., Kumar, D., Kilburn, H. and Chassin, M.R. 1995, 'The decline in coronary artery bypass graft mortality in New York State', *Journal of the American Medical Association*, vol. 273, no. 3, pp. 209-13

Hannan, E.L., Stone, C.C., Biddle, T.L. and DeBuono, B.A. 1997, 'Public release of cardiac surgery outcomes data in New York: What do New York State cardiologists think of it?', *American Heart Journal*, vol. 134, no. 6, pp. 55-61

Hannan, E.L., Vaughn Sarrazin, M.S., Doran, D.R. and Rosenthal, G.E. 2003, 'Provider profiling and quality improvement efforts in coronary artery bypass graft surgery: The effect on short-term mortality among Medicare beneficiaries', *Medical Care*, vol. 41, no. 10, pp. 1164-72

Henderson, A.J. and Henderson, S.T. 2007, 'Provision of a surgeon's performance data for people considering elective surgery' (Protocol), *The Cochrane Library*, no. 1, <www.thecochranelibrary.com>, accessed 16 December 2008

Hughes, C.F. and Mackay, P. 2006, 'Sea change: Public reporting and the safety and quality of the Australian health care system', *Medical Journal of Australia*, vol. 184, suppl. 10, pp. S44-47

Jewett, J.J. and Hibbard, J.H. 1996, 'Comprehension of quality care indicators: Differences among privately insured, publicly insured, and uninsured', *Health Care Financing Review*, vol. 18, pp. 75-94

Kaiser Family Foundation and Agency for Health Care Research and Quality 2004, *National Survey on Consumers' Experiences with Patient Safety and Quality Information*, Kaiser Family Foundation, Washington, DC

Lanier, D., Roland, M., Burstin, H. and Knottnerus, J.A. 2003, 'Doctor performance and public accountability', *The Lancet*, vol. 362, no. 9393, pp. 1404-8

Marasco, S. and Ibrahim, J. 2007, 'Is the reporting of an individual surgeon's clinical performance doing more harm than good for patient care?' in *Informed Consent and Clinician Accountability: The Ethics of Report Cards on Surgeon Performance*, eds S. Clarke and J. Oakley, Cambridge University Press, Cambridge, pp. 197-211

Marshall, M.N. and Brook, R.H. 2002, 'Public reporting of comparative information about quality of healthcare', *Medical Journal of Australia*, vol. 176, no. 5, pp. 205–6

Marshall, M.N., Shekelle, P., Leatherman, S., Brook, R. and Owen, J.W. 2000, *Dying to Know: Public Release of Information about Quality of Health Care*, RAND Corporation/Nuffield Trust, Los Angeles and London

Neil, D.A., Clarke, S. and Oakley, J.G. 2004, 'Public reporting of individual surgeon performance information: United Kingdom developments and Australian issues', *Medical Journal of Australia*, vol. 181, no. 5, pp. 266–8

Oakley, J. 2007a, 'An ethical analysis of the defensive surgery objection to individual surgeons report cards', in *Informed Consent and Clinician Accountability: the Ethics of Report Cards on Surgeon Performance*, eds S. Clarke and J. Oakley, Cambridge University Press, Cambridge, pp. 243–54

—— 2007b, 'Patients and disclosure of surgical risk', in *Principles of Health Care Ethics,* 2nd ed., eds R. Ashcroft, A. Dawson, H. Draper and J. McMillan, John Wiley, London, pp. 319–24

Omoigui, N.A., Miller, D.P., Brown, K.J., Annan, K., Cosgrove, D., Lytle, B., Loop, F. and Topol, E.J. 1996, 'Outmigration for coronary bypass surgery in an era of public dissemination of clinical outcomes', *Circulation*, vol. 93, no. 1, pp. 27–33

Peterson, E.D., De Long, E.R., Jollis, J.G., Muhlbaier, L.H. and Mark, D.B. 1998, 'The effects of New York's bypass surgery provider profiling on access to care and patient outcomes in the elderly', *Journal of the American College of Cardiology*, vol. 32, no. 4, pp. 993–9

Schneider, E.C. and Epstein, A.M. 1996, 'Influence of cardiac-surgery performance reports on referral practices and access to care—a survey of cardiovascular specialists', *New England Journal of Medicine*, vol. 335, no. 4, pp. 251–6

Schwarze, M.L. 2007, 'The process of informed consent: Neither the time nor the place for disclosure of surgeon-specific outcomes', *Annals of Surgery*, vol. 245, no. 4, pp. 514–15

Semmens, J.B., Aitken, R.J., Sanfilippo, F.M., Mukhtar, S.A., Haynes, N.S. and Mountain, J.A. 2005, 'The Western Australian Audit of Surgical Mortality: Advancing surgical accountability', *Medical Journal of Australia*, vol. 183, no. 10, pp. 504–8

Swan, N. 2004, 'Choosing the right surgeon', *The Health Report*, ABC Radio National, 27 September, interviewing Dr Russell Stitz, President of the Royal Australasian College of Surgeons, <www.abc.net.au/rn/healthreport/stories/2004/1208621.htm>, accessed 3 April 2009

—— 2008, 'Public release of health care performance data', *The Health Report*, ABC Radio National, 3 November, interviewing Professor Martin Marshall.

<www.abc.net.au/rn/healthreport/stories/2008/2405760.htm>, accessed 3 April 2009

Vass, A. 2002, 'Performance of individual surgeons to be published', *British Medical Journal*, vol. 324, no. 7331, p. 189

UK Healthcare Commission 2007, 'Rates of survival after heart surgery in the UK', <http://heartsurgery.healthcarecommission.org.uk/Survival.aspx>, accessed 15 December 2008

Werner, R.M. and Asch, D.A. 2007, 'Examining the link between publicly reporting healthcare quality and quality improvement', in *Informed Consent and Clinician Accountability: The Ethics of Report Cards on Surgeon Performance*, eds S. Clarke and J. Oakley, Cambridge University Press, Cambridge, pp. 212–225

NOTES

1   Mortality rates of (de-identified) cardiac units in public hospitals have been published on the internet by the Victorian Department of Human Services since 2002 (see <www.health.vic.gov.au/specialtysurgery/cardiac.htm>). The National Surgical Mortality Audit model developed by the Western Australian branch of the Royal Australasian College of Surgeons has been adopted nationally (see Semmens et al. 2005). See also the dynamic approach to hospital monitoring and public reporting in Queensland Health's annual public hospital performance reports, described in Duckett et al. (2008).

2   The trial of surgeon Dr Jayant Patel may accelerate moves towards public reporting of performance data about health care providers.

3   Referred to as the 'Butcher of Bega' on SBS-TV *Insight: Losing Patients*, 15 April 2008.

4   Also, the Australasian College of Cosmetic Surgery requires cosmetic surgeons to reveal to patients how many times the surgeon has carried out a particular procedure if it is fewer than 100 (see *The Age*, 1 November 2008, p. 6).

5   See the focus group discussions conducted with Melbourne cardiac surgeons during 2004–05, as part of the NHMRC-funded project 236877, *An Ethical Analysis of the Disclosure of Surgeons' Performance Data to Patients Within the Informed Consent Process*.

6   There is also the question of whether publishing unit-level data vs. surgeon-specific data does more to improve patient safety. This question remains unresolved, but we see these as complementary initiatives. Certainly this is how they have been regarded by the UK Healthcare Commission.

7   Note, however, that UK public patients might indirectly 'surgeon-shop' through 'hospital-shopping'; after all, this is part of the point of the Dr Foster

hospital reports for most surgical procedures. These reports are published quarterly as newspaper supplements to *The Times*, and are also available online at: <www.drfosterintelligence.co.uk>.

8   Thanks to an audience at the Oxford–Mt Sinai Consortium on Bioethics, Annual Conference, University of Oxford, 2008. Some of the research for this chapter was supported by National Health and Medical Research Council Project Grant 236877.

11

DISCLOSURE OF MEDICAL INJURY

David Studdert

INTRODUCTION

The global patient safety movement is young. A decade ago, neither health policy-makers nor members of the general public were focused on the problem, and it was a small boutique corner of health services research. In the 1990s, researchers in the United States and Australia, through clinical reviews of large random samples of medical records, estimated rates of inpatient adverse events (Brennan et al. 1991; Wilson et al. 1995; Thomas et al. 2000). The rates were alarmingly high. In 1999, the Institute of Medicine's[1] report, *To Err is Human* (Kohn et al. 2000), recast the United States figures in terms of preventable deaths, famously declaring that between 44,000 and 98,000 Americans died each year as a result of preventable medical errors. With that, the global patient safety movement set sail.

Around the world, numerous public inquiries, a steady drumbeat of media interest and hundreds of millions of dollars in research funds followed. Countries that did not have their own national adverse event estimates sought them, largely replicating the methodology used in the United States and Australian studies. States and hospitals scrambled to establish surveillance systems for tracking injuries, usually in the form of adverse event reporting mechanisms, as the Institute of Medicine's report had strongly urged. Today, efforts to prevent medical injury have assumed a place among the health policy priorities of many countries and the World Health Organization (World Health Organization 2008).

In retrospect, it is clear that the imagery of preventable deaths captured the public imagination in ways that the broader quality of care movement—despite being decades older, methodologically more sophisticated, and arguably more important in public health terms— never could (Brennan et al. 2005). The equation of mortality from medical error to daily jumbo jet crashes (Leape 1994) scared people and prompted immediate government action. Surveys soon showed that patient experiences with adverse events were common (Blendon et al. 2002); if patients were not attuned to the problem of medical error before the waves of publicity hit, they became so afterwards.

That the 'secret' burden of medical injury should be 'unlocked' through random patient chart review studies was, in some respects, as startling as the discovery itself. To many observers, it signalled a fundamental failure in transparency and accountability by the medical establishment (Gibson and Singh 2003; Banja 2005). To some, medicine's time-honoured risk-management strategy for mishaps—straight bat, say as little as possible—now seemed less an understandable medico-legal response to isolated events than a systemic cover-up operation.[2] At any rate, a divide clearly existed between standard clinical practice and what most patients expected to be told when care did not go as planned, especially when they had sustained injury due to error (Gallagher et al. 2003).

This divide has been interpreted by many regulators in the health care sector as a call to arms. Over the last five years, legislators, government agencies, accreditation organisations, professional bodies and hospitals around the world have sought to better align professional practice around disclosure with public expectations (Gallagher et al. 2007). This chapter overviews that activity. Although the focus is on Australia, comparisons are made with developments in other countries, particularly the United States, which sits beside Australia at the vanguard of countries regulating to promote disclosure.

WHY DISCLOSE?

Available evidence suggests that the vast majority of patients want and expect to be told of things that go wrong in their care (Witman et al. 1996; Vincent et al. 1994; Hingorani et al. 1999; Hobgood et al. 2002). But what rationale besides populism justifies disclosure as a socially desirable practice, one deserving of the force of regulation to advance it? There are two main rationales, one grounded in considerations of justice and medical ethics, the other in considerations of injury prevention and public health.

The ethical imperative

Respect for patient autonomy is a guiding ethical principle in modern medical practice (Beauchamp and Childress 1994). Informed consent, decision-making by families at the end of life and the sharing of prognostic information with patients are all manifestations of a broad consensus that competent adults are best placed to make their own health care choices. To impose another's views—a clinician's, hospital's, government's—in deciding what happens to a patient's body would be to treat patients like children or animals.

Concerns to ensure patient autonomy usually emphasise measures at the front end of care. The doctrine of informed consent, for example, dictates disclosure of treatment risks and options in comprehensible form before a patient signs on to a particular treatment. But respect for autonomy is not restricted to particular parts of the care continuum. The immediate aftermath of care remains part of the course of treatment, especially when the clinician–patient relationship remains intact. Notions of both autonomy and justice dictate that patients continue to have strong interests in receiving information about their care after it has been rendered, including any information the provider may have that explains how treatment has affected the patient's well-being.

Several other more pragmatic considerations bolster the ethical case for disclosure. A climate in which clinicians are not forthright with patients about what happens during care may damage trust, which is increasingly recognised as a critical ingredient of a successful therapeutic relationship (Hall 2002). In addition, an adverse event is often the starting point in a new process of care. Therefore, failure to disclose it may limit patients' opportunities to make informed decisions about future treatments.

The public health imperative

Medicine is a latecomer to the science of accidents, but decades of experience accumulated in other industries, such as aviation and nuclear power, indicate that openness about error is critical to prevention (Perrow 1984; Reason 1997). 'Every defect a treasure' goes the mantra in quality improvement circles (James 1997). Burial of that treasure is a foregone opportunity to identify vulnerable points, or 'latent errors', in systems of care; it is also indicative of a culture lacking the ingredients necessary for error prevention strategies to succeed (Reason 1990).

Calls for transparency usually focus on the need for better reporting of adverse events and near-misses. The need to establish new reporting systems and invigorate existing ones was a key recommendation of *To Err is Human* (Kohn et al. 2000), and called for by many patient safety experts (Berwick and Leape 1999). The industry has responded. Surveillance through reporting systems provides valuable raw material for identifying causal factors behind common and serious errors. Insights from those analyses may then be used to shape and implement prevention strategies.

What has any of this got to do with disclosure? Adverse event reporting and disclosure are two sides of the transparency coin. A provider who does not report is unlikely to disclose, and vice versa. Thus, promotion of disclosure reflects and promotes a culture of openness on which successful prevention activities hinge.

REGULATORY APPROACHES

It is too soon to anticipate the range of regulatory strategies that will be deployed to advance the policy goal of increasing the frequency and effectiveness with which providers disclose unanticipated outcomes of care to patients. To date, however, policy-makers have favoured two main strategies.

The first strategy involves development and promulgation of standards to guide practice. Although they are voluntary and exhortative in nature, these standards typically contain fairly detailed 'how to' information aimed at improving the quality and timeliness of disclosure (see Chapter 4).

The second strategy consists of attempts to stimulate providers' willingness to disclose by mitigating perceived barriers to the practice. Survey data and anecdotal evidence suggest clinicians and hospital leaders fear that information conveyed in disclosure conversations will increase their medico-legal exposure (Gallagher et al. 2003; Lamb et al. 2003). To combat this fear, and thus remove an ostensibly important obstacle to disclosure, policy-makers have enacted or strengthened laws protecting certain parts of disclosure conversations from use in legal proceedings against providers; they have also looked to existing 'qualified privilege' laws for further safeguards.

VOLUNTARY STANDARDS

Modest beginnings

Historically, providers have had little or no guidance on when and how to discuss adverse events and errors with patients. The conventional risk-management response of saying no more than was absolutely necessary essentially quashed interest in developing such expertise. Some medical professional organisations nodded to disclosure as an ethical obligation, but they neither emphasised its importance nor armed members with the tools needed to conduct disclosure effectively (Gallagher et al. 2007).

The first formal attempt to regulate disclosure appeared in the United States in 2001. The Joint Commission on Accreditation of Healthcare Organizations[3] issued a requirement that patients be informed about all outcomes of care, including 'unanticipated outcomes' (Joint Commission 2001). It was a modest start. The standard did not specify the content of a disclosure conversation, nor did it compel an explanation that the unanticipated outcomes were due to error, partly out of concern that the standard not force admissions of liability (Gallagher et al. 2007). Nonetheless, the Joint Commission's move was groundbreaking; it heralded a shift from mere endorsement of the importance of disclosure to a requirement with some teeth, linked as it was to the accreditation status of hospitals.

Australia's National Open Disclosure Standard

Australia was next. The Australian Council for Safety and Quality in Health Care, established in 2000, quickly designated disclosure as a priority area. The Council presciently cast disclosure as general quality improvement issue rather than as a problem area in need of special oversight. The National Open Disclosure Standard (NODS) was developed in 2002, and endorsed by the Australian Health Ministers in July 2003 (Australian Commission on Safety and Quality in Health Care 2008).

NODS is a substantive document. Its stated intention is to facilitate open communication with patients and their families about adverse events in health care.[4] NODS specifies the main elements of a disclosure as: an expression of regret; a factual explanation of what happened; and an outline of the consequences of the event, including steps being taken to manage it and prevent a recurrence. Importantly, the standard also outlines a process through which disclosure should occur. One limitation, which comes through the description of the various steps and resources involved in the process, is that the standard is geared primarily towards disclosure in hospital settings.

The standard has been disseminated widely through the Australian health care system. Some states have adopted policies aimed at increasing its uptake (see, for example, New South Wales Health 2007; Queensland Health 2006). A recent evaluation of the standard's implementation at 21 of 40 pilot sites around Australia suggested a reasonable degree of enthusiasm for it among both patients and providers (Iedema et al. 2008). However, uncertainty remains about the feasibility of incorporating NODS into the care process, particularly about how the additional burdens it creates will be resourced.

Other standards

Following the lead of the United States and Australia, several other countries have issued disclosure standards. The United Kingdom's *Being Open* policy, modelled on NODS, was established in 2006 and accompanied by an ambitious educational campaign (National Patient Safety Agency 2005). The Canadian Patient Safety Institute released formal guidelines in 2008 after extensive consultation (Patient Safety Institute 2008). In New Zealand, disclosure has been endorsed in principle, and district health boards must have disclosure policies in place by 2010 (Malcolm and Barnett 2007).

Common themes

Looking across this collection of disclosure standards and guidelines, several common features are evident. First, all are voluntary in nature and eschew heavy-handed enforcement. Second, there are tensions and ambiguities in the standards about whether acknowledgment of error is appropriate or desirable. Most standards are studiously vague on this point, although the Canadian guidelines go so far as to explicitly disavow the use of the term 'error'.

Third, on the question of whether an apology should form part of disclosure, tensions and qualifiers are evident. The UK policy is unusually direct in stating that: 'Patients and/or their carers should receive an apology . . . and staff should feel able to apologise on the spot' (National Patient Safety Agency 2005: 6). NODS, however, includes an 'expression of regret' as an appropriate element of a disclosure, defining it as 'an expression of sorrow for the harm experienced by the patient'. The Canadian guidelines use the same term, noting that:

In principle, apology as part of disclosure of an adverse event ... [is] the right thing to do. In practice, apology as part of disclosure is complex because of the ambiguity of commonly used apology language. There is a belief that apology implies blame for providers, which is often inconsistent with a just patient safety culture. There is also a widely expressed concern that an apology could be taken as a confession or admission of legal responsibility, exposing health care providers, organisations and others ... to potentially unwarranted risk. (Patient Safety Institute 2008: 23)

Thus, whether standards should encourage providers to apologise, and what form such apologies ought to take, remain vexed questions. They are questions, as the Canadian guidelines highlight, that feed directly to a larger debate about the impact of disclosure on medico-legal risk.

DOES DISCLOSURE INCREASE PROVIDERS EXPOSURE TO LIABILITY?

Clear tensions exist between the push for greater transparency about adverse events and the traditional risk-management view that revelation increases clinicians' vulnerability to liability (Studdert and Brennan 2001). In the United States, where most of the research on disclosure has been conducted to date, surveys of doctors have consistently identified fear of increased liability as one of the main reasons they are reluctant to communicate with patients about adverse events (Gallagher et al. 2003). Unfortunately, no strong evidence exists there or elsewhere on whether openly communicating about unanticipated outcomes increases liability exposure, decreases it or leaves it unaffected.

There is some anecdotal evidence that open communication about unanticipated outcomes of care may not increase the total compensation costs borne by self-insured hospitals. The best known example is the experience reported by officials from the Veterans Affairs Medical Center in Lexington, Kentucky (Kraman and Hamm 1999). Similar reports are beginning to accumulate from other US health care facilities, suggesting that adoption of progressive disclosure policies does not have negative liability consequences, and may actually have beneficial ones. For example, the University of Michigan Health System recently reported that, since adopting a policy of encouraging physicians to disclose errors and apologise, annual attorney fees and legal actions had decreased by over 50 per cent (Tanner 2002; Boothman 2006).

Despite these promising anecdotes, population-level evidence on the medico-legal implications of disclosure is not yet available, and may not be for some time (Kachalia et al. 2003). Moreover, the Australian litigation environment is quite different from that in the United States: rates of claim and payout levels are markedly lower in Australia, particularly following the round of tort reforms in the early 2000s, which makes it difficult to extrapolate from American experience. Research into the litigation impact of disclosure in Australia is needed but, due to the 'long tail' of litigation and the difficulty of tracking disclosure in real time, this evaluation will not be quick or straightforward.

In the meantime, I believe the cautious view is that disclosure may not have the kind of chilling effect in litigation that some advocates have projected, and may in fact lead to an increase in litigation. The explanation lies in recognising that disclosure may have a claim-inhibiting effect in some circumstances, but a claim-prompting effect in others (Studdert et al. 2007). In other words, although disclosure may quell some patients' interest in litigating, it will ignite interest in others, particularly those who would not have learned of their injury in the absence of the disclosure. The net impact of disclosure on the size and cost of litigation ultimately depends on the balance between these two effects.

But, regardless of whether perceptions about the medico-legal implications of disclosure match the reality, the fact is that many providers remain wary, and this wariness undercuts enthusiasm for disclosure. In response, policy-makers have taken two steps: passage of apology laws, and invigoration of qualified privilege laws as they relate to disclosure activities. The next two sections discuss developments on each of these fronts.

APOLOGY LAWS

Rationale

As alluded to earlier, apology has emerged as probably the most controversial issue in the disclosure debate. Some commentators argue that an apology is no less than a moral imperative, and that providers who do not apologise after a harmful error are behaving unethically (Berlinger 1995; Studdert et al. 2007). Providers' resistance to disclosure in general, and apologies in particular, appears to be rooted in medico-legal concerns, yet apology advocates counter that this move actually *reduces* medico-legal activity (Wojcieszak et al. 2007; Boothman 2006).

The energy and forcefulness with which adherents to the latter view have pressed their case is remarkable, particularly in the United States where they have coalesced into something approaching a political movement (Wojcieszak et al. 2007; Clinton and Obama 2006).

The laws

As stakeholders in the medical, patient safety and legal communities thrash out these issues, legislators have quietly gone about passing laws aimed at encouraging apologies and softening provider resistance by attempting to reduce perceived medico-legal risks. So called 'apology laws' have been enacted in approximately 35 American states (Gallagher et al. 2007 and in every Australian state and territory.

Australian apology laws share several common features. An 'apology' is defined as an expression of regret or sorrow made orally or in writing. The laws pertain to apologies made after 'incidents' occur and laws are directed towards restricting the inferences that may be drawn from apologies, the uses to which apologies may be put in civil proceedings, or both. The laws generally relate to personal injury and civil proceedings, not specifically to medical injury or medical negligence litigation.

Although all (or nearly all) apology laws share the above features, they also vary in several aspects of their structure and breadth. All but two jurisdictions (the Northern Territory and Queensland) declare that an apology is not an admission of fault or liability. Four jurisdictions explicitly state that apologies are not relevant to determinations of fault or liability. And the laws in all but two jurisdictions (South Australia and Victoria) include what is probably the most potent statement: an apology is inadmissible in civil proceedings.

How much protection?

There are many reasons why these apology laws may not be sufficient to mollify anxiety about disclosure among providers (Madden and Cockburn 2007; Iedema et al. 2008). Two potential 'holes' are apparent in the protections themselves. First, in every jurisdiction except the Australian Capital Territory and New South Wales, an admission of fault or liability is explicitly excluded from the definition of an apology; in other words, if a *mea culpa* statement forms part of the disclosure conversation, the apology law's protections may be lost.

Second, an apology is merely one element in a comprehensive disclosure, as the NODS makes clear. When the apology law protections apply, this aspect of the disclosure conversation may not be indicative of fault nor admissible in civil proceedings, but other aspects of the conversation could be—for example, accompanying information related to causality ('Our care caused your injury') or fault ('This should not have happened').The extent to which those other aspects of disclosure attract protection depends largely on the reach of a second body of law: statutory provisions relating to qualified privilege.

QUALIFIED PRIVILEGE FOR QUALITY ASSURANCE ACTIVITIES

Rationale

Qualified privilege is a legal doctrine that springs from common law and statute. It protects documents and communications from demands to disclose them—usually in the context of legal proceedings—provided specified conditions are met. The rationale for the special protection of qualified privilege is to encourage candidness and the free flow of information in circumstances in which that is regarded as socially beneficial.

Governments in Australia have long taken the view that information produced as part of activities and procedures aimed at improving quality of care in health care facilities may warrant qualified privilege. The general rationale applies. Improving quality and safety depends on a high degree of openness and honesty about failures. Health professionals must be willing to step forward to identify, discuss and analyse those failures. Without some confidence that the communications around these activities enjoy protection, there would be little enthusiasm for undertaking them. Indeed, the health professionals partaking in the activities could be forgiven for fearing that they were engaged in building a case against themselves.

The laws

All states and territories deal with qualified privilege in the health care context by statute. Four states (New South Wales, Queensland, Tasmania and Victoria) and both territories anchor the privilege provisions in an entity referred to as the Quality Assurance Committee (QAC). Western Australian law refers to a Quality Improvement Committee and the wording of a new law in South Australia (not yet in force) focuses on the group undertaking an 'authorised quality improvement activity'. The QAC, or its equivalent, is defined as a body engaged in quality assurance work, and declared by the relevant minister to be deserving of qualified privilege protections.

In sum, there is a fair degree of consistency in the structure and content of qualified privilege laws related to health care. New legislation in South Australia and Queensland is poised to bring the states further into line.

Relationship to disclosure

How does qualified privilege law intersect with disclosure? In some instances, the adverse event that triggers the disclosure process may also be, or may become, the subject of a QAC's work. This situation of overlap raises a couple of distinct questions: Do the *protections* provided to the QAC communications by qualified privilege laws extend to the contents of the disclosure conversation? And are there *prohibitions* (as opposed to protections) on the release of information introduced by qualified privilege law, which may inhibit the ability of persons conducting disclosure from conveying information to patients about what has happened to them?

How much protection?

A thorough examination of Commonwealth, state and territory laws relating to qualified privilege is needed to answer the questions posed above, and that has not been conducted for purposes of this review.[5] However, several general observations have relevance for both questions. First, many adverse events (defined broadly as unexpected outcomes) do not become the focus of work by a QAC; for those events, the qualified privilege laws will not be relevant. Second, for many adverse events, disclosure processes will be initiated very soon after the event has occurred—well before it has time to become the formal subject of a QAC's work. Thus, real-world temporal realities may obviate the applicability of privilege laws to disclosure conversations, even in situations in which the event goes on to become a QAC concern.

Third, the principal focus of QAC activities tends to be on the causes of adverse events, particularly organisational factors that have high potential for repetition. Why an adverse event occurred and what is being done to prevent its recurrence are undoubtedly important elements of a disclosure conversation. But they are not the only elements. Therefore, even if information about the event is deemed to fall under the umbrella of QAC privilege, it is not clear that the privilege would extend to all aspects of the disclosure conversation.

In summary, privilege laws aimed at QAC activities may extend some protections to the contents of disclosure conversations, but these protections appear to be neither broad nor strong in relation to disclosure. Limits on the protection they provide appear to stem primarily from their inapplicability to the disclosure process.

For similar reasons, claims that privilege laws inhibit or circumscribe the conveyance of information to patients as part of a disclosure process are probably overblown. In a few jurisdictions, most notably New South Wales and the Northern Territory, it is conceivable that certain types of information that health professionals may wish to draw into disclosure conversations may cross into the work of QACs, and thereby be restricted from release to patients. But, for the most part, disclosure conversations are not touched. Moreover, this use of the privilege provisions does not fit with their intended purpose.

MANDATES

Although policy-makers in Australia have discussed various mechanisms of motivating clinicians and hospitals to disclose more often and more effectively, there have been no strong moves in Australia to date to mandate the practice. By contrast, seven American states—Nevada, Florida, New Jersey, Pennsylvania, Oregon, Vermont and California—have enacted laws compelling health care institutions disclose serious unanticipated outcomes to patients. Pennsylvania's 2002 law was the first and arguably stands as the sternest.[6] It requires hospitals to notify patients in writing within seven days after a 'serious event'. To counteract concerns about litigation exposure, the law includes a provision prohibiting the use of the content of such communications as evidence of liability for the disclosed event.

CONCLUSION: WHAT FUTURE FOR DISCLOSURE AND ITS REGULATION?

A transformation is underway in how the medical profession communicates with patients about injuries and errors. One recent review predicted that 'full and frank disclosure of these events to patients is likely to be the norm rather than the exception' (Gallagher et al. 2007: 2718). To reach the point at which disclosure is business as usual, however, clinicians, risk managers and leaders in health care will need to undergo an attitudinal and practice transformation within their own professional ranks. Old habits die hard in medicine.

Disclosure is unlikely to become part of standard practice without a mix of coaxing, incentives and, most importantly, up-skilling to prepare clinicians to engage in these tremendously difficult conversations with patients. Regulation of disclosure thus looks set to continue, and quite possibly expand.

Changing entrenched professional practice, especially in medicine, is notoriously difficult. The favoured regulatory approaches to date— voluntary standards and measures aimed at reducing providers' medico-legal apprehensions—have been relatively meek and limited. It seems likely that they will not be sufficient to effect widespread changes in practice. Yet the appetite of the public and policy-makers for greater transparency about adverse events is unlikely to abate. This combination portends movement toward stiffer regulation and enforcement efforts in the future.

However, disclosure poses considerable challenges for command-and-control forms of oversight. Enforcement is nearly impossible. Without comprehensive adverse event reporting systems, as well as the substantial resources needed to audit patient medical records and to contact patients, it will be very difficult for regulators to monitor whether disclosures have occurred in appropriate circumstances, much less the quality of those disclosures. The actual content of disclosures is an especially elusive target for regulation. Disclosures are complex and subtle discussions, and should be tailored to the nature of the event, the clinical context and the patient–provider relationship; they are not amenable to 'cookbook' rules specifying precisely what information to disclose, and how.

For all of these reasons, the potential for top-down regulation to have a meaningful effect on disclosure conversations is limited. It is instructive that none of the US states that have enacted mandates have attempted serious enforcement, and only Pennsylvania even specifies the sanctions for non-compliance. The most successful disclosure initiatives are likely to be those that emerge locally, are driven by an institutional leadership and a workforce committed to transparency, and are underpinned by educational campaigns that provide front line clinicians with the needed skills.

What forms of regulation are best suited to ensure initiatives with those features flourish? If the current approaches are unlikely to achieve this end, and more traditional command-and-control approaches also have dim prospects, the path forward is unclear. It is an area ripe for creativity. The array of pressures and sensitivities that surround efforts to ensure openness with patients around injury and error are distinct, but not unique; other realms of patient safety face more or less similar challenges. Thus, what works best for disclosure may well turn out to borrow from, inform and ultimately resemble what works best elsewhere.

REFERENCES

Australian Commission on Safety and Quality in Health Care 2008, *Open Disclosure Standard*, <www.safetyandquality.gov.au/internet/safety/publishing.nsf/Content/former-pubs-archive-disclosure-progress>, accessed 5 November 2008

Banja, J. 2005, *Medical Errors and Medical Narcissism*, Jones and Bartlett, Sudbury, MA

Beauchamp, T. and Childress, J. 1994, *Principles of Biomedical Ethics*, Oxford University Press, Oxford

Berlinger, N. 1995, *After Harm: Medical Error and the Ethics of Forgiveness*, Johns Hopkins University Press, Baltimore, MD

Berwick, D.M., Leape, L.L. 1999, 'Reducing errors in medicine: It's time to take this more seriously', *British Medical Journal*, vol. 319, no. 7203, pp 136-7

Blendon, R.J., DesRoches, C.M., Brodie, M., Benson, J.M., Rosen, A.B., Schneider, E., Altman, D.E., Zapert, K., Herrmann, M.J. and Steffenson, A.E. 2002, 'Views of practicing physicians and the public on medical errors', *New England Journal of Medicine*, vol. 347, no. 24, pp. 1933-40

Boothman, R. 2006, 'Apologies and a strong defence at the University of Michigan Health System', *Physician Executive*, vol. 32, no. 2, pp. 7-10

Brennan, T.A., Gawande, A., Thomas, E. and Studdert, D. 2005, 'Accidental deaths, saved lives, and improved quality', *New England Journal of Medicine*, vol. 353, no. 13, pp. 1405-9

Brennan T.A., Leape L.L., Laird N.M., Hebert, L., Localio, A.R., Lawthers, A.G., et al. 1991, 'Incidence of adverse events and negligence in hospitalized patients: Results of the Harvard Medical Practice Study I', *New England Journal of Medicine*, vol. 324, pp 370-6

Clinton, H.R. and Obama, B. 2006, 'Making patient safety the centerpiece of medical liability reform', *New England Journal of Medicine*, vol. 354, no. 21, pp. 2205-8

Gallagher, T.H., Studdert, D.M., and Levinson, W. 2007, 'Disclosing harmful medical errors to patients: Recent developments and future directions', *New England Journal of Medicine*, vol. 356, no. 26, pp. 2713-19

Gallagher, T.H., Waterman, A.D., Ebers, A.G., Fraser, V.J. and Levinson, W. 2003, 'Patients' and physicians' attitudes regarding the disclosure of medical errors', *Journal of the American Medical Association*, vol. 289, no. 8, pp. 1001-7

Gibson, R. and Singh, J.P. 2003, *Wall of Silence: The Untold Story of the Medical Mistakes That Kill and Injure Millions of Americans*, Lifeline Press, Washington, DC

Hall, M.A. 2002, 'Law, Medicine and Trust', *Stanford Law Review*, vol. 55, no. 2, pp. 463-527

Hingorani, M., Wong, T. and Vafidis, G. 1999, 'Patients' and doctors' attitudes to amount of information given after unintended injury during treatment: Cross sectional, questionnaire survey', *British Medical Journal*, vol. 318, no. 7184, pp. 640-1

Hobgood, C., Peck, C.R., Gilbert, B., Chappell, K. and Zou, B. 2002, 'Medical errors—what and when: What do patients want to know?', *Academic Emergency Medicine*, vol. 9, no. 11, pp. 1156-61

Iedema, R.A.M., Mallock, N.A., Sorensen, R.J., Manias, E., Tuckett, A.G., Williams, A.F., Perrott, B.E., Brownhill, S.H., Piper, D.A., Hor, S., Hegney, D.G., Scheeres, H.B. and Jorm, C.M. 2008, 'The National Open Disclosure Pilot: Evaluation of a policy implementation initiative', *Medical Journal of Australia*, vol. 188, no. 7, pp. 397-400

James, B.C. 1997, 'Every defect a treasure: Learning from adverse events in hospitals', *Medical Journal of Australia*, vol. 166, no. 9, pp. 484-7

Joint Commission on Accreditation of Healthcare Organizations 2001, *Standard RI.1.2.2*, 1 July 2001

Kachalia, A., Shojania K.G., Hofer, T.P., Piotrowski, M. and Saint, S. 2003, 'Does full disclosure of medical errors affect malpractice liability? The jury is still out', *Joint Commission Journal on Quality and Patient Safety*, vol. 29, no. 10, pp. 503-11

Kohn, L.T., Corrigan, J.M. and Donaldson, M.S., eds 2000, *To Err is Human: Building a Safer Health System*, National Academy Press, Washington, DC

Kraman, S.S. and Hamm, G. 1999, 'Risk management: Extreme honesty may be the best policy', *Annals of Internal Medicine*, vol. 131, no. 12, pp. 963-7

Lamb, R.M., Studdert, D.M., Bohmer, R.M.J., Berwick. D.M. and Brennan, T.A. 2003, 'Hospital disclosure practices: Results of a national survey', *Health Affairs*, vol. 22, no. 2, pp. 73-83

Leape, L.L. 1994, 'Error in medicine', *Journal of the American Medical Association*, vol. 272, no. 23, pp. 1851-7

Madden, B. and Cockburn, T. 2007, 'Bundaberg and beyond: Duty to disclose adverse events to patients', *Journal of Law and Medicine*, vol. 14, no. 4, pp. 501-27

Malcolm, L. and Barnett, P. 2007, 'Disclosure of treatment injury in New Zealand's no-fault compensation system', *Australian Health Review*, vol. 31, no. 1, pp. 116–22

National Patient Safety Agency (UK) 2005, 'Safer practice notice—being open when patients are harmed', <www.clingov.nscsha.nhs.uk/Default.aspx?aid=2710>, accessed 5 November 2008

New South Wales Health 2007, 'Policy directive: Open disclosure', NSW Health, Sydney, <www.health.nsw.gov.au/policies/pd/2007/pdf/PD2007_040.pdf>, accessed 20 January 2008

Patient Safety Institute (Canada) 2008, 'Canadian Disclosure Guidelines', <www.patientsafetyinstitute.ca/Disclosure.html>, accessed 5 November 2008

Perrow, C. 1984, *Normal Accidents: Living with High-Risk Technologies*, Basic Books, New York

Queensland Health 2006, 'Clinical incident management implementation standard', Queensland Health, <www.health.qld.gov.au/patientsafety/documents/cimist.pdf>, accessed 21 January 2009

Reason, J.T. 1997, *Managing the Risks of Organizational Accidents*, Ashgate, Aldershot

Reason, J.T. 1990, *Human Error*, Cambridge University Press, New York

Studdert D.M. and Brennan T.A. 2001, 'No-fault compensation for medical injuries: The prospect for error prevention', *Journal of the American Medical Association*, vol. 286, no. 2, pp. 217–23

Studdert, D.M., Mello, M.M., Gawande, A.A., Brennan, T.A. and Wang, Y.C. 2007, 'Disclosure of medical injury to patients: An improbable risk management strategy', *Health Affairs*, vol. 26, no. 1, pp. 215–26

Tanner, L. 2002, '"Sorry" seen as magic word to avoid suits', *Seattle Post-Intelligencer*, 11 November

Thomas, E.J., Studdert, D.M., Burstin, H.R., Orav, E.J., Zeena, T., Williams, E.J., Howard, K.M., Weiler, P.C. and Brennan, T.A. 2000, 'Incidence and types of adverse events and negligent care in Utah and Colorado', *Medical Care*, vol. 38, no. 3, pp. 261–71

Vincent, C., Young, M. and Phillips, A. 1994, 'Why do people sue doctors?', *Lancet*, vol. 343, no. 8913, pp. 1609–13

Wilson, R.M., Runciman, W.B., Gibberd, R.W., Harrison, B.T., Newby, L. and Hamilton, J.D. 1995, 'The Quality in Australian Health Care Study', *Medical Journal of Australia*, vol. 163, no. 9, pp. 458–71

Witman, A.B., Park, D.M. and Hardin, S.B. 1996, 'How do patients want physicians to handle mistakes?', *Archives of Internal Medicine*, vol. 156, no. 22, pp. 2565–9

Wojcieszak, D., Saxton, J.W. and Finkelstein, M.M. 2007, *Sorry Works! Disclosure, Apology, and Relationships Prevent Medical Malpractice Claims*, AuthorHouse, Bloomington, IN

World Health Organization 2008, 'Patient safety', <www.who.int/patientsafety/en>, accessed 5 November 2008

NOTES

1   Part of the National Academies in the United States, the pre-eminent advisory body to government on science, engineering and medicine.

2   Like most grand conspiracy theories, this view almost certainly missed the mark: during our work in Utah and Colorado (Thomas et al. 2000), it became evident that, unfortunately, hospitals themselves had little or no systematic knowledge of where and how often adverse events were occurring within their facilities.

3   This organisation is now called the Joint Commission

4   An adverse event is defined in NODS as 'an incident in which unintended harm resulted to a person receiving health care'.

5   Work along these lines is underway, in a research project the author has recently been engaged to conduct for the Australian Commission on Safety and Quality in Health Care.

6   See Pennsylvania's *Medical Care Availability and Reduction of Error Act (Mcare)* 2002, Act 13, Sec. 302, <www.psa.state.pa.us/psa/lib/psa/act_13/act_13.pdf>, accessed 21 January 2009.

12

DOES LITIGATION AGAINST DOCTORS AND HOSPITALS IMPROVE QUALITY?

David Hirsch

While the incidence of iatrogenic injury is alarmingly high, the number of patients who ever seek, let alone receive, compensation for those injuries is surprisingly low. Despite the 'disconnect' between these numbers, there is considerable interest in the question of whether litigation against doctors and hospitals improves patient safety.

Early studies of this question have been anecdotal and of questionable quality. They have been used selectively by the opposing medical and legal protagonists during the 'medical indemnity crises' since the mid-1990s to argue for or against tort reform. As other chapters in this book amply demonstrate, an increasing body of scholarly literature has been emerging in recent years which is more rigorous in its analysis of medical error and its causes and the strategies for risk-reduction (for example, see Mello and Zeiler 2008). Measurable, empirical evidence of the effect of litigation on patient safety remains scant, however. Despite the lack of clear evidence, this chapter aims to show that there are good reasons to believe that litigation against doctors and hospitals in our fault-based tort law system does have a salutary effect on medical practice.

Broadly speaking, there are two ways in which litigation can promote quality and safety. First, litigation can impose *sanctions* where there are breaches of protocols and guidelines that have been developed by the medical profession itself to define and maintain an acceptable standard of care. The regulatory pyramid model holds that health care regulation moves upwards from 'soft' to 'hard' strategies—that is, from voluntarism up through the self-regulation by the professions, to command and control (Braithwaite et al. 2005). Equally basic to effective regulation are the twin principles of transparency and accountability, which both legitimate regulation and help drive changes in behaviour. In the responsive regulation model, litigation may be seen as the ultimate command and control mechanism. A public trial leading to a verdict against a wrongdoer both identifies and proscribes unacceptable conduct, and also satisfies the need for transparency and accountability.

Second, and more contentious, is whether litigation provides any effective *deterrent signal* that prevents poor practice and encourages good practice. It has been argued that in some limited circumstances litigation can have this desired effect, but that the complexities of medical error and the perceived inflexibility of legal principles make litigation a generally dubious driver of behaviour change (Mello and Brennan 2002). Most of the criticisms of fault-based tort law (which is the litigation system at issue) are, I suggest, a more or less thinly veiled attempt at insulating the medical profession from legal accountability, and also an attack upon lawyers—who are, after all, soft targets in a climate that saw insurance premiums rise sharply from the mid-1990s.

It is important to appreciate that, to the extent there is literature critical of medical litigation, it emanates almost exclusively from the United States or else relies heavily on American findings. The litigation landscape in the United States is, in many ways, unique and differs markedly from the situation in Australia. The 'arguments' against the benefits of litigation rely on anecdotes of unfairness and supposedly baseless decisions always seen from the doctors' point of view. These are coupled with the reflexive but largely discredited belief that the surge in medical indemnity premiums that led to the 'medical negligence crisis' and tort reform was driven by greedy lawyers and patients with unrealistic expectations (Mello et al. 2005).[1]

This chapter will discuss the role of litigation as the ultimate regulatory tool in promoting better health care by sanctioning against the breach of guidelines and protocols. It will then consider the deterrent signal of litigation. I argue that the oft-repeated criticisms, while attractive to those with an in-built bias against litigation, are largely without substance. I suggest that critics of litigation ignore the importance of legal accountability and the indirect benefits that flow from a compensation system which holds that avoidable iatrogenic injuries should have consequences for the doctors and hospitals responsible for causing them, and not simply for the patients who are left to suffer from them.

Before considering these two themes, it is important to address some misconceptions and practical realities about medical litigation in Australia, and also to consider the multiple objectives behind the tort law system. An appreciation of these will hopefully lead to a better understanding of whether, and to what extent, litigation can, and can be expected to be, an effective regulatory tool, a deterrent to poor practice and an impetus to better practice. At the very least, this discussion should lead to a more critical evaluation of the 'studies' that aim to promote the anti-litigation sentiment that pervades discourse in this area.

COMPARISONS WITH THE UNITED STATES

There are significant differences between medical litigation in the United States and Australia.

First, medical negligence trials in the United States are almost exclusively heard by juries, whereas in Australia almost all cases are decided by judges alone.[2] Critics often claim that juries ignore the evidence and vote on sympathy grounds, or that they cannot understand or do not apply the law. These criticisms are probably overstated even in the United States, where in about two-thirds of cases juries find for the doctors and, in general, award very modest compensation. This issue is irrelevant in Australia. Further, decisions made by judges must provide reasons, to which an appeal for clarification may be made, to ensure that the facts were properly understood and the law properly applied. Juries do not give reasons for their decision and their verdicts are, by and large, not subject to appeal.[3]

Second, an Australian litigant who loses a case will ordinarily be ordered to pay the legal costs of the winner. This costs penalty is a strong disincentive against making a claim in the first place. In the United States, where a person's right to advance a claim (meritorious or not) is nearly sacrosanct, there are no costs penalties if the claimant loses. This encourages more speculative claims and can account for more litigation than is seen in Australia.

Third, supposedly extravagant American jury awards of millions of dollars for 'pain and suffering' are thought to be a principal driver of rising claims costs and insurance premiums. Such awards are rare, even in the United States, but in Australia they are unheard of. Even in the unregulated environment before the tort reforms of recent years, the highest awards that Australian judges would give for pain and suffering would be around $400,000 (in New South Wales) and about half of that in other states (such as Queensland and Tasmania). In other words, in Australia before tort reform, a quadriplegic, ventilator-dependant 18-year-old, with full awareness of her circumstances and a normal life expectancy, was awarded no more than $400,000 for a life of misery and pain. Subsequent tort reforms have capped the already modest (and arguably inadequate) damages for pain and suffering in a reflexive response to the situation in the United States.

Fourth, American juries can award punitive damages in addition to compensatory damages. Punitive damages are, self-evidently, designed to punish the wrongdoer for 'high-handed, insolent, vindictive or malicious conduct' (see *Uren v John Fairfax & Sons Pty Ltd* 1966), and such damages are meant to assuage the desire for revenge. In Australia, punitive (or 'exemplary') damages in medical litigation historically were almost unheard of,[4] and tort reform has now eliminated the possibility of punitive damages altogether.

Finally, US lawyers charge contingency fees that entitle them to a percentage of the client's award (in medical negligence claims, usually around 40 per cent). This may account for the 'greedy lawyer' descriptions, although in a country wedded to free enterprise, such a criticism seems disingenuous. Such contingency fees are, however, illegal in Australia, where barristers and solicitors are generally engaged on the basis of hourly or daily rates, and cannot charge fees based on the value of the outcome. Whereas a US lawyer can expect to earn, say, $2 million from a successful $5 million claim, Australian lawyers would receive only a fraction of this, and the fee is based entirely on the value of the work actually done.

This is not an exhaustive list of the differences between the US and Australian litigation picture, although it aims to demonstrate that whatever perceived 'excesses' exist in the United States, they do not apply equally here. The literature that takes aim against US litigation therefore needs to be read with these differences in mind because medical litigation in Australia is more limited and measured.

PRACTICAL REALITIES

One of the practical barriers to litigation by aggrieved patients and their families is limited access to experienced lawyers willing to take on a case. Some believe that the speculative 'no win, no fee' arrangements that prevail in medical litigation in Australia encourage litigation, however, it is not that simple. First, the costs penalty rule remains, so if a patient sues a doctor and loses he will still pay the doctor's legal costs, even if his own lawyer gets nothing. Second, these speculative arrangements select against marginal or difficult cases because lawyers, hopeful of getting paid, tend to pursue only the clearest cases of negligence. This helps to explain why most cases settle out of court and few are ever heard by a judge.

In addition to caps on damages for pain and suffering, tort reform in many states has imposed thresholds to ensure that only claims involving the most severe injuries are worth pursuing. Because the vast majority of medical errors lead to relatively modest rather than catastrophic injuries, most cases of medical error never see the light of day as a legal claim.

Having eliminated smaller claims and capped recovery for serious injuries, tort reform in some states has thrown up a further barrier to litigation by limiting costs recovery for lawyers in cases where the damages recovered are below a certain value (e.g. $100,000 in New South Wales). This creates a disincentive for lawyers to take on cases with a value below the costs recovery threshold. In the end, even cases of medium value may not be financially worth pursuing from the plaintiff's point of view, or from a lawyer's point of view, and so these cases never see the light of day either.

All of this has been a boon to the insurance industry and to doctors whose risk of being sued—which was small to begin with—is even smaller now. For the present purposes, a practical consequence—intended or not—of tort reform is that whatever power litigation might have to 'police' and 'proscribe' medical errors is significantly reduced because fewer people are able to make claims and almost nobody is 'brought to book'.

The decrease in numbers is reported in the 'Medical Indemnity Insurance Report', published by the Australian Competition and Consumer Commission (ACCC) annually. The 2008 report (see Figure 12.1) demonstrates the decline in claims frequencies.[5] It can be seen that from 2002 the claims frequency has dropped relative to the ultimate number of claims expected to be paid. This demonstrates not only that fewer patients make claims but also that insurers expect to pay more of those that are made. This may be related to the merit of those claims but the trend has also been driven by the claims being cheaper to resolve than they were before the effects of tort reform, thus encouraging resolution.

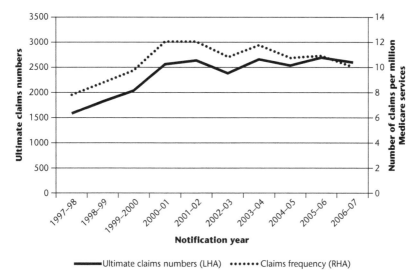

Figure 12.1 Ultimate claim numbers and claims frequency by year of notification, 1997–98 to 2006–07

Source: Australian Competition and Consumer Commission (2008: 25).

THE OBJECTIVES OF TORT LAW

Before any critical assessment is made of the value of medical litigation in improving patient safety, it behoves us to consider the objectives of tort law.

It is neither possible nor desirable to compensate everybody for every misfortune suffered from cradle to grave. Indeed, the over-arching principle of the common law is to let the loss lie where it falls, unless there is a *good reason* to shift the burden of loss from the injured person to somebody else.

Tort law aims to provide a coherent and workable system for compensating injured people. It holds that a *good reason* to shift the burden of loss exists where the damage complained of is caused by the fault of another. Every legal claim for compensation involves a determination of *fault, causation and damage.* If the plaintiff can prove, on the balance of probabilities, that her *damage* (the injuries and the losses) was *caused* (in a legal sense) by the *fault* (negligence) of the defendant, then she or he will be awarded compensation. The amount received is intended to restore the plaintiff, as far as money can, to the position he or she was in before the injury occurred.

Corrective justice and distributive justice are other objectives of tort law (see generally Balkin and Davis 2004: Chapter 1). Corrective justice holds that a person who injures another by his fault should be made responsible for the damage done. There is a subtle, but important, difference between *responsibility* (accepting 'ownership' of the wrong done) and *blame* (fixing moral culpability). Critics routinely and glibly complain that tort law is about blame; it is not.

Distributive justice aims to ensure a fairer distribution of the burdens and benefits of risky activities (Keating 2000). Essential to this objective is the availability of insurance. From the perspective of distributive justice, insurance should be viewed not as a burden about which to complain (as it has been during the 'indemnity crisis' years), but rather as the necessary cost of entitlement to practise a sometimes risky and often very lucrative profession.

Finally, and by no means paramount, is the objective of deterrence. On this point, some understanding of the difference between tort and crime is important. Historically, the prosecution of wrongdoers was a private matter where the aggrieved party brought an action seeking both compensation and retribution. Vengeance, moral culpability, punishment and immediate deterrence animated these private prosecutions. For reasons too complex to discuss here, private prosecutions diminished and the state, through its criminal laws, took over the business of defusing private vengeance by prosecuting and punishing the criminal in the name of the community at large, and, through sentencing, supposedly sending the deterrent signal far and wide.

In contrast to the public criminal law, tort law developed as a means for individuals to obtain private, civil redress from a wrongdoer. The test of wrongdoing was negligence, not criminal conduct. The objective was compensation for losses suffered, not punishment for moral culpability,[6] although certain vestiges of the historical private prosecution remained. Tort claimants seek 'vindication' in the sense of recognition of wrong-doing, and they expect the wrongdoer to 'learn a lesson' from a finding of negligence. They also expect that by publicly declaring what negligent conduct is, the law will force others to 'lift their game' and prevent injury to other innocent victims in the future.

It is in this small corner of tort law—its ability to declare what the standard of reasonable care is—that the question of the ability of litigation to improve patient safety arises. In the context of the overall aims of tort law, the deterrence objective is not prominent. Yet, in the arguments about medical litigation, and whether it should be preserved or replaced by a bureaucratic 'no fault' system, the ability of tort law to achieve deterrence is often seen as a touchstone of its relevance. I argue that medical litigation generates a strong, if sometimes indirect, deterrent signal. Even if the deterrent signal is weak, as the critics say, tort law needs to be preserved as a coherent compensation system *grounded in theories of corrective and distributive justice*, with the benefits of transparency of process and accountability for those whose lack of reasonable care caused avoidable injury.

LITIGATION AND REGULATION

Regulation is all well and good, but what happens when, despite the implementation of guidelines and protocols, these are ignored or flaunted? Few would disagree that there needs to be a mechanism to enforce compliance in these circumstances.

Internal sanctions like dismissal or deregistration exist, and may be engaged by employer hospitals as part of clinical governance, or by professional bodies to maintain public confidence and high standards. Unfortunately, there is no reason to think that these sanctions are systematic, and every reason to believe that they are not. Complaints by patients, whether to the hospital or a complaints commission, are managed with a view to conciliation and making the problem go away. Very few result in disciplinary action. Sometimes poor practice is discovered or reported internally. Laws have recently been passed that effectively force the medical profession to become whistleblowers against their own in some circumstances (see *Medical Profession Amendment Act* 2008 (NSW)). However, it is too early to tell whether this will have any effect other than to increase hostility towards the law and discourage doctors from disclosing their problems to their colleagues.

As will be seen, litigation can also sanction wrongdoing, but its application is even more haphazard than the internal sanctions noted above. With so few injured patients willing or able to bring a compensation claim, it is very easy to avoid the legal consequences of poor practice. With almost nobody 'getting caught', litigation may be considered irrelevant as a regulatory tool. This said, in those few cases where litigation is commenced, the existence of guidelines and protocols can be cogent evidence of what the profession itself considers to be the standard of reasonable care. The injured patient, who has the legal onus of proving fault in order to succeed, can be assisted significantly by demonstrating that there was no compliance with a rule designed to reduce the risk of harm, and iatrogenic injury has followed.

This is not to say that guidelines and protocols usurp the role of expert opinion; they do not. There may be cases where expert evidence shows that these are outdated or not relevant to the peculiar circumstances of the particular case, but by and large guidelines and protocols provide useful signposts for judges when deciding what a doctor should or should not have done.

The question of who sets the standard of reasonable care—the law or the medical profession—was decided in Australia in the well known 1992 High Court case *Rogers v Whitaker.* The case involved the failure to warn a patient with one good eye and one bad eye of a very small risk of total blindness due to sympathetic ophthalmia if she had an operation on the bad eye. The doctor admitted that no warning was given, and the court accepted that the patient would have declined the operation on her bad eye if she was aware of the risk of total blindness. The doctor's defence was that other doctors would have also failed to warn of the risk of sympathetic opththalmia because the risk was so slight. The doctor urged the High Court to follow the English approach set out in the 1957 case of *Bolam v Friern Hospital.* The *Bolam* test says that *a doctor* is not negligent if he acts in accordance with a practice accepted at the time as proper by a responsible body of medical opinion, even though other doctors adopt a different practice.

The High Court rejected the *Bolam* test for Australia, and maintained that judges, not doctors, will set the standard of reasonable care. While medical opinion—including best-practice guidelines and protocols—is important and often decisive, ultimately the question of negligence is for the law to decide and not for doctors to rule on themselves.

To be an effective regulatory tool, however, litigation must exert an influence beyond the particular case. This can only happen if and when the medical profession, and not just the persons directly involved, appreciates that breaches of guidelines and protocols can have legal consequences that involve public and professional scrutiny and perhaps financial pain. It is the awareness of those consequences and the desire to avoid them that lead to the next and more vexed question of the deterrent effect of litigation.

LITIGATION AND DETERRENCE

Arguments for and against the utility of litigation as a deterrent to bad practice and an impetus to good practice take as their starting point the proposition that people, being 'rational economic agents', will act to limit any adverse financial consequences of their actions. This economic theory makes two assumptions, both of which require closer examination. First, it assumes that people will alter their behaviour in response to perceived litigation risks. Second, it requires that that people 'internalise' the costs of errors, thus giving them a direct economic incentive to avoid making them.

In a careful review of the literature, Mello and Brennan (2002) examined the evidence for and against the *deterrent signal* of tort law. They found very little hard evidence that the threat of economic penalty was an incentive to behaviour change, at least in some contexts. In the areas of motor vehicle accidents, a comparison of fault-based tort compensation and no-fault compensation did not point to a strong deterrent signal for tort law; the number of accidents and fatalities did not significantly change. Mixed results were also found in the area of workers' compensation, although there did appear to be some relationship between experience-rated premiums and fatality rates. Mixed results were also found in the product liability area, with some manufacturers being prepared to continue to make and market dangerous products despite exposure to class actions for compensation.

One of the arguments often advanced against the utility of tort law as a deterrent is that insurance blunts the pain of any compensation claim, removing whatever economic 'sting' a claim might inflict. The idea is that if individuals had to directly pay for the consequences of, say, a motor vehicle accident where a pedestrian was rendered a quadriplegic, then each of us would drive more carefully. This is a facile argument. It is in the nature of most accidents that they occur because of innocent inadvertence and not reckless indifference to risk. If the latter were the case, criminal charges could be brought. Making individuals pay for the potentially catastrophic consequences of momentary inadvertence will not prevent these kinds of accidents.

It has also been argued that the only effect that litigation has against doctors and hospitals is that it encourages 'defensive medicine'—care provided for the sole or principal purpose of avoiding litigation. Mello and Brennan explain that, properly understood, this is over-deterrence or excessive precaution-taking; it does not actually deter substandard care.

Central to the process is the notion that a significant number of medical errors are preventable, and that enterprises can actually be active in their prevention. It is a truism that, in the context of health care delivery, most errors involve systems rather than isolated acts of inadvertence. A safe hospital is not one that employs perfect staff who never make mistakes (which is impossible), but rather one which puts checks and balances and procedures in place that anticipate and address errors before they spiral into catastrophic outcomes for patients.

What is true of medical enterprises is not, however, true of individual doctors. First, the likelihood of an individual doctor not aligned with an enterprise (for example, a general practitioner or private specialist) being sued is far lower than the likelihood of an enterprise being sued. For individuals, a lawsuit it a rare aberration whereas for enterprises it is a fairly common occurrence: the threat of litigation, and the costs involved, are therefore more 'real' for enterprises than for individual doctors. Second, individual doctors are well insulated by insurance from the direct economic effects of a compensation claim. Not only does general risk rating (as opposed to individual risk rating) ensure that their premiums will not increase if they are sued, they do not even have to pay an excess to access their insurance (what Americans call an 'insurance deductible') in the event of a claim.

The effectiveness of litigation as a deterrent to poor practice lies not in the reality of claims numbers and costs but *in their perception*. It is true that most individual doctors will never be sued, despite there being a widespread belief, fomented largely to encourage doctors to 'get on board' with the tort reform programs pushed by their insurers, that they will be. The fear of litigation far outstrips the reality. In this context, fear can have a salutary effect on behaviour. Although few doctors will feel any direct financial pain from having to pay damages to an injured patient, nor will their insurance coverage be jeopardised or their premiums increase because of a claim, the strongly promoted and held belief that this will occur has not altered.

It follows from the above that the economic argument for deterrence is more strongly felt in the enterprise context than at the level of the individual doctor. Larger claims numbers, internalisation of the costs of errors and the means to improve care through improved systems all support the view of an effective deterrent signal for medical enterprises. The economic argument for deterrence of errors made by doctors not aligned to an enterprise is, at least theoretically, much weaker. Does this mean that the threat of litigation does not exert any meaningful effect on the conduct of individual doctors?

In my view, the effect of the threat of litigation against individual doctors should not to be under-estimated. Although the economic consequences of error are not strong, those who would argue against the effectiveness of a deterrent signal on individual doctors fail to recognise that doctors, perhaps more than most people, are not 'rational economic agents'. Doctors have far more at stake than simple monetary loss in any possible litigation.

As any doctor who has been involved in a legal claim will tell you, the situation is enormously stressful, and the consequences (whether the doctor is found negligent or not) can be damaging to a doctor's hard-earned reputation. I believe it is these factors, and not money, which are at the root of doctors' anxieties about litigation. It is these less tangible, although arguably more important, consequences that provide a significant stimulus for individual doctors to do whatever they can to improve the way they practise.

While hospitals are more organic and web-like than an individual doctor's surgery, doctors also have systems which can be improved. In one case, a doctor was successfully sued for failing to properly convey abnormal test results to a woman who had breast cancer (see *Kite v Malycha* 1998). In another, a doctor failed to inform the partner of a man who had tested positive for HIV, despite the fact that both had attended the doctor for joint counselling about sexually transmitted diseases before embarking on a sexual relationship (see *PD v Harvey* 2003). Each of these cases involved isolated incidents and unusual facts, but the cases were widely reported. There is little doubt that doctors across Australia took note and reviewed their systems for reporting test results and counselling patients about sexually transmitted diseases.

OTHER CRITICISMS OF TORT LAW AS A REGULATORY MECHANISM

It will be seen from the foregoing that there are good reasons to believe that tort law can, and does, deter poor practice and promote patient safety. Litigation against medical enterprises is internalised by those organisations. A feedback loop sends a deterrent economic signal to improve systems. Litigation against doctors can also improve patient care, not so much because of the volume of claims against them and the costs of compensation, but because of the desire of doctors to avoid the legal process altogether.

Despite evidence of positive effects, arguments are still advanced against tort law and in favour of a no-fault compensation system. It is beyond the scope of this chapter to comprehensively analyse the arguments for and against each system, although it is worth looking at some of the criticisms in a general way.

Proof of negligence

Retrospective file reviews have shown that in many cases the medical reviewers would not have found negligence where judges or juries have, and conversely, they would have been critical of practices even though no negligence was found (Brennan et al. 1996). It is easy to conclude that success in a legal claim has little to do with actual negligence and more to do with other factors like sympathy and the quality of advocacy, ignoring some of the realities of medical litigation (Rice 2004). These conclusions should not be accepted uncritically.

First, it is artificial to simply review hospital records and determine whether there was negligence or not. Many cases involve events not recorded, or a conflict between what was recorded and what actually happened. Records are only part of the story. A trial where the facts can be tested by cross-examination is needed in order to arrive at a clear appraisal of events and incidents.

Second, sympathy and advocacy do not displace evidence in a court of law. Judges do not decide the negligence question out of thin air. In medical cases, negligence is virtually impossible to prove unless there is expert evidence that the conduct in question fell below the standard of reasonable care expected in the circumstances. As noted above in the discussion on the *Rogers v Whitaker* case, in Australia doctors do not have the 'last word' on negligence in the sense that a judge must accept the expert's view.

Third, critics of tort law often claim that experts are really 'hired guns', in that they are picked to support the case of the side by which they are chosen. To the extent that some experts are partial to one party's cause, it is my experience that this is seen more often in the defence camp than in the plaintiff's camp. It is undeniable that experts will have their own perspectives, based on unique knowledge and experience. This is not a reason to reject the tort system as some kind of lottery. On the contrary, the tort system permits these various positions to be tested in court.

Finally, if the standard of reasonable care is to improve over time and not remain static and mired in the practices of the past, it is necessary from time to time to bring cases that challenge the *status quo*. Most doctors would prefer the English *Bolam* test of negligence by which a doctor should not be found negligent if he or she did what others might have done in the circumstances. Australian law rejects this self-policing of the profession. As was once famously said: 'It is not the law that, if all or most of the medical practitioners in Sydney habitually fail to take an available precaution to avoid foreseeable risk of injury to their patients, then none can be found guilty of negligence' (see *Albrighton v Royal Prince Alfred Hospital* 1980, per Reynolds JA).

Where does the fault lie?

Another criticism of tort law is that it lays the blame on individual actors and individual events, when in fact most medical errors are related to complex systemic problems involving many factors and many people. It is certainly true that many, if not most, medical errors involve inadequate systems, or breakdowns in systems that were otherwise adequate. When errors occur, there is almost always at least one person who failed to do what he or she ought to have done. Two observations can be made.

First, many legal claims are directed at hospitals and not individuals. In some cases, the hospital is named as the employer of a staff member whose actions are in question (which lends some support to the argument that tort law still targets individuals), but in many cases the allegation of negligence involves the inadequacy of a system, or the failure to ensure that a system already in place was working properly. The issue in dispute, therefore, is not always the actions of one person but the overall management of the hospital.

Second, even where the actions of an individual working in a hospital are singled out in a legal claim, the underlying issue is usually inadequate experience or training. Neither of these needs to reflect poorly on the individual (although either may), and the message sent by a finding of negligence is that hospitals should ensure that staff are properly trained and have sufficient experience to handle a given situation.

It may be said that, since litigation often names individuals or focuses on the actions of individuals, it is an impediment to improved practice because it discourages reporting of errors due to the fear of blame. If this reluctance to disclose errors and learn from them is as pervasive as some say it is, it is more a reflection of the culture of the medical profession than the fear of litigation. Indeed, studies have shown that doctors and nurses are erroneously trained to believe that they can practise without error. When error does occur, they experience fear of punishment and disapproval by their colleagues (Leape 1997). Litigation, a rare event, cannot realistically be blamed for the reticence of doctors and nurses to disclose error.

Causation

One of the most difficult aspects of any medical negligence claim is proving that negligence caused the injuries complained of. It needs to be remembered that people engage with the medical profession because they already have a medical problem, and often a poor medical outcome is the result of the underlying condition rather than anything done or not done by doctors or hospitals. Another difficulty is that a specific poor outcome can be the result of many interventions, only one of which may have involved negligence. The criticism that usually emerges in this context is that the law is fixated on 'linear' causation, whereas in reality medical events occur in a 'causal web'.

The fundamental problem is that legal causation is not the same thing as medical causation. It is not the function of the law to tease out every strand of the web of medical causation and lay this out as if in a peer-reviewed medical journal. The question for the law is about *responsibility* and who ought to bear the burden of the loss—the patient on the one hand or the doctor or hospital on the other. The proper question is not 'What caused the plaintiff's poor outcome?' but rather 'Is negligence the cause of the poor outcome?'

The legal question involves two aspects. First, would the outcome have occurred even without the negligence (the factual causation question)? Second, if not, should the doctor or hospital be responsible for the outcome (the normative question)? The issue was put succinctly by the High Court of Australia in *March v Stramare (E & MH) Pty Ltd* (1991: 509 per Mason CJ):

> In philosophy and science, the concept of causation has been developed in the context of explaining phenomena by reference to the relationship between conditions and occurrences. In law, on the other hand, problems of causation arise in the context of ascertaining or apportioning legal responsibility for a given occurrence. The law does not accept John Stuart Mill's definition of cause as the sum of the conditions which are jointly sufficient to produce it. Thus, at law, a person may be responsible for damage when his or her wrongful conduct is one of a number of conditions sufficient to produce that damage.

When it is understood that medicine and law approach causation differently, the force of the criticism that the law lacks scientific rigour falls away. This is not to say that the law is unconcerned with the science of medical causation. On the contrary, most medical cases involve a vigorous contest over the cause or causes of a poor outcome. But it is sufficient for the purposes of assigning *legal responsibility* to establish that negligence was *a contributing factor*, even if there were many other factors that conspired to produce the damage of which the injured patient has complained.

CONCLUSION

The question of whether litigation against doctors and hospitals improves patient safety is one that has generated more heat than light. In order to answer the question, it is necessary to strip away the myths and misconceptions about medical litigation that pervade the discourse. It is also imperative to appreciate the differences between the litigation landscape in the United States and Australia. Most of the perceived excesses of the American system have been seized upon to make the case for tort reform in Australia as if the situation in the two countries were the same; it is not.

The small number of compensation claims previously brought against doctors and hospitals in Australia has diminished still further. Additionally, the effect of litigation on the delivery of health care needs to be understood in the light of the fact that, whatever force litigation is able to exert, it is not overwhelming, nor is it destructive of the medical profession.

Litigation remains an important and effective regulatory tool, since it can sanction, in a public and transparent way, guidelines and protocols that the medical profession itself believes should be followed. As such, litigation stands at the apex of the regulatory pyramid.

Litigation has also proven to be an effective deterrent to poor practice and an incentive to improve systems. The economic model of deterrence is especially apposite in the context of medical enterprises that can internalise the costs of compensation claims and are thus given a strong incentive to improve systems. Individual doctors, who are well insulated from the economic consequences of their mistakes by insurance, are less influenced by economic concerns than they are by concerns about personal anxiety and loss of reputation. For them, the perceived threat of litigation—even if unrealistic and exaggerated—is incentive enough to take steps to improve their own practices.

Criticisms of the law, especially on questions of the proof of negligence, the assignment of responsibility and the establishment of causation, are largely ill-informed, and derive from a failure to appreciate the realities of medical litigation and the objectives of tort law.

There is every reason to believe that litigation can, and does, improve the delivery of health care. By what means, and to what extent, should be the object of further study.

ACKNOWLEDGMENT

The author wishes to thank Ngaire Watson, Barrister, for her assistance in the writing of this chapter.

REFERENCES

Australian Competition and Consumer Commission (ACCC) 2008, *Medical Indemnity Insurance: Fifth Monitoring Report*, Commonwealth of Australia, Canberra

Baker, T. 2005, *The Medical Malpractice Myth*, University of Chicago Press, Chicago

Balkin, R. and Davis, J. 2004, *Law of Torts*, 3rd ed., LexisNexis Butterworths, Sydney

Braithwaite, J., Healy, J. and Dwan, K. 2005, *The Governance of Health Safety and Quality*, Commonwealth of Australia, Canberra

Brennan, T.A., Sox, C.M. and Burstin, H.R. 1996, 'Relation between negligent adverse events and the outcomes of medical-malpractice litigation', *New England Journal of Medicine*, vol. 335, no. 26, pp. 1963-7

Ipp Report 2002, *Review of the Law of Negligence Report*, Commonwealth of Australia, Canberra

Keating, G. 2000, 'Distributive and corrective justice in the tort law of accidents', *Southern California Law Review*, vol. 74, no. 1, pp. 193-224

Leape, L. 1997, 'A systems analysis approach to medical error', *Journal of Evaluation in Clinical Practice*, vol. 3, no. 3, pp. 213-22

Mello, M. and Brennan, T. 2002, 'Deterrence of medical errors: Theory and evidence for malpractice reform', *Texas Law Review*, vol. 80, no. 7, pp. 1595-1637

Mello, M., Kelly, C. and Brennan, T. 2005, 'Fostering rational regulation of patient safety', *Journal of Health Politics, Policy and Law*, vol. 30, no. 3, pp. 375-426

Mello, M. and Zeiler, K. 2008, 'Empirical health law scholarship: The state of the field', *Georgetown Law Journal*, vol. 96, no. 2, pp. 649-702

Rice, B. 2004, 'Malpractice: How to neutralize the sympathy factor', *Medical Economics*, vol. 81, no. 4, pp. 80-2

CASES

Albrighton v Royal Prince Alfred Hospital (1980) 2 NSWLR 542, 562-3
Backwell v AAA [1997] 1 VR 182
Bolam v Friern Hospital Management Committee [1957] 1 WLR 582
Kite v Malycha (1998) 71 SASR 321
March v Stramare (E & MH) Pty Ltd (1991) 171 CLR 506
PD v Harvey [2003] NSWSC 487
Rogers v Whitaker [1992] HCA 58; (1992) 175 CLR 479
Uren v John Fairfax & Sons Pty Ltd (1966) 117 CLR 118

NOTES

1   It is beyond the scope of this paper to discuss the origins of the 'medical indemnity crisis', either in the United States or Australia. But it is sufficient that most of the reasons for the increase in insurance premiums generally through the 1990s—especially in Australia—had little to do with increases in claims numbers and costs and were mostly related to poor management of the largest medical indemnity provider, United Medical Protection, together with a poor investment climate and a number of factors outside of the control of insurers. Following the recommendations of the Ipp Report (2002), all Australian jurisdictions enacted legislation that curbed the frequency and economic effect of liability litigation. Tort reform has reduced claims numbers and costs considerably but not medical indemnity premiums. For a critical evaluation of the situation in the United States, see Baker (2005).

2   Jury trials in medical cases are still widely used in Victoria.

3   In the United States, jury verdicts are sometimes appealed and high damages awards are reduced. Such an appeal does not disturb the jury's findings on liability.

4   The only successful case, *Backwell v AAA* (1997) involved a fertility clinic that threatened a client who was going to expose negligence in IVF treatment.

5   *Claims frequency:* This is the ultimate number of claims expected by year of notification expressed as a proportion of the total number of Medicare services provided in the corresponding year.
    Ultimate number of claims: This is the total number of notifications that the insurers expect will eventually become claims and be paid.

6   This is a distinction routinely lost in polemics against tort law. Most doctors consider a negligence claim to be tantamount to a criminal charge, and they

see themselves as being punished when in truth it is about responsibility for conduct that, while unintended, fell below an acceptable standard of care and caused injury. In the American context, however—where punitive damages can still be awarded against a negligent doctor—it is perhaps more understandable that medical litigation is seen as punishment, a view not supportable in Australia.

13

HOSPITAL LICENSURE, CERTIFICATION AND ACCREDITATION

Jenny Berrill and Judith Healy

THE REGULATORY MAZE

The aim of hospital inspection schemes run by external bodies is to ensure that hospitals are well-designed and well-run facilities that provide good working environments for staff and high-quality health care for patients. A review by an external body is an investment in quality assurance on the part of both regulators and hospitals—and a big investment for those hospitals that are subject to multiple inspections of their structure, equipment and performance. A key regulatory issue is whether benefits are produced for patients in terms of better and safer care. The multiple hospital inspection schemes, with their overlaps and gaps, reflect the fragmented health sector and federal system of government in Australia; over 30 bodies are variously engaged in setting standards, licensing, certifying and accrediting hospitals (Australian Commission on Safety and Quality in Health Care 2006). A manager of a large acute care hospital thus must manage multiple reviews with associated documentation and on-site inspections, as well as many additional reporting requirements. For example, state and territory governments license private hospitals; the Australian Council on Healthcare Standards (ACHS) accredits hospitals; the National Association of Testing Authorities (NATA) certifies pathology services; Food Standards Australia audits food safety; and professional colleges accredit medical training positions.

There are three forms of external inspection schemes: licensure, accreditation and certification. This chapter focuses on acute care hospitals and examines the evidence on the impact of these three types of inspection schemes on the quality and safety of health care for patients. (We use the generic term 'inspection' interchangeably with 'review' in this chapter and without pejorative intent.)

Inspection schemes in changing times

Acute care hospitals have changed dramatically over the last few decades in their structures, the procedures they undertake and their patient management systems. This has occurred in response to advances in knowledge and technology, changing population structures and disease patterns, constraints on resources and rising public expectations (McKee and Healy 2002). For example, hospitals are much busier places, where increasingly specialised professionals use complex procedures to treat sicker patients more intensively in shorter stays. In the Australian federal system of government, the states and territories have the primary responsibility for the provision of public hospital services. Hospitals dominate the health system and consume a large portion of state and territory government budgets; they are highly political in that they dominate health policy, and their activities (particularly their failures) attract considerable media interest, especially around election time.

Australia in 2006 had 1290 hospitals, including 736 public acute hospitals, 284 private hospitals and 252 private free-standing day hospitals (nearly double the number of day hospitals compared with 1996) (Australian Institute of Health and Welfare 2008: 347). Hospital inspection schemes must keep pace with the changes underway in hospitals, and respond appropriately to the varied nature of the hospital sector with its mix of public and private hospitals, as well as their case mix of patients. The three main types of hospital inspection schemes, while overlapping to some extent, have somewhat different functions and philosophies.

Licensure refers to the legal recognition of an organisation or practitioner, the aim being to ensure basic standards of public health and safety (Shaw 2004). Each state and territory has its own legislation relating to the licensure of private hospitals (including free-standing day hospital facilities), as well as legislation relevant to the operation of public hospitals. State and territory licensure schemes date from the 1950s and vary considerably across jurisdictions. The legislation usually has a number of requirements. These include compliance with recognised national codes such as building design (for example, new and refurbished facilities need to comply with the Building Code of Australia), occupational health and safety, infection control, reporting and accountability, as well as basic standards for staffing, facilities and equipment, emergency procedures and, more recently, patient care and clinical practice. A hospital, or its licensee, is usually granted a licence by the state or territory government when compliance with the requirements is demonstrated.

Certification refers to a guarantee by a certification body, through an evaluation process, that an organisation has capacity or technology in a certain field and meets certain design standards. Certification may be voluntary or mandatory, and applies more to technical aspects of health care, such as equipment or a laboratory. Certification schemes originated in the late 1940s at the international level to ensure industries standardised their processes and systems to guarantee a standard of quality of product or service.

Accreditation is a mechanism where an independent body evaluates the degree of compliance by an organisation with previously determined standards and, if deemed adequate, the organisation is awarded a compliance certificate (Scrivens 1998). The aim is to move performance beyond a minimal level towards optimal and achievable standards (Australian Council for Safety and Quality in Health Care 2003). In many countries, hospital accreditation by an NGO has become a major mechanism for regulating hospitals and an accepted alternative to direct government quality control.

A framework of schemes

A large number of bodies are involved in hospital regulatory schemes. A top tier of international-level organisations accredits the national-level bodies, develops standards, devises assessment procedures and promotes its own networks of members. In relation to the Australian hospital sector, the main bodies are the International Society for Quality in Healthcare (ISQua), the International Organization for Standardization (ISO) and the Joint Accreditation System–Australia and New Zealand (JAS–ANZ).

The national tier has two main hospital accreditation organisations, both independent 'not-for-profit' bodies: the Australian Council on Healthcare Standards (ACHS) and the Quality Improvement Council (QIC), plus various certification bodies.

State and territory government licensure schemes, based on their respective legislative regulations and arrangements, inhabit the third tier.

The fourth tier has a growing number of bodies, including 'for profits', who assess on behalf of accreditation or certification agencies, including the Australian Auditing and Certification Service Pty Ltd, Benchmark Certification, Institute for Healthy Communities of Australia Ltd, International Standards Certification Proprietary Ltd, Quality Management Certification, Quality Management Services and SAI Global.

Changing public policies

Over the last few decades, Australian governments have supported the principle of regular external inspections, mostly voluntary on the part of hospitals rather than mandatory, and carried out as a review by an independent agency. Accreditation, in particular, became the norm for hospitals from the late 1990s, and thus developed as a major regulatory mechanism for ensuring that hospitals meet basic standards and aspire to continuing quality improvement.

In 2003, the Australian Health Ministers served notice that the accreditation field was due for an overhaul (Australian Council for Safety and Quality in Health Care 2003). In June 2006, the Australian Health Ministers' Advisory Council (AHMAC) requested the Australian Commission for Safety and Quality in Health Care to review accreditation reform options and to propose 'an alternative model'. The Commission engaged in extensive consultations and put out several discussion papers. Its final report, released in February 2008, proposed a series of reforms intended to offer a uniform national approach to assessment, simplification of the system, reduced duplication of effort, greater efficiency, a better balance between improvement and compliance, more emphasis on preventing risks to patients, more outcome-focused standards, improved assessor reliability, and the collection and analysis of safety and quality data (Australian Commission on Safety and Quality in Healthcare 2008b: 2–3).

The Health Ministers endorsed the proposed principles at their April 2008 AHMAC meeting (Department of Health and Ageing 2008). A group was set up to advise the ministers on how to implement the new accreditation model, to devise a preliminary set of standards, and to undertake a review of state and territory government licensure schemes.

The new accreditation model was to include the following elements:

- Australian Health Standards to apply to all health services;
- a Quality Improvement Framework to set out principles;
- expanded scope of accreditation to all health services;
- national data collection and reporting to measure outcomes and progress;
- mutual recognition in order to minimise the compliance burden;
- obligations to comply with requirements and consequences for non-compliance; and
- a 'national entity' (a new or existing body) to lead and coordinate reform (Australian Commission on Safety and Quality in Health Care 2007c).

Three main issues for public policy emerged from these discussion papers and consultations. The first was accountability. Government (Commonwealth, state and territory) proposes to make accreditation bodies more accountable to government and the public and less the captive of industry and the professions. Proposals for strengthening public accountability include separating standard-setting from inspections, making procedures and decisions more transparent, moving from voluntary to mandatory inspections and standards, and requiring minimum standards across the health sector.

The second issue to emerge was effectiveness. There is to be more emphasis upon efforts to improve the validity and reliability of assessments, and to track the relationship between accreditation outcomes for hospitals and safety and quality outcomes for patients.

The third policy issue is efficiency. The Council of Australian Governments (COAG) seeks to harmonise arrangements across the various inspection schemes, develop national standards, weigh up the benefits against the costs and minimise the regulatory burden. The latter has also become an issue in other health systems: for example, the United Kingdom has announced the development of a 'concordat' to deliver smarter, more joined up inspection programs that reduce the burden of inspections, and with the goal to reduce inspectorates (Healthcare Commission 2006).

HOSPITAL LICENSURE

In countries with private health care services, there is a need for governmental oversight to ensure citizens will not be harmed, exposed to hazards, or at risk of injury. All Australian state and territory governments have established their own licensure schemes to regulate the private hospital sector. Legislation differs in relation to what is licensed (e.g. the facility, the type of service, the procedure, the beds, the owners), other requirements (e.g. the extent of local demand), the licensing procedure (e.g. documentation, on-site inspection), and re-licensing requirements (e.g. a one-off licence, a renewal fee or another inspection).

For example, in Queensland the *Private Health Facilities Act* 1999 requires, amongst other things, persons proposing to operate a private health facility to be approved. In New South Wales, the *Private Health Facilities Act* 2007 requires private hospitals to meet general licensure standards. There are also some specific standards (e.g. on cardiac catheterisation, emergency services, intensive care, dialysis, neonatal special care and open-heart surgery) which apply to each class of facility and specialist service, including general, surgical, obstetric, psychiatric and rehabilitation. In the Australian Capital Territory, the *Public Health Act* 1997 focuses on procedures that put patients at risk. These include the administration of a general, spinal, epidural or major regional block anaesthetic or intravenous sedation for the purposes of a procedure, including endoscopy, dialysis, haemofiltration or perfusion, administration of cytotoxic agents or cardiac catheterisation.

In most countries, hospital licensure is granted by an officer with delegated authority under the legislation, after receiving advice from a government-authorised officer that minimum standards are met, and a hospital must maintain its licence to continue to function and care for patients (Hafez 1997). Continued licensure may be renewed upon payment of a fee, assuming no problems have been reported, or else may require an inspection and/or submission of documentation (Rooney and Van Ostenberg 1999). Most Australian licensure systems undertake initial and subsequent assessments of compliance against standards, and may require licensees to submit regular reports, including data on patient diagnosis and outcomes (Australian Commission on Safety and Quality in Health Care 2008a: 39–40). Licensure schemes include the ability to apply sanctions where there is non-compliance. There also is a focus on continuous improvement in order to rectify problems when detected, rather than simply removing the licence (Australian Council for Safety and Quality in Health Care 2003).

The self-monitoring and evaluation of government regulatory agencies and their licensure schemes was found, at least in the United States, to be poor (Rooney and Van Ostenberg 1999). Ongoing evaluation of government regulatory schemes is an important component of transparency and accountability to the public, and demonstrates whether the investment in the regulation of hospitals is cost effective.

One commentator argues that hospital licensing schemes in the United States could be reinvigorated on the grounds that these schemes already cover most hospitals, and that licensure should become more like accreditation schemes, with a baseline review, problem analysis, tailored regulation and oversight revision (Blum 2008).

The Australian context is different in that licensure mainly applies only to the private hospital sector (while the US hospital sector is highly privatised). Private hospitals in Australia are subjected to additional regulation through mandatory licensing as well as the requirements of other inspection schemes, such as accreditation.

Harmonisation reform is needed in Australia, as licensure requirements differ across the jurisdictions as well as across the public and private sectors. This has particular impact on health care organisations that own private hospitals located in multiple states and territories. One solution may be for the jurisdictions to agree upon common legislation. One difficulty with a legal approach to regulation in the rapidly changing health sector, however, is that legislation is inherently inflexible and difficult to change.

HOSPITAL CERTIFICATION

Certification refers to a guarantee by a certification body that an organisation meets certain design standards in its equipment, processes or systems. Certification is usually voluntary rather than mandatory and, in relation to a hospital, can apply to the whole or a component of a hospital.

The best known certification scheme, the International Organization for Standardization (ISO), is a worldwide federation of national standards bodies from over 90 countries. ISO 9000 standards apply to the service industry, which includes health, and focus on design specifications for processes and products, rather than an assessment of service outcomes; they do not incorporate continuous improvement concepts (Rooney and Van Ostenberg 1999: 7). ISO itself does not certify organisations as meeting its standards, rather ISO-recognised external auditors use the standards in their certification reviews.

The Joint Accreditation Scheme–Australia and New Zealand (JAS–ANZ) is a quasi-government scheme that uses ISO and other international standards, and accredits bodies that certify management systems, products and personnel. JAS–ANZ health care standards were developed in consultation with the hospital industry, including the Private Healthcare Industry Quality and Safety Committee. The JAS–ANZ Healthcare Sector Scheme accredits a network of certification bodies whose audit teams undertake annual audit visits. Approximately 100 health care providers, including Australian Defence Forces hospitals and private hospitals, are certified under this scheme (JAS–ANZ 2008), although the Australian Defence Forces now allow their hospitals a choice of approved accreditors.

HOSPITAL ACCREDITATION

Accreditation is regarded as a key regulatory mechanism for improving the quality of hospital care. After rapid growth during the 1990s, accreditation schemes now exist in over 40 countries around the world (Shaw 2003). The origins of hospital accreditation lie in the 'hospital standardization' program begun in 1917 by the American College of Surgeons, whose surveyors inspected hospitals against agreed standards with the aim of improving widely varying hospital conditions. The hospital accreditation model was initially embraced by the United States, Canada, New Zealand and Australia (Scrivens 1995). There are two main philosophical approaches to accreditation. The first views accreditation as a developmental process that aims to produce continuous quality improvement, with all organisations receiving some level of accreditation. The second views accreditation as an outcome of an assessment against minimum standards that must be met and preferably surpassed.

Accreditation is generally conducted by an independent national agency, usually a quasi-government agency or non-government agency (NGO). An accreditation agency may apply agreed standards, or may set the standards, and conducts regular reviews of applicants against these standards. Accreditation began as a voluntary scheme but increasingly is expected or required by governments and insurance funds. The developmental approach is giving way to compulsory minimum standards, and there is increasing pressure to make accreditation reports public rather than confidential.

An accreditation cycle generally involves an intensive sequence of activities over a three- to four-year period. Initially, the applicant conducts a self-assessment against standards devised by a standard-setting body and then develops a quality action plan; the accreditor undertakes a desk audit of the outcome of the submitted material; a survey team of two or three people (often health professionals from other hospitals) undertakes an arranged site visit to seek evidence documented in the self-assessment through interviews, observations and document review; the survey team writes a summary report for the accreditation body's consideration; and finally, a decision is made and, if positive, an accreditation certificate is issued. The accredited organisation will be required to report on quality activities during the cycle in order to retain accreditation, or may receive unannounced inspection visits. The cycle begins again after perhaps three years.

Accreditation agencies are mostly NGOs and governed by a board that represents the key stakeholders. This promotes acceptance since an accreditation scheme must devise standards that are feasible and acceptable to the field, but it also raises the issue of 'regulatory capture'. This dilemma is particularly acute for voluntary accreditation schemes that depend upon fees from members.

The Australian Council on Healthcare Standards (ACHS) was established in 1974 and is by far the biggest accreditation provider for hospitals in Australia. It is also active in the growing Asian market. Most revenue ($8.06 million operating budget in 2006–07) comes from member fees. The 30-plus member Council comprises representatives of national health bodies, professional associations, government, peak industry groups and the Consumers Health Forum of Australia (CHF). Over half of its 350 surveyors are volunteers whose time is provided by ACHS member organisations.

Surveyors assess achievement against 58 criteria set out in the ACHS manual, the Evaluation and Quality Improvement Program (EQuIP), now in its fourth edition. The ACHS has four levels of recognition based on the duration of accreditation: four years of accreditation; two years with corrective action required on some criteria within twelve months; conditional one year accreditation where there is a high priority recommendation for improvement within 60 days; and non-accreditation.

The Quality Improvement Council (QIC), a national non-profit body, has twenty years' experience and mainly accredits, through licensed providers, community services and some rural hospitals against a two-tier system of core and service-specific standards. These standards are in their fifth edition. About 400 agencies were enrolled in QIC accreditation procedures in 2007. The QIC applies a developmental model of continuous quality improvement, with accreditation awarded for three years; no organisation has been refused accreditation.

POLICY ISSUES FOR HOSPITAL INSPECTION SCHEMES

The philosophy of hospital inspection schemes is in the process of changing as part of broader and more patient-centred health sector reforms, and in the wake of public alarm after a series of hospital scandals and inquiries. This scrutiny began with a focus upon accreditation schemes but has widened to cover licensure. Moving from accountability to the accreditation organisation's members, to accountability to the public requires a philosophical shift, since accreditation and certification agencies were initially established to provide confidential reviews to their members. It also requires a shift in emphasis from a 'well-run organisation' fit for professionals to work in, to a hospital fit for patients to be treated in (Scrivens 1995). The trend to mandatory schemes and standards raises the stakes for accreditation agencies, with more pressure to base a decision on valid and reliable measures of compliance against standards, and to establish the links between quality standards, accreditation outcomes and quality outcomes.

Mandatory or voluntary schemes and standards

Accreditation has become the norm in the Australian hospital sector since virtually all large public hospitals and all private hospitals now seek accreditation. In 2004–05, 83 per cent of all public hospitals were accredited (Department of Health and Ageing 2006: 11). The ACHS had 1048 member organisations in its accreditation program at 31 December 2006, of which 58 per cent were public organisations and 42 per cent private; over half the inpatient facilities had fewer than 100 beds; and 13 per cent of organisations were day-only or community centres (Australian Council on Healthcare Standards 2007: 13).

State and territory governments expect, or require in some cases (e.g. Victoria and the ACT), their public hospitals to be accredited with an approved accreditation organisation. Smaller numbers of small public hospitals are accredited, however, possibly because they lack the funds and capacity to engage in the complex accreditation process. Accreditation is set to become mandatory across the health sector as the Australian Health Ministers in 2008 agreed that all health facilities, including day hospitals, would be required to seek some form of accreditation.

The private hospital sector has embraced accreditation over the last two decades. This has been driven by private health insurance funds that require hospitals to be accredited in their 'preferred provider' contracts, while other hospitals must be approved by the Commonwealth Minister of Health in order to receive at least a minimum level of payments (so-called 'second-tier default benefits payments'). In addition, the Australian Private Hospital Association requires its members to be accredited.

Health insurance legislation is being used to reinforce accreditation status among private hospitals. From July 2008, under the *Private Health Insurance Act* 2007 (Cth) (s 121.5(6)), the Commonwealth minister recognises (declares) a private hospital eligible for claims from health insurance funds, one of the conditions being that the hospital be accredited with an approved ISQua or JAS-ANZ provider.

Setting and measuring standards

A standard is the expected level of capacity or performance against which an organisation, activity or product is assessed. Standards Australia defines a standard as 'a published document which sets out specifications and procedures designed to ensure that a material, product, method or service is fit for its purpose and consistently performs in the way it was intended' (Standards Australia 2007). A standard thus represents a view by a competent authority on what represents an acceptable or sometimes an optimal level of performance.

The assumption was (and is) that a well-organised hospital structure will create an environment in which professional standards can flourish and where patients will receive good health care (Scrivens 1995: 90). Standards originally focused on structure and process; they have now broadened to include outcomes, including clinical outcomes. Health care standards are usually developed by expert consensus, reflect current thinking about health policy and care quality, respond to advances in technology and treatments, and are built around structure (facilities, equipment), work processes (clinical guidelines, staff supervision) and outcomes (infection rates, fatality rates).

A proposal to separate the development of standards from their assessment met an equivocal response in consultations with stakeholders (Australian Commission on Safety and Quality in Health Care 2007b). Supporters of separation claimed a dual body has no incentive to fail those that do not meet standards; opponents claimed separation would add to the costs, sideline the industry and the professions from standards development, and allow government to capture the process and exert undue external regulatory pressure.

In 2008, the Health Ministers called for uniform Australian Health Standards with patient safety and quality requirements at their core. The aims are to reduce duplication and conflict between sets of standards, ensure consistency of key safety and quality items, and produce greater clarity and certainty for health services. Considerable technical effort has been devoted to making the measurement of standards valid (sound) and reliable (repeatable), as well as to the politics of agreeing on standards with a range of stakeholders (Australian Commission on Safety and Quality in Health Care 2006: 9). Can a standard be defined in measurable terms, and does the measure indicate quality performance?

Standards vary on the level of detail and achievement expected. Australian standards tend to be framed in broad terms so that virtually all organisations can show compliance and progress. In contrast, the United States Joint Commission in Healthcare sets detailed and extensive standards that its surveyors tick off in site visits. The drive to improve measurement leads to more standards and more specificity— the downside being the checklist approach of 'regulatory ritualism' (Braithwaite et al. 2007). For example, the ACHS EQuIP in 2006 introduced greater complexity by expanding to 58 criteria with five levels of achievement ($58 \times 5 = 290$ items).

The stakes were raised for accreditation schemes and standards by the Health Ministers in 2008 with their call for 'obligations to comply ... and consequences for non-compliance' to be imposed upon health care facilities. Standards become more important if hospitals incur serious sanctions for non-compliance. Hospital inspection schemes depend upon credible and competent surveyors and inspectors and their variability in rating organisations against standards is a common concern (Australian Commission on Safety and Quality in Health Care 2008b). Licensure inspectors and accreditation surveyors must interpret standards, and there is often a subjective element in supposedly objective standards. Standards can be ambiguous, while scores depend on the experience of the individuals undertaking the inspection. There are problems of inter-surveyor reliability (the extent to which two surveyors operating independently assign the same value for the attribute they are measuring), and also intra-surveyor reliability (the degree to which a single surveyor assigns the same value when measuring the same attribute at different times) (Morrissey 2002;

Crisp 2006; Australian Commission on Safety and Quality in Health Care 2006: 17). Accreditation bodies try to reduce surveyor variation and have proposed more training programs for accreditation surveyors. For example, ISQua recently awarded the ACHS surveyor training program a four-year accreditation.

A shift from a developmental to mandatory approach changes the role of a surveyor from an educator to a regulator. Different inspection schemes have somewhat different philosophies and hence surveyor styles. An auditor in a government licensure scheme is usually a government employee, deemed an 'authorised officer' under respective state or territory legislation, and many are nurses with expert knowledge in quality and safety (infection control, safety systems), and skills in regulatory enforcement (Morrissey 2002: 8–9). In contrast, accreditation surveyors are usually peers, often employees of another hospital and mostly volunteers, who see themselves as peer educators; they evaluate progress against standards, and recommend but do not enforce decisions.

Encouraging or enforcing standards

Hospital accreditation agencies take a developmental approach, and thus issue conditional and short-term accreditation, even to health services that do not meet compulsory standards. Government licensure bodies also are loath to revoke a hospital licence if they do not meet the requirements, as they must balance the need to protect patients versus the need to ensure an adequate supply of services (Zeribi and Marquez 2005). An escalation to severe sanctions, such as withdrawing accreditation or licensure, has major ramifications politically, as well as a major impact on public access to services. Hospitals, therefore, are very seldom refused a license, certification or accreditation. For example, the ACHS gave conditional registration pending compliance with standards to six hospitals in 2005 but did not revoke accreditation from any facilities in 2005 or 2006. The number of health facilities assessed as making 'little achievement' on mandatory criteria decreased from ten in 2003 and 2004 to two in 2005 and none in 2006. Non-accreditation followed serious failures for a few: fewer than 1 per cent of organisations in 2003 and 2004, and none in 2005 and 2006 (Australian Council on Healthcare Standards 2005, 2007). Should this be interpreted as progress by facilities in meeting standards over time or as growing leniency? While the Health Ministers intimated in 2008 that they expected a tougher approach in future with 'consequences for non-compliance', Health Ministers may be less inclined to support a tough line if 'consequences' are applied to one of their public hospitals.

Withdrawal of accreditation, a sanction from the top of the regulatory pyramid, might be viewed as a failure of the accreditation process. Accreditation agencies have an array of supports and sanctions at their disposal before recourse to revocation of recognition. A regulator must have the capacity to escalate the strength of sanctions, however, if regulation is to have force (Braithwaite et al. 2007). Similarly, withdrawal of licensure could be seen in the same light; as a result, most legislation includes soft sanctions such as fines, but also support systems. Responsive regulation calls for regulatory discussions at the base of the regulatory pyramid, before escalating to serious sanctions in the few cases of non-compliance.

Regulators need to undertake a range of creative interventions, and combinations of interventions, since multiple interventions are more effective than single interventions (Marquez 2001). Hospital accreditation surveyors and licence inspectors treat an onsite visit partly as a peer review process, where they discuss with hospital staff how best to make improvements, for example, in infection control. This is a particularly valuable learning opportunity for people who work in professionally isolated situations, such as in day hospitals or small rural hospitals. Successful regulatory mechanisms include discussion between peers, repetition of messages and reinforcement of improved practice (Marquez 2001).

One regulatory approach could be to concentrate on the high performers, with the intention being to promote continuing quality improvement (CQI) and publicise the successes of industry leaders in order to prompt laggards to lift their standards. The counter approach is to concentrate on the poor performers in order to ensure that minimum standards are met. In this view, inspection schemes should concentrate on 'weeding out the bad apples'. For example, one hospital licensee commented that '99 per cent of licensees are excellent; the licensure system is needed for the 1 per cent of cowboys'. For example, the United Kingdom Department of Health now pays more attention to poor performers by sending remedial teams to work with 'failing hospitals' (Healthcare Commission 2007). If the aim is to bring all hospitals up to a certain standard, would inspection schemes do better to concentrate more effort on the minority of health services assessed as poor performers?

Costs of hospital review schemes

Inspection schemes involve substantial direct costs and time on the part of hospitals. The main income of Australian accreditation and certification agencies is from membership fees. For example, ACHS fees are based on size, complexity and geographical spread, and accreditation charges range from $8000 for a small rural hospital and $15,000 for a medium metropolitan hospital to $40,000 for a large hospital. ISO accreditation charges range from $6000 to $30,000 for small to medium-sized hospitals (Appleyard and Ramsay 2008: 18–19). License fees are significantly less—for example, the annual licence fee for a health care facility in New South Wales is $750 (New South Wales Government 2008) and in the Australian Capital Territory ranges from $1000 down to $200 for large to small hospitals (ACT Department of Health 2001).

There are also substantial indirect costs to a hospital in complying with the relevant standards, providing documented evidence, arranging and hosting an onsite survey, and actioning any recommendations. While the costs for licensure are considerably less than for accreditation, the roles are very different. Accreditation compliance is costly in terms of having in place a continuous quality improvement (CQI) scheme, since a hospital must assign highly paid professionals to the accreditation process, as well as to developing and managing CQI activities. Compulsory accreditation for small health facilities with limited budgets, particularly rural hospitals, would therefore have significant cost implications. A move to a mandatory and national accreditation scheme may put pressure upon government to contribute to the costs, especially if government is involved in setting and raising the standards.

Consumer views

Increasingly, health consumers are no longer content to be treated as passive recipients of what is deemed to be good for them. They want to be partners in decision-making about their own health, and to be involved in designing, managing and delivering hospital care, in order to ensure hospitals are safe, effective and appropriate to community needs. The move towards greater consumer empowerment has occurred at the same time as an erosion in the trust relationship between the health system and patients, partly in response to the well-publicised adverse incidents that have occurred at Australian hospitals (Department of Health and Aged Care 2000: 39).

The participation by consumers in health care policy and practice is now sought as a means of improving the quality of care and making the system more accountable. For example, both the ACHS and QIC promote the use of consumer reviewers as part of the survey team in mental health services (Mental Health Council of Australia 2008). A growing number of governments and care providers actively seek consumer views. For example, the Department of Health and Aged Care developed a Consumer Health Strategy and has funded a range of projects to strengthen consumer participation (Department of Health and Aged Care 2000).

Despite a nod to the concept, the accreditation field has not embraced a patient-centred approach. The Consumers Health Forum (CHF) complains that discussions on quality revolve around the views of health care providers rather than consumers (Consumers Health Forum of Australia 2007). The CHF points out that consumers want holistic health care, and cites the indicators on quality care identified by consumers and published by the Picker Institute in Europe, which include access, effectiveness, communication and participation, care and physical comfort, continuity of care, human needs, efficiency, information, and involvement of family and friends (Health Care Consumers Association of the ACT 2003: 21). Patient satisfaction ratings, accepted in principle as a valid quality measure, are seldom included in an accreditation procedure (Australian Commission on Safety and Quality in Health Care 2006: 28). Nor are they routinely sought in the licensure procedure.

Consumers probably assume that hospitals are regularly inspected, and that these inspections guarantee that the hospital provides safe and good quality care. But given the lack of information in the public domain, few health consumers know the results of hospital inspection schemes. A patient in Australia can find out more from websites about the standards of hospitals in the United Kingdom and the United States than about Australian hospitals.

While consumers believe that accreditation could help to prevent mistakes by ensuring that health services have standards in place, there is also a perception that currently 'accreditation is a bit of toothless tiger' (Consumers Health Forum of Australia 2007: 5). In an editorial in *The Australian Health Consumer*, McCallum (2002) has suggested questions (some rhetorical) that consumers should ask in encounters with the health system: Did you kill me? Did you damage me? Did you fix me? Did you care for me? Did you involve me in what was going on? Did you make me comfortable?

Jeffrey Braithwaite, at the National Forum on Safety and Quality in Health Care in Adelaide in 2008, urged patients to realise that 'it's partly their responsibility to advocate for themselves and monitor their situation while in hospital ... I'm not saying people shouldn't trust the health system—many people receive excellent care—but be vigilant, don't go it alone. You need relatives, friends or colleagues to speak up for you and monitor your progress.'

Transparency

Accreditation is moving from being an internal industry arrangement, to one more open to external scrutiny by those who pay for it (government and private funders) and by those it is designed to assist (patients). Accreditation schemes are caught between the preference of their members for confidential review and the transparency demands of the public and the state. The Patterson review of safety and quality arrangements in Australia identified transparency issues for, first, decision-making processes; second, reporting the outcomes of the process; and third, public access to information (Patterson 2005).

Public reporting of performance is widely used in the United States to drive quality improvement. Hospital performance records have been disclosed publicly in several states in the United States—for example, in New York, California and Pennsylvania—since the early 1990s. The Californian Office of Statewide Health Planning and Development provides web-based 'quality data reports' on such things as preventable hospitalisations, heart attack outcomes and intensive care outcomes. The Office states that the reports are intended to encourage all Californian hospitals to improve their care, give credit to the leaders, and help insurers, employees and consumers to select hospitals that offer good quality care (Office of Statewide Health Planning and Development 2009). The US federal Agency for Healthcare Research and Quality also reports scores on hospital performance indicators with comparisons against state and national averages. The Joint Commission, in response to public pressure, publishes a 'quality report' with accreditation scores for each hospital, and an online comparison with state and national scores (Scrivens 1995: 118).

Research shows that quality improvement efforts follow public reporting, since hospitals that report performance to the public engage in more quality improvement activities (Fung et al. 2008; Hibberd et al. 2003; Scholle 2006). The main motivation among doctors and hospitals for demonstrating quality improvements is concern for one's reputation among one's peers, although public reporting so far has not had a significant impact on consumer and purchaser behaviour (Marshall et al. 2000).

Compared with the United States and the United Kingdom, much less information is published on the performance of Australian hospitals. For example, the ACHS did not name the 26 hospitals given only provisional accreditation in 2003. The ACHS website lists accredited hospitals (the list is buried in the 'members' section) and their accreditation expiry date. The ACHS asks hospitals to lodge their accreditation report or a short statement, but few have done so, showing voluntarism to be a weak mechanism in promoting greater transparency. Although Victoria puts considerable emphasis upon accreditation, only about 42 out of 170 Victorian health facilities had lodged an accreditation statement on the ACHS website (as at 4 December 2008). The QIC website provides the names of accredited organisations and the expiry dates. Government licensure information, where it does exist on websites, usually lists only the name of the licensed hospital and the licensee's name.

The media's approach of 'naming, shaming and blaming' in response to public reports by hospitals on their performance means that Health Departments and hospitals are loath to report and very defensive. In Australia, the Queensland government has attempted to reconceptualise public reporting, and to refocus on the action taken to improve performance through the public reporting on investigations and their outcomes (Duckett et al. 2008: 616; see also Chapter 6, this volume).

DO EXTERNAL REVIEWS IMPROVE QUALITY AND SAFETY?

The Australian Council for Safety and Quality in Health Care claims that 'Australia has benefited enormously from systems for standards setting and accreditation in health' (Australian Council for Safety and Quality in Health Care 2003: 26). In its series of consultations with stakeholders in the accreditation field, the Commission also found a consensus view that accreditation is an important regulatory mechanism for promoting organisational compliance with standards, and that accreditation schemes have improved the quality of health and aged care (Australian Commission on Safety and Quality in Health Care 2007a). There is some evidence from accreditation data that organisations, over time, do improve their structures and procedures and do meet minimum standards; however, hard evidence of the impact of accreditation upon patient outcomes remains elusive. While accreditation (and licensure) arguably achieve the goal of ensuring that hospitals meet minimum standards, there is little empirical evidence on whether accreditation is a cost-effective strategy for raising performance towards maximum standards (Scrivens 1998). Uncertainty about the extent of quality improvement continues, as do calls for more research to compare the costs of accreditation with its benefits (Shaw 2003). A systematic review of the accreditation research literature found little rigorous evidence to support claims of positive impacts on quality outcomes, although there are consistent findings that accreditation promotes change in organisations and supports professional development (Greenfield and Braithwaite 2007). Uncertainty about the extent of benefits in terms of patient outcomes is problematic given concern about the administrative burden of many inspections (Australian Commission on Safety and Quality in Health Care 2007c).

A reasonable assumption, despite the absence of rigorous evidence, is that well-designed and well-run hospitals produce good patient outcomes (Robinson 1995). Thus an ACHS professional noted that: 'There is documented evidence of improved management and numerous examples of improved patient outcomes … It is appropriate to expect that if the "environment" is ordered and safe then patient outcomes are more likely to be desirable ones.' (Collopy 2000: 211)

Does accreditation improve quality outcomes for patients?

Accreditation agencies are looking to realign their standards with outcome measures, both in order to improve these measures and to focus more attention on patient outcomes (Brennan 1998). A review of studies on the relationship between accreditation and quality measures, however, found inconsistent results and generally no relationship between a specified quality measure and an accreditation outcome (Greenfield and Braithwaite 2007). In the absence of both good outcome measures of quality for hospitals and outcomes trend data, there is little hard evidence on whether accreditation improves health outcomes for patients (Øvretveit 2003). The challenge is to align hospital quality outcomes measures with accreditation measures.

Hospital performance in relation to quality is now being measured. Internationally, the identification and measurement of indicators on hospital performance has progressed over the last decade, with the United States the leader in the field. The Agency for Healthcare Research and Quality publishes quality indicators for hospitals; the Organisation for Economic Cooperation and Development publishes quality indicators for national health care systems; and the United Kingdom's NHS is working on a 'new generation' of quality indicators (UK Department of Health 2008).

The US National Committee for Quality Assurance has identified some improvements in quality indicator trends—for example, more than 96 per cent of cardiac patients are prescribed beta blockers after a heart attack compared with 62 per cent in 1996 (Scholle 2006). However, a survey of US hospitals by the Hospital Consumer Assessment of Healthcare Providers and Systems found little improvement in some areas that have long been the target of quality improvement initiatives, including pain management and hospital discharge arrangements (Ashish et al. 2008).

Accreditation agencies collect a huge amount of data, but this is generally not used to evaluate the effectiveness of accreditation. For example, process standards lack validation, such as whether an information system actually improves patient care. There is also little analysis of the relationship between accreditation and health outcomes for patients, such as 30-day post-hospital mortality. If accreditation improves quality, one would expect a correlation with performance indicators. Since most health facilities are accredited, the question is not a binary yes or no as to the success of accreditation, but rather relates to the extent of the relationship between accreditation measures and clinical performance measures. Research is hindered because accreditation agencies generally do not publish overall accreditation scores, partly because there is no weighting on the separate standards. For example, the ACHS does not produce a total score given the problems of aggregation in a multivariate scoring system. A more realistic cause and effect comparison would be between a specific standard, such as the presence of an infection team within the hospital, and the reduction of rates of hospital-acquired infection.

The ACHS clinical indicator database has collected data since 1998 on 308 clinical indicators from 689 hospitals. This offers an opportunity to track progress on patient safety and quality and to relate clinical performance measures to accreditation measures. Of the 108 indicators with sufficient data from 2001 to 2007 to show statistically significant trends, 77 show improvements (Australian Council on Healthcare Standards 2008).

The ACHS also has reported trend data on the performance of hospitals against accreditation standards over the period 2003–06. For example, the number of organisations awarded 'four-year accreditation status' rose from 34 per cent in 2004 to 82 per cent in 2006, and Outstanding Achievement scores were awarded to seventeen organisations in 2004 and 26 in 2006 (Australian Council on Healthcare Standards 2007: 2).

However, some of this improvement could perhaps be attributed to accreditation applicants becoming more familiar with the ACHS standards first introduced in 2003.

ACHS survey teams also comment on high-performing organisations that they regard as leaders in their field (Australian Council on Healthcare Standards 2007: 29–40). These comments indicate the creativity and energy of highly motivated professionals in these health organisations. For example, in relation to 'improved structure and process', the Portland and District Health (Victoria) was described by surveyors as a leader in touch-screen information technology, while the waste management system of the Royal Brisbane and Women's Hospital (Queensland) was recognised in local and national awards. The Eastern Heart Clinic (New South Wales) had improved its quality of clinical services and had published its analyses of care outcomes; and Gambro Healthcare (Queensland) compared well on dialysis outcomes against similar clinics.

The absence of hospital performance data against which to compare accreditation results is not a problem that accreditation agencies can solve alone, since this requires national coordination by governments to gather hospital performance and outcomes data. Australia has stepped up its development on hospital performance indicators through work underway at the Australian Institute of Health and Welfare, and through the inclusion of performance indicators in the 2009 intergovernmental hospital funding agreement (the Australian Health Care Agreements). The Health Ministers also have endorsed national data collection, including safety and quality, to track progress among accredited hospitals (Australian Commission on Safety and Quality in Health Care 2007c).

Does accreditation improve safety outcomes for patients?

Hospital review schemes now include measures of patient safety in their standards. For example, ACHS standards expect a hospital CEO 'to ensure the provision of quality, safe services' and, under clinical criteria, safe practice procedures are expected in several areas: medications, infection control, pressure ulcers, falls, blood, and correct patient procedures. However, the ACHS standards currently do not require a hospital to report adverse events, or to have a response procedure in place to reduce the risk of further incidents (unlike United States accreditation criteria).

Of the organisations surveyed by the ACHS in 2003–04 and two years later, while 61 per cent had improved in quality and safety, many had not improved in crucial areas such as infection risks, credentialling staff and fire safety (Australian Council on Healthcare Standards 2007: 6). It is alarming that some hospitals do not have in place risk-management procedures that have been part of hospital best practice for many years.

A review of the international literature found no convincing research evidence on whether accredited hospitals have fewer adverse events (Trowbridge and Wachter 2001). In Australia, health departments require hospitals to report adverse events, and many have established legislatively protected reporting systems; however, adverse events remain a problematic indicator of patient safety given substantial under-reporting. Do more reports mean that a hospital is taking the issue seriously, or that more errors are being made?

While an entire accreditation scheme should not be dismissed because of a few failures, accreditation has failed to detect patient safety problems in some notable cases. The US Joint Commission was criticised for accrediting several hospitals that later were revealed to be seriously substandard in some areas (Gaul 2005). In Australia, the Bundaberg Hospital was accredited by the ACHS in mid-2003, two months after Dr Patel began as Director of Surgery, while public inquiries later revealed serious failures of hospital management (Davies 2005). Three other accredited hospitals have been embroiled in medical scandals (Camden and Campbelltown Hospitals in Sydney, the Canberra Hospital and King Edward Memorial Hospital in Perth), where whistleblowers were forced to go public after hospital managers failed to address problems reported to them (Faunce and Bolsin 2004).

CONCLUSION: THE FUTURE OF THE REGULATORY MAZE

Australian public health policy now seeks to harmonise the multiplicity of hospital inspection arrangements by external bodies. The schemes are under pressure to become more patient-centred and to demonstrate their contribution to strengthening the quality and safety of health care for Australians. The reform process has commenced and is engaging a multiplicity of stakeholders, while pressure from the public for greater transparency is likely to grow.

REFERENCES

ACT Department of Health 2001, 'Explanatory Memorandum of the ACT Health Care Facilities Code of Practice 2001 declared under the *Public Health Act 1997*', ACT Health, Canberra

Appleyard, G. and Ramsay, J. 2008, *Cost Analysis of Safety and Quality Accreditation in the Australian Health System*, Australian Commission for Safety and Quality in Health Care, Sydney

Ashish, K.J., Orav, E.J., Zheng, J. and Epstein, A.M. 2008, 'Patients' perception of hospital care in the United States', *New England Journal of Medicine*, vol. 359, no. 18, pp. 1921–31

Australian Commission on Safety and Quality in Health Care 2006, *Discussion Paper: National Safety and Quality Accreditation Standards*, Australian Commission on Safety and Quality in Health Care, Sydney

—— 2007a, *Consultation Paper: An Alternative Model for Safety and Quality Accreditation of Health Care*, Australian Commission on Safety and Quality in Health Care, Sydney

—— 2007b, *Draft Report on the Review of National Safety and Quality Accreditation Standards*, Australian Commission on Safety and Quality in Health Care, Sydney

—— 2007c, *Draft: An Alternative Model for Safety and Quality Accreditation*, Australian Commission on Safety and Quality in Health Care, Sydney

—— 2008a, *Proposals on an Alternative Model for Safety and Quality Accreditation and Matters Relating to Costs and Duplication of Accreditation Processes*, Australian Commission on Safety and Quality in Health Care, Sydney

—— 2008b, *Final Report on the Review of National Safety and Quality Accreditation Standards*, Australian Commission on Safety and Quality in Health Care, Sydney

Australian Council for Safety and Quality in Health Care 2003, *Standards Setting and Accreditation Systems in Health: Consultation Papers*, Commonwealth of Australia, Canberra

Australian Council on Healthcare Standards 2005, *National Report on Health Services Accreditation Performance 2003 and 2004*, Australian Council on Healthcare Standards, Sydney

—— 2007, *National Report on Health Services Accreditation Performance 2003–2006*, Australian Council on Healthcare Standards, Sydney

—— 2008, *ACHS Clinical Indicator Report for Australia and New Zealand 2001–2007*, Australian Council on Healthcare Standards, Sydney

Australian Institute of Health and Welfare 2008, *Australia's Health 2008*, Australian Institute of Health and Welfare, Canberra

Blum, J. 2008, 'A revisionist model of hospital licensure', *Regulation & Governance*, vol. 2, no. 1, pp. 48–64

Braithwaite, J., Makkai, T. and Braithwaite, V. 2007, *Regulating Aged Care: Ritualism and the New Pyramid*, Edward Elgar, Cheltenham

Brennan, T. 1998, 'The role of regulation in quality improvement', *Milbank Quarterly*, vol. 76, no. 4, pp. 709–31

Collopy, B. 2000, 'Clinical indicators: An effective stimulus to improve patient care', *International Journal of Quality in Health Care*, vol. 12, no. 3, pp. 211–16

Consumers Health Forum of Australia 2007, *Safety and Quality Project 2007-08: It is All About Communication*, Information Paper May 2007, Consumers Health Forum of Australia, Canberra

Crisp, H. 2006, 'Training surveyors for consistency', paper presented at the ISQua Conference, London, 22–25 October

Davies, G. 2005, *Commissions of Inquiry Order (No. 2) 2005*, <www.qphci.qld.gov.au/final_report/Final_Report.pdf>, accessed 3 December 2008

Department of Health and Aged Care 2000, *Education and Training for Consumer Participation in Health Care*, Commonwealth of Australia, Canberra

Department of Health and Ageing 2006, *The State of Our Public Hospitals*, Commonwealth of Australia, Canberra

—— 2008, *Media Release and Summary of Australian Health Ministers Meeting April 2008*, Commonwealth of Australia, Canberra

Duckett, S., Collins, J., Kamp, M. and Walker, K. 2008, 'An improvement focus in public reporting: The Queensland approach', *Medical Journal of Australia*, vol. 189, nos 11/12, pp. 616–17

Faunce, T. and Bolsin, S. 2004, 'Three Australian whistle blowing sagas: Lessons for internal and external regulation', *Medical Journal of Australia*, vol. 181, no. 1, pp. 44–7

Fung, C.H., Lim, Y.W., Mattke, S., Damberg, C. and Shekelle, P. 2008, 'Systematic review: The evidence that publishing patient care performance data improves quality of care', *Annals of Internal Medicine*, vol. 148, no. 2, pp. 111–23

Gaul, G.M. 2005, 'Accreditors blamed for overlooking problems', *Washington Post*, 25 July, Washington, DC

Greenfield, D. and Braithwaite, J. 2007, *A Review of Health Sector Accreditation Research Literature*, Centre for Clinical Governance Research, University of New South Wales, Sydney

Hafez, N. 1997, *Technical Report Number 15: International Comparative Review of the Health Care Regulatory Systems*, Partnerships for Health Reform, United States Agency for International Development, Bethesda

Hibberd, J., Stockard, J. and Tusler, M. 2003, 'Does public hospital performance reporting stimulate quality improvement efforts', *Health Affairs*, vol. 22, no. 2, pp. 84–94

Healthcare Commission 2006, *The Concordat: Working in Partnership*, <www.concordat.org.uk/homepage.cfm>, accessed 7 January 2009

—— 2007, *The Concordat Website: Key Achievements*, <www.concordat.org.uk/progress?keyachievements.cfm>, accessed 7 January 2009

Health Care Consumers Association (HCCA) of the ACT 2003, *Discussion Paper: Response to the Consumer Health Forum and Submission to the Consumer Participation Project in the Australian Council for Safety and Quality in Health Care Planning Process*, August, HCCA, Canberra

JAS-ANZ 2008, <www.jas.anz.com.au>, accessed 15 September 2008

Marquez, L. 2001, *Helping Healthcare Providers Perform According to Standards*, Operations Research Issues Paper 2(3), US Agency for International Development by the Quality Assurance Project, Bethesda

Marshall, M., Shekelle, P., Leathman, S. and Brook, R. 2000, 'The public release of performance data. What do we expect to gain? A review of the evidence', *Journal of the American Medical Association*, vol. 283, no. 14, pp. 1866–74

McCallum, L. 2002, 'Consumer participation in accreditation', Editorial, *The Australian Health Consumer*, vol. 2002, no. 2, pp. 4–6

McKee, M. and Healy, J., eds 2002, *Hospitals in a Changing Europe*, Open University Press/Buckingham, Philadelphia, PA

Mental Health Council of Australia 2008, Network of Consumer and Carer Surveyors, <http://mhca.org.au>, accessed 7 January 2009

Morrissey, J. 2002, 'Eyeing the watchdog', *Modern Healthcare*, vol. 32, no. 16, pp. 8–9

New South Wales Government 2008, *Private Hospital Licensing*, <www.nsw.gov.au/hospital/phc/licensing>, accessed 3 November 2008

Office of Statewide Health Planning and Development 2009, Healthcare Information Division—Data Products, Office of Statewide Health Planning and Development, State of California, <www.oshpd.ca.gov/HID/DataFlow/HospQuality.html>, accessed 9 January 2009

Øvretveit, J. 2003, *What are the Best Strategies for Ensuring Quality in Hospitals?*, Health Evidence Network, World Health Organization Europe, Copenhagen

Patterson, R. 2005, *National Arrangements for Safety and Quality of Health Care in Australia: The Report of the Review of Future Governance Arrangements for Safety and Quality in Health Care*, Commonwealth of Australia, Canberra, <www.health.gov.au/internet/wcms/publishing.nsf/content>, accessed 6 July 2006

Robinson, R. 1995, 'Accrediting hospitals', *British Medical Journal*, vol. 310, no. 6982, pp. 755–6

Rooney, A. and Van Ostenberg, P. 1999, *Licensure Accreditation and Certification: Approaches to Health Services Quality*, Quality Assurance Methodology Refinement Series, US Agency for International Development, Bethesda

Scholle, H.S. 2006, 'Transparency: Does public reporting help or hinder quality?' paper presented at the ISQua Conference, London, 22–25 October

Scrivens, E. 1995, *Accreditation: Protecting the Professional or the Consumer?* Open University Press/Buckingham, Philadelphia, PA

—— 1998, 'Policy issues in accreditation', *International Journal for Quality in Health Care*, vol. 10, no. 1, pp. 1–5

Shaw, C. 2003, 'Editorial: Evaluating accreditation', *International Journal of Quality in Health Care*, vol. 15, no. 6, pp. 455–6

—— 2004, *Toolkit for Accreditation Programs*, International Society for Quality in Health Care, Melbourne

Standards Australia 2007, *What is a Standard?*, <www.standards.org.au>, accessed 29 January 2007

Trowbridge, R. and Wachter, R. 2001, 'Legislation, accreditation, and market-driven and other approaches to improving patient safety', in *Making Health Care Safer: A Critical Analysis of Patient Safety Practices*, eds K. Shojana, B. Duncan, K. McDonald and R. Wachter, Agency for Healthcare Research and Quality, Rockville, MD

UK Department of Health 2008, *Quality Indicators*, <www.hsj.co.uk/news/2008/11/dh_sets_out_framework_for_improving_quality_of_care.html>, accessed 18 November 2008

Zeribi, K. and Marquez, L. 2005, *Approaches to Health Care Regulation in Latin America and the Caribbean: Regional Experiences and Challenges*, LACHSR report number 63, United States Agency for International Development Quality Assurance Project, Bethesda

14

CONNECTING HEALTH CARE THROUGH INFORMATION TECHNOLOGY

Peter Sprivulis

Health care has long recognised the first-order benefits of investment in information technology to improve the timeliness and quality of clinical information access, to automate repetitive health care tasks and to allow the extraction of structured data to support evaluation of health care performance. In the face of an overwhelming chronic disease epidemic, investment in more sophisticated technologies (e-health systems) that empower health consumers to manage their own care and enable the sharing of clinical information and clinical decision-making between a multidisciplinary team and the health consumer is urgently required.

This chapter addresses the role of e-health in delivering these health care reforms, and examines the technical, clinical and organisational regulatory challenges associated with the implementation of a national e-health system.

THE CHALLENGES FACING AUSTRALIAN HEALTH CARE

Australian health care is faced with daunting challenges during the first half of the twenty-first century. Relentless growth in demand for health care services, where every year will be harder, will be the norm. Australian government health expenditure is projected to nearly double as a proportion of GDP, from 3.8 per cent in 2006–07 to 7.3 per cent in

2046–47 (Commonwealth Department of Treasury 2007: 47). This rise in demand is fuelled by population ageing, increasing rates of chronic disease, and rising health consumer expectations and health care technology costs. An increasing gap between health services supply and demand is developing. This is illustrated by the fact that, despite the real growth in health care expenditure in Australia exceeding 5 per cent per annum between 1995–96 and 2005–06 (Australian Institute of Health and Welfare 2007: 8), Australian health consumers are experiencing increasing delays and difficulty in accessing the most basic health care services, such as access to primary care, access to chronic disease prevention, access to planned elective surgery and access to Emergency Department care (Australian Institute of Health and Welfare 2006). Access is particularly poor for Australians residing in rural and regional communities and for those with the poorest health in Australia—that is, Indigenous Australians (Commonwealth Department of Treasury 2007; Mooney 2003; Humphreys et al. 2002; Australian Bureau of Statistics 2005).

Australia, in common with most OECD economies, has recognised the need to radically alter the delivery of health care if access is to improve and Australia's currently excellent health outcomes are to be maintained. The main thrust of reform is an increased emphasis on prevention of chronic disease and, where chronic disease is present, earlier identification and more aggressive management and monitoring in order to delay or prevent complications that often require expensive hospital-based management (National Health and Hospitals Reform Commission 2008a). The National Health and Hospitals Reform Commission has been charged with the responsibility of developing the blueprint for Australia's health care system reform by the national government (National Health and Hospitals Reform Commission 2008b).

Fractured health care

Amongst the many challenges the national health reform agenda faces, the fragmented, even fractured, nature of health care delivery in Australia has been recognised as a significant reform barrier. Australian health care is delivered in a wide range of community- and hospital-based settings. At present, the ability to share information between these settings is limited and fragmented. Communication failures and disconnects result in delays in care, and duplication of procedures and investigations, forcing poorly informed health care providers to 'reinvent the wheel'. This fractured system results in the inefficient use of valuable resources, reduces quality of care, impairs continuity of patient care and threatens patient safety. An analysis of 'sentinel events' (events that potentially or actually lead to serious harm to patients) in Australian public hospitals in 2004–05 reported that the most common contributing factor was lack of, problems with, or breakdown in rules/policies/procedures in information/documentation. This was mainly due to a breakdown in communication (Australian Institute of Health and Welfare, and Australian Commission on Safety and Quality in Health Care 2007). Fractured health care causes significant harm to patients through medication errors, omissions and errors in care delivery due to unreliable and inadequate processes of communication and information sharing, both within organisations and across different health care service providers. Medical errors have been estimated to cost between one and two billion dollars annually, despite many of them being potentially preventable (Richardson and McKie 2007; Wilson et al. 1995).

The chronic disease 'merry-go-round'

Figure 14.1 illustrates the experiences of a typical health consumer with chronic disease attempting to negotiate the chronic disease 'merry-go-round'. The figure shows a 58-year-old woman with diabetes attempting to negotiate a round of referrals in order for health professionals to work out whether her diabetes is damaging her kidneys and, if so, what should be done about it.

The figure illustrates that poor information-sharing results in inefficiencies and less than optimal care. This manifests as unnecessary repetition of diagnostic tests and increased patient risk. Unfortunately for the patient, the kidney damage that gave rise to the referral could have been dealt with months or years earlier—if only her general practitioner (GP) had been able to detect a subtle deterioration in her kidney function amongst the paper 'blizzard' of results and reports generated by the chronic disease merry-go-round. No matter how good the actual quality of care is at any particular point in the referral cycle (or how talented the individual doctor), unless there is high-quality information recording, sharing and use, patient risk is increased.

In a system with poor information-sharing and a high degree of patient movement between providers (10 per cent of all GP consults are with a patient that they have never seen before), the accumulation of inefficiencies in the health care system can be very costly. It is estimated that 25 per cent of clinicians' time may be spent collecting data and information (Australian Audit Commission 1995). Similarly, up

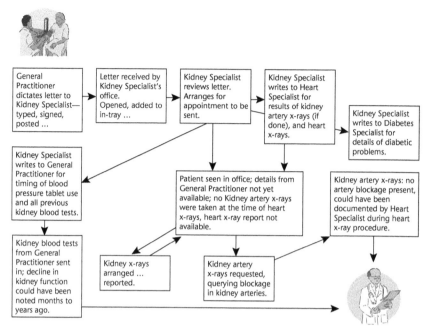

Figure 14.1 Information flow for a 58-year-old woman with diabetes referred to a kidney specialist—if all goes well

Source: Peter Sprivulis

to 35 per cent of referrals to hospitals are considered inappropriate (Elwyn and Stott 1994). The inability of a health professional to detect or discover what medications a patient may be taking can lead to diagnostic confusion and adverse drug reactions. The inappropriate use of medicines in Australia is estimated to be costing $380 million per year, just in direct costs, in the public hospital system alone (Australian Council for Safety and Quality in Health Care 2002).

ROLE OF E-HEALTH IN SUPPORTING AUSTRALIAN HEALTH CARE REFORM

Information technology has made a substantial impact on the timeliness and quality of clinical information access and the extraction of structured data to support evaluation of health care performance inside the walls of a single health care institution, such as a hospital, a pathology laboratory or a general practice clinic. The benefits of investment in more sophisticated technologies are increasingly recognised. These technologies empower health consumers to manage their own care, enable the sharing of clinical information and clinical decision-making between a multidisciplinary team and the health consumer (irrespective of physical location of the team members or health consumer), guided by the implementation of shared clinical knowledgemanagement and decision-support tools (Chaudhry et al. 2006).

The forms of e-health investment that appear likely to yield the largest benefits by supporting health care reform to improve chronic disease management, the appropriateness and safety of health care delivery, improved demand management and increased health care workforce productivity are summarised below.

Improving appropriate use of health care services via e-referral

The key to accessing appropriate 'upstream' care, prior to the development of complications requiring hospitalisation, is referral of the right patient to the right health care service at the right time. Reform of referral processes, enabled by e-health investment, provides an opportunity for state and territory jurisdictions to intervene in the course of a chronic illness and to reduce the requirements for hospitalisation for the management of complications. Referrals may be made more accurate using a combination of appropriate referral guidelines and access to better information when triaging incoming referrals.

Supporting better use of medicines via e-prescribing and medication management

Electronic prescribing decision support, when properly integrated with prescribing workflows, has consistently been demonstrated to improve the appropriateness of prescribing, with increased rates of prescription of the most appropriate, effective and least expensive prescribing option, in a wide range of clinical settings. Prescribing decision support is also associated with substantial reductions in the rates of adverse drug events.

In addition, the current national investment in e-health infrastructure via the National E-Health Transition Authority (NEHTA) can be used for the development of medication management monitoring systems in order to detect problems associated with medication adherence or incorrect and unsafe dosing for all Australians taking prescribed medication.

Enabling self-managed care through online self-managed care services and e-consultation

Self-managed care, where the health consumer is given the tools, education and support to effectively manage their chronic disease themselves, yields better health outcomes than paternalistic models of chronic disease management (see Sarol et al. 2005). The widespread penetration of broadband internet services into the households of ageing Australian baby boomers with chronic diseases offers an important opportunity to reform the default model of care for stable chronic disease, such as high blood pressure, diabetes, asthma and high cholesterol.

Self-managed care requires a shared electronic health record and e-consultation tools (that have the form, function and are as intuitive and familiar as email). Together, these enable health consumers to share important changes in their clinical condition, or discuss important questions concerning the management of their condition with their primary health care provider in a timely and cost-effective way.

Improving the management of complex health problems through shared care

The principal objective of shared care is to enhance the day-to-day monitoring of health consumers with complex or potentially unstable clinical conditions, in order to improve the timeliness and effectiveness of interventions to reduce the severity of complications of these conditions. Shared care is critically dependent upon the daily capture and recording of patient observations and symptoms, and the sharing of this information between a range of health care providers, some of whom are engaged in the direct delivery of care, and others who provide advice and guidance to the care process. Shared care works most effectively when the shared care team accesses and uses a common information platform—the shared electronic health care record—and a common set of decision-support tools. These ensure that there is a shared understanding between all team members, regarding the appropriate initial treatment, and routes of referral and escalation of clinical problems as they arise, in order that timely, knowledgeable and appropriate interventions can be initiated to restore the patient's health.

Making use of national shared electronic health record data to evaluate the effectiveness of health spending, and medical product and device safety

A significant proportion of health care funding is wasted because its effect cannot be measured due to a lack of relevant data. Harmonising the identifiers and terminologies used in national health care information stores, and linking this information to national shared electronic health record health care outcome data, accelerates evaluation of the effectiveness and safety of new health care products, services, policies and expenditure.

AUSTRALIAN E-HEALTH INVESTMENT

A substantial investment in e-health infrastructure to assist healing of the information fractures is currently underway within Australia. It is estimated that Australian federal, state and territory governments have spent approximately $2 billion on e-health infrastructure during the period 1999–2008. This includes direct investment in a range of mechanisms such as national e-health identifiers, terminologies and standards via NEHTA, information technology adoption incentives to community providers, and expenditure within state/territory public health systems. The existing investment is necessary, but not sufficient, to fully enable the level of information-sharing required to support effective chronic disease management.

The requirement for further coordinated e-health investment has been recognised by the recent publication of a national e-health strategy (Department of Health and Ageing 2008). The strategy describes an evolutionary, rather than revolutionary, approach to e-health development, and acknowledges the need for national infrastructure, such as a universal provider, and individual health consumer identifiers. The strategy emphasises the need to develop core information services that are nationally scalable, such as a common connectivity 'stack' that allows any provider to exchange information with any other in the country or an e-consultation service. As the national e-health agenda matures, there will be a need to balance the desire to achieve national alignment/participation with the value and knowledge gained through smaller scale 'cutting edge' systems implemented locally by smaller regions, such as an area health service or GP division.

The strategy recognises the pivotal role of shared health records in implementing the e-health reforms described above. Investment in national shared electronic health records logically and naturally builds on the investment in foundation national e-health services (including universal health care identifiers, clinical terminologies, interoperability and messaging standards) by Australian governments via NEHTA. These enable sharing of health care information between community provider records (e.g. general practitioner, pharmacy, residential care, personal health consumer records, pathology, imaging and medical specialist reports) and hospital provider records (e.g. discharge summaries, procedure and outpatient consultation reports).

Shared electronic health records allow the distillation and assembly of information that represents the distinctive features or state of an individual's health at a point in time, relevant to ongoing health care delivery or clinical decision-making, and collation in a form that can be made ubiquitously available and interpretable by other e-health services. It is important to observe that the form of national shared records is not likely to be a single vast data 'bucket' containing every scrap of electronic information concerning an individual's health. Rather, national shared records are likely to be brought together in a manner similar to the folios of a compendium, bound by the use of common identifiers and information specifications, with different folios added over time, according to health care priority and having due regard for individual privacy (e.g. beginning with summary health profile information and information available in existing national registers, such as the Australian Childhood Immunisation Register).

REGULATORY CHALLENGES

The Australian e-health strategy recognises the need for an ongoing coordination and orchestration entity, most likely leveraging Australia's existing investment in NEHTA, operating under the stewardship of a national e-health governance board. This entity faces a number of formidable challenges in delivering the national e-health specifications and information services that comprise the 'railroad tracks' of national health reform. If the *current* Australian e-health architecture is likened to a railway system, it would be apparent that the trains do not currently share the same timetable and run on a variety of incompatible rail gauges. Significantly, many of the carriages can't be connected to the available engines and are not properly designed to carry confidential freight safely. In addition, there is significant uncertainty about the best route via which to send the freight, and little knowledge of whether the freight (that is, confidential health information) ever arrives at its intended destination.

Interoperability challenges

This disconnectedness is a consequence of the failure to recognise the importance of interoperability in strategic e-health investment, noting that—as with many complex, abstract concepts—this is far easier to do in hindsight. Information system interoperability is the ability of information systems to exchange information and to use the information that has been exchanged (Institute of Electrical and Electronics Engineers 2001). Interoperability is familiar to all of us through the national and international electronic banking system, where every credit card is the same shape and size and can be swiped and read by any credit card reader in any shop in the world. Further, the local e-commerce network behind the card reader can find and communicate, via an interoperable electronic banking network, with your bank, check whether you have the funds available to complete your transaction, and request that your bank initiate the transfer of funds to the shop owner's bank account on your behalf. The creation of this worldwide interoperable network is a stunningly successful example of networked regulation (see Figure 2.2 in Chapter 2). This regulatory network is driven largely by the enormous transactional efficiencies that stem from banking transaction automation enabled by interoperability for each actor within the network, including us as customers, the shop owners from where we purchase, and our banks and credit card providers.

From the above railway system analogy, it should be apparent that Australia's past e-health investments have created significant technical, business process and organisational interoperability challenges. From these challenges flow equally important challenges for adoption, change management, governance and coordination, that must be overcome if health care is to emulate the interoperability of the international banking system.

Technical challenges

A naïve but intuitive classification usefully classifies technical interoperability into four broad levels (see Table 14.1).

Information exchange between Australian health care institutions (e.g. hospital to general practice and vice versa) currently occurs at all four levels. Most current Level 4 interoperability initiatives are focusing

307

Table 14.1 Definitions of four levels of sophistication and standardisation of health information exchange interoperability

Level number	Interoperability	Definition	Example
Level 1	Non-electronic data	Minimal use of information technology to share information	Mail, telephone
Level 2	Machine-transportable data	Transmission of non-standardised information via basic information technology; information within the document cannot be electronically manipulated	Fax or exchange of documents in other image formats such as scanned documents transmitted as portable document format (PDF) files
Level 3	Machine-organisable data	Transmission of structured messages containing non-standardised data; requires interfaces to translate data from the sending organisation's vocabulary to the receiving organisation's vocabulary	E-mail of free text, exchange of files in incompatible/proprietary file formats
Level 4	Machine-interpretable data	Transmission of structured messages containing standardised and coded data; systems exchange information using the same formats and vocabularies	Automated exchange of coded results from external laboratories into an electronic medical record, automated exchange of the patient's 'active problem' lists between providers

Source: Adapted from Walker et al. (2005).

on specific, high-volume, structured information domains (such as pathology result messaging), in order to reduce information exchange transaction costs, (similar to the banking example described above) by increasing the automation of message creation, exchange and filing, rather than being driven by genuine reform to the model of Australian health care.

An important role for the national e-health entity that supersedes NEHTA will be the creation of a national certification and conformance accreditation process. This would ensure that future e-health investments conform to the specifications developed by NEHTA for the use of technical standards for electronic information exchange, including the specifications concerning:

- secure messaging standards;
- clinical terminology standards;
- electronic clinical document structure standards;
- interoperability with national e-health infrastructure, such as national health provider and individual identifiers; and
- technical architecture.

In many ways, technical interoperability is the 'easiest' of the e-health interoperability challenges to manage and regulate (from a position about halfway up the responsive regulation pyramid). Many of the standards specified by NEHTA already exist, and testing conformance with them is a well-defined and relatively straightforward process that is well accepted within the international information technology industry. While the rail gauges can be standardised, what may be more important is what freight is being carried by them.

Business process challenges

While the technical interoperability issues deal with whether or not electronic information is transported (i.e. one machine can talk to another machine), it does not address issues of health information quality, or the extent to which shared information can be trusted by all actors who may need to rely upon it in a particular health care microsystem. The extent to which information can be trusted requires the recognition and adoption of common, safe, reliable clinical business processes by clinicians (business process interoperability), so that apparently similar types of information from different clinical sources can confidently be reconciled with each other, allowing the maintenance of a trustable 'source of truth'.

High-priority examples of health information that has high value for clinical decision-making, and carries high risks if not properly reconciled, include an individual's list of current and past clinical problems, their medications and known adverse drug reactions/drug allergies. This information comprises the kernel of an individual's 'summary health profile'. Summary health profile information is often updated during individual episodes of care, such as during a general practice consultation or hospital admission. Any shared electronic health record system will necessarily contain copies of an individual's summary health profile, even if only in serial event summaries (such as hospital discharge summaries, referral documents produced by GPs and specialist medical reports), although preferably as a structured information service. The accuracy of summary health profile information depends on the hospital doctor, general practitioner and specialist all understanding the importance of the summary health profile, and upon multiple actors having an interest in its content, currency and accuracy. Crucially, all must use the same business process to verify the information at the commencement of an episode of care, and to document and communicate changes to the information at the end of the episode of care.

Development of standard business processes for summary health profile reconciliation is a complex undertaking. In the absence of such processes, the accuracy of shared records may be called into question, substantially reducing their informational value.

Standard business processes are required for most health information-handling and sharing scenarios. These processes must cover relatively simple processes, such as patient identification (to ensure that at the onset of an episode of care, the correct universal patient identifier is allocated to the patient's clinical record). More challenging are the complexities of summary health profile reconciliation and pathology messaging, where pathology results require acknowledgment and action, to ensure a pathology laboratory can be confident an abnormal result (e.g. a positive Pap smear) has been acknowledged and the patient appropriately referred for gynaecological follow-up. Electronic prescribing in the era of electronic prescribing decision support is another critical example of a business process that, if not implemented correctly, can result in far more harm than good (Coiera and Westbrook 2006).

The fragmentation of Australia's health care community makes it highly unlikely that safe and reliable business process standards will emerge by self-regulation alone. Few actors within the community currently appreciate the importance of standard processes for information-handling. Experience with shared record trials in the Northern Territory, however, illustrate a fairly rapid appreciation of the need to contribute accurate and up-to-date information to health records within a local shared record environment.

Increasing awareness of the need for standard business processes for health information handling, and translating this awareness into active participation in the coordinated development of nationally scalable business processes, will require the creation of a new 'line of business' by the national e-health entity that supersedes NEHTA, in conjunction with Australia's leading health care quality and safety agencies.

On the positive side, one of information technology's great assets is the capability to 'hard wire' a desired business process as a default process, once that business process has been defined. Software is much easier and less expensive to develop, and the implementation risks are greatly lowered, once appropriate standard business processes have been identified and translated into software requirements.

Organisational challenges

While the presence of technical interoperability and common business processes will ensure that accurate, valuable and transportable health information is *available*, it does not guarantee that valuable health inform-ation will be *shared* when needed. A significant set of issues that frequently hamper health information sharing initiatives is a failure of organisational interoperability. The differences in organisational policies concerning health information custodianship, access, review, amendment and sharing between different health care organisations within Australia's diverse health care community, preclude sharing, or the acknowledgment of the validity of shared electronic health information.

A simple example of an organisational policy standing in the way of e-health connectivity is the story of electronic prescribing. Despite the spending of several hundred million dollars of federal provider incentives, and near world-leading uptake of prescribing software technologies in Australia's general practice community over a twenty-year period, legislative barriers (that were only removed in 2008) pre-cluded pharmacy acceptance of digitally signed prescriptions. This has meant that all Australian electronically generated prescriptions, until very recently, needed to be printed and signed by hand, stifling the development of e-health connectivity between primary care and community pharmacy.

A common and general organisational interoperability problem in e-health is the management of an individual's right to privacy, when one health care provider or organisation seeks to share health information with another for the primary purpose of continuing clinical care (e.g. sharing of a clinical report written by specialist in private with another specialist working in an acute hospital). Differences in organisational approaches to the management of privacy often drive the development of non-interoperable organisational information-sharing policies, which can result in valuable information not being shared when needed.

The magnitude of the problem has been recognised by specifically charging NEHTA, and the entity that will supersede NEHTA, with responsibility for supporting the development of a national blueprint for the management of privacy in the e-health era, that takes into account and balances often conflicting goals, principles and legislation in an attempt to ensure important information is available when needed in the interests of the clinical care, while ensuring the individual's right to privacy and control of their privacy are maintained.

Adoption and change management challenges

In stimulating the adoption of interoperability, there are several critical considerations. These include the most appropriate change management tools to apply, the structure of incentives and engagement strategies to engage the hearts and minds of both clinicians and health consumers, recognition that the ultimate goal of the strategy implies profound reform of health care delivery, and the importance of avoiding unilateral e-health investment strategies that run counter to the information-sharing paradigm supporting the overall health care reform objectives.

The costs associated with change management and adoption are typically an order of magnitude *higher* than the costs associated with the acquisition of the technology. There is little point in trimming the technology acquisition budget if it is likely to result in a solution that is more difficult to integrate into workflows, or if it will not fully support the desired health care reform. Equally, there is little point in investing in technology if there are major structural obstacles that will prevent adoption and uptake. An example of the latter is e-consultation where, until such time as an appropriate remuneration model is designed, it is highly unlikely that general practitioners will support the use of email-style consultations to support self-managed care of chronic disease, if the general practice remuneration model only funds in-person face-to-face consultations.

In designing the appropriate change-management and adoption model, there is no substitute for experimentation and prototyping (rapidly, and on a small scale) to inform model development. Prototyping provides an instance of an implementation that can be touched, felt and engaged with by all stakeholders. Prototyping teaches us that we usually know less than we assume we know about what will work in the real world, as well as what features of an implementation are important or not to users of the technology. Prototyping should be a collaborative exercise and conducted to take advantage of grassroots knowledge of process, while keeping in mind the goals of national scalability, interoperability and sustainable architecture.

Again, one of e-health's greatest benefits is in 'hard wiring' the desired clinical decision or action as the *default* decision or action. If the prototype reveals that the technology/business process solution does not result in making the right thing the easiest thing to do, the solution must be reconsidered or redesigned.

Governance and coordination challenges

The potential benefits from investment in e-health are considerable. However, investment in e-health won't yield benefits by itself, but rather should be seen as an investment in the railway system needed to carry health reform. The realisation of benefits will require a high level of cooperation between all Australian health care stakeholders, and the development and implementation of a coordinated approach to the financial, policy and clinical change management. Careful consideration of the most appropriate governance structure is needed, given the requirement to integrate policy, financial, clinical and e-health investment across both state, territory and federal spheres of health care operations, and the need to adequately consider and represent the interests of all stakeholders, including health care professionals, health consumers, private insurers and private health care providers.

The national e-health strategy is critical of current e-health governance arrangements, noting:

> The current national E-Health governance arrangements have supported improved coordination between Commonwealth and the State and Territory Governments in the oversight of their respective health information management responsibilities. However, the current arrangements are not sufficient to provide effective governance of the national E-Health agenda. This is due to factors such as a lack of

organisational capability or capacity to deliver the national E-Health strategy and work program, a high reliance on collaboration between disparate committee, sub-committee and working groups, and the relatively limited representation of key health stakeholders in decision making processes. (Department of Health and Ageing 2008: 18)

The strategy enunciates a number of governance principles that should underpin the design of a national e-health governance structure. These principles include greater clarity of accountability, transparency and appropriate stakeholder representation that is not unduly influenced by the rapidity of change at the political level, in order to drive greater collaboration between all stakeholders in working towards the common long-term e-health and health-reform objectives.

The strategy document recommends that a national e-health governing board, comprising an independent chair and a breadth of cross-sectoral stakeholder representation, reporting to the Australian Health Ministers' Advisory Council, takes accountability for setting overall national e-health direction and priorities, for reviewing and approving e-health strategy and funding decisions, and for monitoring progress against national e-health strategy deliverables and outcomes. The board would be supported by and oversees an ongoing national e-health entity, superseding NEHTA, to coordinate and oversee the e-health strategy, investment and the execution of the national components of the e-health work program.

The challenge for such an independent and consolidated structure, which supersedes a byzantine array of committees and entities with fragmented responsibility, will be to maintain an outward-looking attitude that is genuinely attentive to the requirements of health reform. The end-game is not a technically beautiful and 'complete' system ready at some point in the future. Rather, the governance structure must provide the coordination for an ongoing journey, and should concentrate on delivering what we currently understand as being the most important e-health technologies, that will enable the most urgently required health reforms, in the full knowledge that both our understanding of what is required and how to deliver it will continue to evolve in the future.

CONCLUSION

Australia is making substantial progress in developing the e-health infrastructure necessary to support the reform of its health care services, in order to meet the challenges of delivering safe and effective health care to an ageing population with high rates of chronic disease, using innovative models of care, in the twenty-first century. The ongoing rate and effectiveness of Australian health reform will be greatly influenced by the availability of national e-health infrastructure, particularly the availability of shared electronic health records. Several e-health steps with the capacity to accelerate reform have been identified, and each will make an important contribution to improving the appropriateness, effectiveness and safety of Australian health care.

As health care organisations implement these more sophisticated and complex systems of health care, the need to collaborate effectively at the organisational, clinical process and information-sharing levels requires all actors in the health care system to give up some autonomy. All actors in the health care enterprise must migrate towards collaboratively maintained and shared sources of 'clinical truth', in order to gain the trust of the health care community expected to rely upon them. These sources must be maintained by common and agreed (i.e. interoperable) business processes for both manual and electronic clinical information handling and reconciliation, and common (i.e. interoperable) technical standards for electronic clinical information exchange.

A logical role for networked regulation follows from this requirement to collaborate effectively at the technical, business process and organisational/model of care levels. This applies not only in the 'propellor head' technical electronic information architecture and exchange domains, but also—and perhaps more importantly—in the recognition and adoption of common, safe, reliable clinical business processes by clinicians, and in the policies for electronic information-sharing, custodianship and access between the diverse array of health care organisations that comprise the Australian health care community.

REFERENCES

Australian Audit Commission 1995, *For Your Information*, Australian Audit Commission, Canberra

Australian Bureau of Statistics 2005, *The Health and Welfare of Australia's Aboriginal and Torres Strait Islander Peoples*, Australian Bureau of Statistics, Canberra

Australian Council for Safety and Quality in Health Care 2002, *Second National Report on Patient Safety Improving Medication Safety*, Australian Council for Safety and Quality in Health Care, Canberra

Australian Institute of Health and Welfare 2006, *Australia's Health 2006*, AIHW cat. no. AUS 73, Australian Institute of Health and Welfare, Canberra, <www.aihw.gov.au/publications/index.cfm/title/10321>, accessed 29 January 2009

—— 2007, *Health Expenditure Australia 2005-06*, AIHW cat. no. HWE 37, Australian Institute of Health and Welfare, Canberra, <www.aihw.gov.au/publications/index.cfm/title/10529>, accessed 29 January 2009

Australian Institute of Health and Welfare and Australian Commission on Safety and Quality in Health Care 2007, *Sentinel Events in Australian Public Hospitals 2004-05*, AIHW cat. no. HSE 51, Australian Institute of Health and Welfare, Canberra, <www.aihw.gov.au/publications/index.cfm/title/10353>, accessed 29 January 2009

Chaudhry, B., Wang, J., Wu, S., Maglione, M., Mojica, W., Roth, E., Morton, S.C. and Shekelle, P.G. 2006, 'Systematic Review: Impact of Health Information Technology on Quality, Efficiency, and Costs of Medical Care', *Annals of Internal Medicine*, vol. 144, no. 10, pp. 742-52

Coiera, E.W. and Westbrook, J.I. 2006, 'Should clinical software be regulated?', *Medical Journal of Australia*, vol. 184, no. 12, pp. 600-1

Commonwealth Department of Treasury 2007, *Intergenerational Report 2007*, Commonwealth Department of Treasury, Canberra, <www.treasury.gov.au/igr/IGR2007.asp>, accessed 29 January 2009

Department of Health and Ageing 2008, *National E-Health Strategy Summary December 2008*, Commonwealth of Australia, Canberra, <www.health.gov.au/internet/main/publishing.nsf/Content/National+Ehealth+Strategy>, accessed 4 April 2009

Elwyn, G.J. and Stott, N.C.H. 1994, 'Avoidable referrals? Analysis of 170 consecutive referrals to secondary care', *British Medical Journal*, vol. 309, no. 6954, pp. 576-8

Humphreys, J., Hegney, D., Lipscombe, J., Gregory, G. and Chater, B. 2002, 'Whither rural health? Reviewing a decade of progress in rural health', *Australian Journal of Rural Health*, vol. 10, no. 1, pp. 2-14, <www.blackwell-synergy.com/doi/abs/10.1046/j.1440-1584.2002.00435.x>, accessed 29 January 2009

Institute of Electrical and Electronics Engineers 2001, *The Authoritative Dictionary of IEEE Standards Terms*, 7th ed., Institute of Electrical and Electronics Engineers, New York

Mooney, G.H. 2003, 'Inequity in Australian health care: How do we progress from here?' *Australian and New Zealand Journal of Public Health*, vol. 27, no. 3, pp. 267-70

National Health and Hospitals Reform Commission 2008a, *Principles for Australia's Health System*, Commonwealth of Australia, Canberra, <www.nhhrc.org.au/internet/nhhrc/publishing.nsf/Content/principles-lp>, accessed 29 January 2009

——2008b, *Terms of Reference*, Commonwealth of Australia, Canberra, <www.nhhrc.org.au/internet/nhhrc/publishing.nsf/Content/terms-of-reference>, accessed 29 January 2009

Richardson, J. and McKie, J. 2007, *Reducing the Incidence of Adverse Events in Australian Hospitals: An Expert Panel Evaluation of Some Proposals*, report no. RP 2007 (19), Centre for Health Economics, Monash University, Melbourne, <www.buseco.monash.edu.au/centres/che/pubs/>, accessed 29 January 2009

Sarol J.N., Nicodemus, N.A., Tan, K.M. and Grava, M.B. 2005, 'Self-monitoring of blood glucose as part of a multi-component therapy among non-insulin requiring type 2 diabetes patients: A meta-analysis (1966-2004)', *Current Medical Research and Opinion*, vol. 21, no. 2, pp. 173–84

Trewin, D. and Madden, R. 2005, *The Health and Welfare of Australia's Aboriginal and Torres Strait Islander Peoples*, AIHW report no. 4704.0, Commonwealth of Australia, Canberra, <www.aihw.gov.au/publications/index.cfm/title/10172>, accessed 29 January 2009

Walker, J., Pan, E., Johnston, D., Adler-Milstein, J., Bates, D. and Middleton, B. 2005, 'The Value of Healthcare Information Exchange and Interoperability', *Health Affairs* Web Exclusive 19 January pp. W5–18

Wilson, R.M., Runciman, W.B., Gibberd, R.W., Harrison, B.T., Newby, L. and Hamilton, J.D. 1995, 'The Quality in Australian Health Care Study', *Medical Journal of Australia*, vol. 163, no. 9, pp. 458–71

15

DO PUBLIC INQUIRIES IMPROVE HEALTH CARE?

Malcolm Masso and Kathy Eagar

Health care services in Australia are regularly subjected to inquiries. These can be variously classified as inquisitorial/investigatory inquiries, system improvement inquiries/reviews (such as have occurred in mental health and maternity care), and 'political' and policy advisory inquiries, such as Senate inquiries.

The focus of this chapter is on inquisitorial/investigatory inquiries. These inquiries don't just happen. They are typically the culmination of a 'scandal' reported very widely in the media, and can be seen to represent a response to perceived regulatory failures. Along with court proceedings, licence suspensions and tribunals, public inquiries are one of the last resorts, a public statement that regulation has failed at lower levels in the regulatory pyramid (see Chapter 1). Yet not every 'scandal' in health care leads to a public inquiry. Indeed, the reality is quite the reverse: the number of inquisitorial/investigatory inquiries in Australia this decade has been minuscule in proportion to the number of systematic errors reported.

This chapter begins by examining the circumstances that have triggered public inquiries in this decade. It then uses these inquiries as case studies to examine whether, and to what extent, public inquiries have a role in improving the quality and safety of health care in Australia, and whether or not the need for public inquiries can be prevented.

TRIGGERS TO PUBLIC INQUIRIES

In Australia, inquisitorial/investigatory inquiries occur:

- regularly (and largely behind closed doors) at the level of the individual clinician (e.g. through the various health care complaints mechanisms);
- occasionally (and again behind closed doors) at the level of multidisciplinary teams of clinicians (again through the various health care complaints mechanisms); and
- infrequently at the organisational and state levels. Inquiries at this level typically, though not always, involve significant media coverage, public hearings and public submissions. They are always established by government.

Table 15.1 lists the major organisational and state level inquiries into patient care in Australia since 2000. All of these inquiries were instigated under state or territory legislation by the relevant minister and reported their findings back to that minister.

These six inquiries in eight years have three important features in common. All were about acute care in public hospitals. With the exception of Royal Melbourne Hospital and New South Wales acute care services, the immediate trigger was allegations raised by staff working at the same hospital. The New South Wales inquiry was triggered by a number of events that occurred around the same time, including a coroner's report, patient complaints and vocal complaints made in the media by clinicians. The role of staff in the events leading up to the inquiry is an important commonality that contrasts most of these inquiries with other methods of regulation—and, indeed, seems the best predictor of the circumstances likely to trigger a public inquiry. While complaints by patients may lead to other actions (such as closed inquiries by health care complaints organisations), public inquiries to date have been triggered by staff and/or organised community or political lobbies speaking out on behalf of patients. This suggests their third commonality—all attracted significant political and media interest.

There are also some important differences between these six inquiries. While all were in the media before the inquiry began, in three of the cases (King Edward Memorial Hospital, Royal Melbourne Hospital and the Canberra Hospital), the major media interest did not begin until the inquiry began or reported. In the other three cases (Camden and Campbelltown Hospitals, Bundaberg Base Hospital and New South Wales acute care services), there had already been intense media interest

Table 15.1 Major public inquiries since 2000

Health service	Abbreviation	State	Year	Trigger
King Edward Memorial Hospital	KEMH	Western Australia	2001	Allegations of unreasonably high rates of adverse clinical outcomes raised by the hospital chief executive
Royal Melbourne Hospital	RMH	Victoria	2002	Allegations of nursing misconduct raised in an anonymous letter to the hospital
Canberra Hospital	TCH	Australian Capital Territory	2003	Allegations of unsafe neurosurgical services raised by a doctor at the hospital
Camden and Campbelltown Hospitals	CCH	New South Wales	2003/04	Allegations of unsafe patient care raised by nurses at the hospital
Bundaberg Base Hospital	BBH	Queensland	2005	Allegations of unsafe surgeon raised by a nurse at the hospital
New South Wales acute care services	NSW	New South Wales	2008	Coroner's recommendation and allegations about two hospitals (Royal North Shore [RNS] and Bega Hospital [BHI]), against a background of concerns in the media about clinicians more broadly

before the inquiry. This media interest no doubt provided at least some of the impetus for the inquiry itself.

While some of the staff who raised the allegations were perceived as 'whistleblowers', not all were. In some but not all cases, the issues had been percolating in the background (sometimes for several years) before a trigger event finally led to the public inquiry. In other cases, the public inquiry was triggered as soon as the issues became public. Four inquiries were triggered by initial concerns about individual clinicians (Royal Melbourne Hospital, the Canberra Hospital, Bundaberg Base Hospital and Bega Hospital), but in two cases (King Edward Memorial Hospital, Camden and Campbelltown Hospitals) the initial allegations were more systemic or general in nature.

INQUIRY PROCESSES AND OUTCOMES

King Edward Memorial Hospital (KEMH)

On 7 December 1999, the hospital chief executive wrote to the chief executive officer of the (then) Metropolitan Health Service expressing significant concerns about the quality of clinical care and resultant patient safety at KEMH. An initial inquiry (the Child and Glover Review) was established by the Western Australia Department of Health and was undertaken in 2000. This was a two-week review. The reviewers spent one week at the hospital, interviewing 41 people and reviewing selected case notes, registers and other documents. The second week was spent writing the report. The review's findings led to significant media coverage and public debate, with individual doctors and the Western Australian branch of the Australian Medical Association opposing the findings publicly through the media.

The Minister for Health established the subsequent 'Douglas Inquiry' in 2001 in consultation with the state premier. It was established under the *Hospitals and Health Services Act* 1927 and the *Public Sector Management Act* 1994 of Western Australia, and led by a lawyer, Neil Douglas. The brief was 'to inquire into the provision of obstetric and gynaecological services at King Edward Memorial Hospital' over a decade (1990 to 2000). The inquiry focused on systemic and organisational deficiencies and considered management and clinical practices, policies and processes.

This inquiry was exhaustive, with evidentiary materials considered in the inquiry including:

- qualitative and quantitative clinical file analysis of 605 KEMH patient records;
- 293 written submissions;
- interviews with 70 former KEMH patients;
- transcripts of evidence from 106 current and former KEMH staff members;
- various consultants' reports; and
- other documents, amounting to over 2.25 million pages, obtained from KEMH and other sources (Douglas et al. 2001).

The extensive five-volume final report, with 237 recommendations, was tabled in parliament in December 2001. The Department of Health established an implementation group chaired by a deputy director of the department to oversee the implementation of the recommendations. The implementation group disbanded in June 2003 after it had agreed that it had 'completed its task given that all recommendations had been implemented, except the four requiring some form of legislative action'.

The Department of Health internal audit branch audited the implementation of the 237 recommendations in several stages for the next three years (until March 2005), at which time it reported that the substantial majority of recommendations had been implemented (Department of Health of Western Australia, 2005).

Royal Melbourne Hospital (RMH)

In October 2001, the Royal Melbourne Hospital received an anonymous letter alleging, among other matters, that two patients had died after being administered non-prescribed drugs by nurses in its neurology unit. The allegations were referred to the Coroner and Victoria Police. The Nurses Board of Victoria suspended the registration of two nurses and deferred investigations about the alleged misconduct pending the outcome of the coroner's investigation. The executive and board of Melbourne Health both conducted separate investigations into issues associated with the allegations.

In the same month as the allegations were made public (in March 2002), the Minister for Health directed that the Health Services Commissioner conduct an independent inquiry. In contrast to the extensive King Edward Memorial Hospital inquiry, the RMH inquiry was conducted over just three months. The inquiry investigated systemic issues, including medications management, incident-reporting systems, standards of documentation related to patient care, nursing management, systems for staff support and opportunities for improvement identified during the course of the review. The Health Services Commission was specifically asked to make recommendations to ensure quality improvements in systems.

The inquiry included a review of the organisational structure, interviews with 33 key staff, five group interviews involving 60 nurses and an audit of 60 patient records. In addition, the inquiry considered a written submission from the Australian Nursing Federation, undertook an inspection of the neuroscience unit and consulted with experts. Due to time constraints, no interviews were conducted with patients, families or carers and there was no public call for written submissions. No public hearings were conducted.

In total, the inquiry made 73 recommendations (Health Services Commissioner 2002). In response, Melbourne Health developed a Melbourne Health Improvement Plan and, in April 2004, hosted a conference to report on progress against recommendations. The Health Services Commissioner concluded that significant progress had been made and her analysis of the inquiry concluded that the process was both speedy and efficient (Health Services Commissioner 2004). Interestingly, a subsequent but unrelated study (Brand et al. 2007) investigating medical practitioner involvement in quality and safety systems at Melbourne Health found that, of 73 medical practitioners surveyed, 37 (50.7 per cent) had never heard of the report, eighteen (24.7 per cent) had heard of it but not read it, and only eighteen (24.7 per cent) had read it.

Canberra Hospital

In December 2000, the Community and Health Services Complaints Commissioner for the Australian Capital Territory received a request from the relevant minister to inquire into concerns about adverse neurosurgical patient outcomes at Canberra Hospital. Concerns had first been expressed by a physician at the hospital in 1998 (nearly two years before the inquiry) about the standard of care provided by the neurosurgeon who was the subject of the inquiry. A clinical review had been initiated in 1999, but did not proceed because of the lack of availability of the proposed international reviewers.

The review consisted of a statistical analysis of adverse outcomes, a review of information provided by other doctors at the hospital and an independent clinical audit of fourteen patients. The process took over two years to complete because of difficulties the Commissioner had in obtaining evidence from health professionals at the hospital. There was no call for written submissions and no public hearings were conducted.

The outcome of the inquiry was that the neurosurgeon in question voluntarily ceased to operate and a small number of recommendations were made about strengthening peer review and clinical governance systems. The final report was not published until December 2003, some nine months after it was completed (Community and Health Services Complaints Commissioner of the ACT 2003).

Camden and Campbelltown Hospitals

A total of 69 cases were initially referred for investigation to the New South Wales Health Care Complaints Commission by the New South Wales Minister for Health in 2002, based on information provided to him by a group of nurses at the hospitals. The investigation took over a year and, according to the Health Care Complaints Commission, was a 'systems' review.

Following the dismissal of the head of the Health Care Complaints Commission for a perceived failure to adequately investigate these initial allegations, a Special Commission of Inquiry into Campbelltown and Camden Hospitals was established. The nurse informants subsequently made additional allegations to this inquiry. These included allegations that went back as far as 1992. In total, the Special Commission investigated 128 allegations, including 126 allegations of poor patient care.

By the end, the two hospitals were the subject of six separate inquiries over almost three years—the Health Care Complaints Commission inquiry, an internal Health Department inquiry known as the Barraclough Inquiry, a New South Wales Upper House Inquiry into Complaints Handling in New South Wales, the Special Commission, and an Independent Commission Against Corruption inquiry. In addition, various cases were referred to the coroner for review, all of which were subsequently dismissed. Public hearings were held during both the Special Commission and the Upper House Inquiry, and submissions were invited. The various investigations attracted significant international and national media attention that continued for nearly two years.

The power of the Special Commissioner (Bret Walker) under New South Wales law was limited to referring practitioners who had a potential case to answer to the (newly revamped) Health Care Complaints Commission for investigation. In total, Walker referred 36 cases for investigation and dismissed 92 per cent of the allegations. The newly constituted Health Care Complaints Commission subsequently investigated the cases referred from the Special Commission, the outcome of which was that the Health Care Complaints Commission referred twelve clinicians for possible prosecution by either a tribunal or professional standards committee. All of these were subsequently dismissed, although a small number were reprimanded or counselled.

At the system level, the Special Commissioner found that, contrary to what had been alleged, there had been 'no cover-up' of inadequate patient care by the administration of the hospitals (Walker 2004: 2), and he made no adverse findings against any manager. He accepted evidence to the inquiry that the death and complication rates at Macarthur Health Service were no higher than at other comparable hospitals (Walker 2004: 9). Likewise, the Independent Commission Against Corruption subsequently dismissed all allegations of corrupt behaviour (Independent Commission Against Corruption 2005).

In addition to recommendations for legislative change to the statutory patient complaints system, the Special Commission made only five recommendations. Four of these were generic and dealt with procedures relating to the use of root cause analysis in investigating complaints. There was also a recommendation that, to the extent that they had not already done so, the area health authority create policies regarding the principles of open disclosure, complaints handling and dealing with concerns about a clinician.

The limited number of recommendations arising from this inquiry is in stark contrast to the outcomes of the King Edward Hospital and the Royal Melbourne Hospital inquiries. This is particularly the case given that Camden and Campbelltown Hospitals are sometimes grouped together with King Edward Memorial, Bristol and others as examples of scandals where an inquiry subsequently led to improved patient care.

Despite this, several important changes arose from the Camden and Campbelltown Hospitals inquiry. These included funding increases for the two hospitals, the establishment of the New South Wales Clinical Excellence Commission and a reorganisation of the area health service structure in New South Wales.

Bundaberg Base Hospital

The trigger for this inquiry was a collection of serious complaints made by a nurse at Bundaberg Base Hospital about Dr Jayant Patel, a surgeon who had been appointed to the hospital in 2003. The nurse,

Toni Hoffman, first raised her concerns internally in February 2004 and formalised them in a letter to the district manager in October 2004. In March 2005, she provided a copy of the letter to a member of parliament who tabled it in parliament that same month.

After a month of extensive media coverage, the Queensland government established the Bundaberg Hospital Commission of Inquiry (the Morris Inquiry) in April 2005. Its terms of reference included investigating specific issues arising from the appointment of Dr Jayant Patel to the hospital, the complaints that had been made and the reported failure of the hospital administration and Queensland Health to address those complaints. The Commissioner was subsequently restrained by the Supreme Court from proceeding with the Inquiry. A Commission of Inquiry (the Public Hospitals Commission of Inquiry or the Davies Inquiry) was established in September 2005 to continue the work of the Morris Inquiry. Both inquiries had terms of reference that allowed them to examine related issues at other hospitals, and both included public hearings and a call for public submissions.

The final report in November 2005 recommended legal proceedings against Dr Patel and these are still proceeding. It also identified system problems not only at Bundaberg Base Hospital but also at Hervey Bay, Townsville, Rockhampton, Charters Towers and Prince Charles Hospitals. The Commissioner identified five common causes:

- an inadequate budget defectively administered;
- a defective administration of area of need registration;
- an absence of credentialling and privileging or any like method of assessment of doctors;
- a failure to implement any adequate monitoring of performance or investigation of complaints; and
- a culture of concealment by government, Queensland Health administrators, and hospital administrators (Davies 2005: 538).

In parallel, a Queensland Health System Review (the Foster Review) had also been established in April 2005 to examine systemic issues. It reported in September that year (Forster 2005) and recommended sweeping changes to the funding, structure and culture of the Queensland health system.

The government responded by releasing its 'Action Plan—Building a Better Health Service for Queensland' the following month, including a commitment to a multi-billion dollar increase in the health budget. Other significant outcomes included a significant reorganisation of the Queensland health system, public reporting of the performance of Queensland hospitals, and the establishment of a central Reform and Development Division (now the Centre for Healthcare Improvement) within Queensland Health to lead and support the reform process. It includes units devoted to clinical practice improvement, patient safety, and workplace culture and leadership (see Chapter 6).

Acute care services in New South Wales

A Special Commission of Inquiry was established in January 2008 under state legislation. The immediate trigger was a coroner's report in the same month on Vanessa Anderson, a 16-year-old girl who had died at Royal North Shore in November 2005. The coroner found that her death had been preventable and was due to systematic errors in her care. The coroner stated that:

> Unfortunately the same issues are invariably identified, not enough doctors, not enough nurses, inexperienced staff, poor communication, poor record-keeping and poor management. These are systemic problems that have existed for a number of years, and regrettably they all surface in the death of Vanessa Anderson.

The coroner went on to state that: 'It may be timely that the Department of Health or the responsible minister consider a full and open enquiry into the delivery of health services in New South Wales.' (Milovanovich 2008)

The coroner's report had been preceded in December 2007 by the report of a New South Wales parliamentary inquiry into the Royal North Shore Hospital, the genesis of which was publication of allegations that poor care had been provided to several other patients. The inquiry made 45 recommendations, most of which were not confined to Royal North Shore.

At around the same time, there was also significant coverage in the media of other events, including allegations about Dr Graeme Reeves, an obstetrician who had been appointed to work at to Bega Hospital in 2002 (see also Chapter 10).

The government responded to these various events by establishing the Special Commission. The first report of the Special Commission concerns the appointment of Dr Reeves to Bega Hospital, and the policies and practices that existed at the time of his appointment. It found significant deficits in the appointment process and made nine recommendations relating to recruitment and credentialling. It also recommended that Dr Reeves be referred to the New South Wales Director of Public Prosecutions. Dr Reeves is currently in prison awaiting trial.

The terms of reference of the inquiry are much broader than the issues covered in the first report. They include identifying any systemic or institutional issues in the delivery of acute care services in New South Wales public hospitals, and recommending any changes required to existing models of patient care. There is a specific focus on case management, supervision of junior clinical staff, clinical note-taking and record-keeping, and communication between health professionals involved in patient care. The final report was delivered in November 2008 and includes 139 recommendations covering a wide range of issues (Garling 2008). At the time of writing, it is too early to assess the impact of the report.

Common themes

While each of the above inquiries dealt with specific issues, there were also some common themes that were repeated with different emphases in most, but not all, of the subsequent reports. These themes were initially identified in the King Edward Memorial Hospital inquiry, which was described as a 'wake-up call for governments, boards, chief executives, managers and clinicians', requiring a move away from 'softer' regulation to regulation with a harder edge:

- effective clinical governance and leadership that supports open disclosure;
- greater accountability for addressing performance problems;
- rigorous third-party accreditation;
- better data-collection systems to facilitate inter-hospital comparisons;
- standardised systems for credentialling;
- reliable and consistent incident and adverse event reporting systems;
- proper systems for reporting and investigating mortality (McLean and Walsh 2003: 23).

PROSECUTORIAL OR SYSTEMS INQUIRIES?

As discussed in Chapter 1, the rhetoric of regulation in the health sector tries to avoid the idea of 'naming, blaming and shaming' with the intent of promoting a 'safety culture' rather than a 'blame culture', to encourage the reporting of adverse events and near-misses. Equally, and as described in other chapters, systematic approaches to improving quality and safety are generally seen to be more effective than approaches that target individual clinicians.

To a greater or lesser extent, four of the inquiries struggled with this issue. The two exceptions were the King Edward Memorial Hospital and the Royal Melbourne Hospital inquiries. In the case of King Edward Memorial Hospital, the inquiry was not established to make findings about particular conduct or events. Its sole purpose was to examine the systemic issues and the inquiry made no formal findings into what had occurred at the hospital. In the case of the Royal Melbourne Hospital, the prosecutorial and systems inquiries were separated, with the coroner and the police investigating the specific allegations.

Given the context of the other high-profile inquiries with the responsibility of deciding whether action should be taken against any clinicians, it is not surprising that they struggled with the concept of 'no blame'. As one example, Bret Walker, in his inquiry into Camden and Campbelltown Hospitals, concluded that 'the chimera of no-fault in health care should be banished. But the equal absurdity of expecting that all adverse outcomes—or even many of them at all—are due to some hapless doctor's or nurse's fault for which they should be blamed or condemned should also be exploded' (Walker 2004: 90).

The Health Care Complaints Commission had claimed that its initial inquiry into Camden and Campbelltown Hospitals was a systems review. Walker rejected that view completely: 'A false dichotomy was created: systemic problems are the fault of middle and senior managers while non-systemic problems are the fault of clinicians. Either way, individuals are at fault. The real systemic issues are lost in the process.' (Eagar 2004: 10).

As a further example, a separate 'systems review' was established in parallel with the Bundaberg Base Hospital inquiry. Nevertheless, the Bundaberg Base Hospital inquiry necessarily dealt with systemic problems. In practice, the distinction between the two is inevitably blurred.

WHAT INQUIRIES TELL US

Three reviews in the literature have examined common themes across inquiries. Walshe and Shortell (2004) reviewed the experience in six countries (the United States, the United Kingdom, Australia, New Zealand, Canada and the Netherlands). A review by Walshe and Higgins (2002) examined 59 inquiries in the United Kingdom between 1974 and 2002. A review by the Clinical Excellence Commission in New South Wales looked at eight inquiries in six countries (Australia, Scotland, England, Slovenia, New Zealand and Canada), and included three from Australia—King Edward Memorial Hospital, Royal Melbourne Hospital and Camden and Campbelltown Hospitals (Hindle et al. 2006).

Walshe and Shortell (2004), relying on documents and interviews with key informants, reported on examples of major failures (defined as breakdowns that do substantial harm to many patients) in health care. The inquiry into King Edward Memorial Hospital was included in their review, which identified some common themes:

- Failures are often long-standing problems.
- It is often evident with hindsight that many key people and stakeholders knew that something was seriously wrong and did nothing about it.
- The harm caused by these failures can be immense.
- These failures often happen in very dysfunctional organisations.
- Some kinds of failure occur again and again, suggesting that lessons are not being learned (e.g. laboratory failures) (Walshe and Shortell 2004).

They also make the important point that, in all likelihood, the major failures that come to public attention are perhaps only a small proportion of those that actually happen (Walshe and Shortell 2004). The work of Walshe and Shortell identified some common barriers to disclosure and investigation:

- There is an endemic culture of secrecy and protectionism in health services.
- Knowledge is often fragmented across many people, who each know part of the problem or failure rather than the full picture.
- In the face of unwelcome information, the capacity for self-deception and rationalisation 'in hindsight' results in problems not being addressed until evidence is quite incontrovertible.
- Informal mechanisms for dealing with problems (the soft base of the regulatory pyramid) can result in those problems simply being moved somewhere else, rather than being rectified.

- Medical negligence claims may be settled with binding non-disclosure agreements, which does not benefit future patients who may be exposed to the same risk.
- There may be multiple investigations into the same event, resulting in confusion and long delays, and there is some evidence which suggests that inquiries can reach mistaken conclusions. (Walshe and Shortell 2004)

The last point is an important one. 'Get it right first time' is one of the mantras of quality improvement and, at face value, an easy concept to grasp. The same is perhaps even more relevant for public inquiries. The first inquiry into Camden and Campbelltown Hospitals by the New South Wales Health Care Complaints Commission pleased nobody, including the Minister for Health who promptly sacked the Commissioner when the report of the inquiry was released. It was subsequently severely criticised by the Special Commission for a lack of procedural fairness. The first inquiry into what happened at Bundaberg was terminated when the Queensland Supreme Court restrained the Commissioner and Deputy Commissioners appointed to the inquiry from further proceeding on the grounds that there was a 'reasonable apprehension of bias' by the Commissioner (Davies 2005).

Both of these examples illustrate the importance of any inquiry being 'above reproach', particularly in terms of who is conducting the inquiry and how it is conducted. Any lack of confidence in an inquiry simply lengthens the process for everyone, and is likely to compromise the findings—or, perhaps more importantly, the credibility of the findings. An inquiry can act as a 'circuit-breaker' to calm down what can be a very emotive, if not hostile, environment for the players—patients, staff, the media or the general public—as happened in several of the inquiries reviewed in this chapter.

The Clinical Excellence Commission literature review was based on inquiries between 1998 and 2004 and identified some common findings:

- The inquiry teams were largely impartial and objective.
- Some health care was far below standard.
- Quality-monitoring processes were deficient.
- Individual care providers and patients raised the concerns.
- Critics were often ignored or abused.
- Teamwork was deficient.
- Patients and families were not informed members of the team. (Hindle et al. 2006)

It is interesting to reflect on these commonalities in light of the evidence referred to elsewhere in this chapter. It would be surprising if the health care, at least in part, was not below standard, given the incidence of adverse events reported in the literature. What inquiries do, however, is assign a human face and human experience to bland statistics about 'adverse events', which is really just a euphemism for avoidable pain, suffering and death.

It would also be surprising if quality monitoring processes were not deficient, given a literature that describes multiple approaches to improving quality but little guidance regarding the best way of doing so. The finding about patients and families being ill-informed is, again, not unexpected given that it is based on reviewing a series of inquiries involving adverse events. There is now an Australian standard for open disclosure (see Chapter 11) which provides a framework for open communication following an adverse event (Australian Council for Safety and Quality in Health Care 2003). However, there is still a long way to go before it is part of everyday practice in hospitals, with recent evidence suggesting, somewhat tentatively, that it 'could become the central component of negotiating bad news in clinical practice' (Iedema et al. 2008). The remaining three findings about individuals raising concerns, the treatment of critics and the deficiency of teamwork are all manifestations of the culture of health services which not only arise during inquiries but are a core issue when seeking to improve the quality of health services more generally (Ferlie and Shortell 2001; Bate et al. 2007).

History suggests that an inquiry, no matter how much emphasis there may be at the beginning on the performance of individuals (for example, Dr Patel at Bundaberg), is very likely to branch out into organisational issues, such as systems, management accountability and governance, and even enter the murky waters of culture. There is a case for any inquiry to be considered as a potential organisational case study, with a strong likelihood of becoming a case study in organisational failure. This requires the inquiry to 'conform to the standards expected of any primarily qualitative methodology' (Walshe and Higgins 2002: 898).

The extraordinary amount of time and resources devoted to a full-scale inquiry begs the question of what would be found if every hospital were subject to the same level of scrutiny. As one clinician observed when commenting on the inquiry into King Edward Memorial Hospital, 'seven million dollars of careful analysis at any Australian tertiary hospital would have yielded the same conclusions' (Siddins 2003: 28).

CAN INQUIRIES BE PREVENTED?

The similarities between the failures in different countries indicate that the problems and potential solutions are embedded in 'the nature of clinical practice, the health care professions, and the culture of health care organisations' (Walshe and Shortell 2004). While inquiries may have a role in identifying what went wrong, the common issues identified across the various inquiries are largely preventable if effective systems are in place at lower levels of the regulation pyramid.

Underpinning much of the discussion about adverse events, improving quality and safety and the impact of public inquiries is what might be referred to as the 'implementation gap'. It is well known that the incidence of adverse events is about one in ten, that a substantial proportion are preventable, and that the majority are operation or medication related (de Vries et al. 2008). The quality literature argues that the solution is 'a more comprehensive, multilevel approach to change', focusing on the individual, the group or team, the organisation, and the larger system or environment (Ferlie and Shortell 2001: 282).

There is a significant literature on what can be done to prevent inquiries by improving quality and reducing adverse events, but many studies focus on 'what' to do rather than explore the issue of 'how' interventions work, or the circumstances in which a particular intervention will work better than others. This has been described as 'a signal failure to consider the special issues posed by the management of change within highly professionalised organisations' (Ferlie et al. 2000: 97).

The 'quality' literature primarily consists of single-site studies with a focus on describing what happened (Iles and Sutherland 2001), and the implementation of quality improvement has been characterised as largely based on intuition and anecdote (Shojania and Grimshaw 2005). The collaborative methodology is widely used to improve quality, and has appeal as a mechanism to address the sort of issues that might arise from an inquiry, particularly the focus on teamwork and learning, but even the evidence to support this methodology is limited (Schouten et al. 2008). This has resulted in a situation where no single strategy for improving quality can be recommended over any other (Øvretveit 2003: 4), with implementation described as the 'weakest link' in turning proposals for change into reality (Bevan et al. 2008) and the design of effective quality improvement interventions considered still to be in its infancy (Bosch et al. 2007).

This is not a recipe for doing nothing to prevent future inquiries. It simply reflects the fact that improving the quality of services is complex and difficult, and without a particularly sound evidence base to guide practitioners. It is no small wonder that problems recur. As Hindle et al. observed when commenting on the King Edward Memorial Hospital inquiry, clinical pathways are a technically simple but culturally difficult idea (Hindle et al. 2006).

Based on their work examining inquiries in the United Kingdom, Walshe and Higgins (2002) concluded that:

> In both health and social care many inquiries produce similar findings, despite addressing failures in the quality of care which on the face of it have little in common. The consistency with which inquiries highlight similar causes suggests that their recommendations are either misdirected or not properly implemented. Certainly there are few formal mechanisms for following up the findings and recommendations of inquiries. However, many of the problems identified by inquiries are cultural and demand changes in attitudes, values, beliefs, and behaviours—which are difficult to prescribe in any set of recommendations. (2002: 899)

This finding echoes the conclusions of Leape and Berwick when they posed the question of why health care was not demonstrably safer and why it was so difficult to implement safer practices, despite a lot of activity to do so. The answer, they say, is:

> found in the culture of medicine, a culture that is deeply rooted, both by custom and by training, in high standards of autonomous individual performance and a commitment to progress through research...creating cultures of safety requires major changes in behavior, changes that professionals easily perceive as threats to their authority and autonomy. (Leape and Berwick 2005: 2387)

The issue of culture is complex, and has generated a voluminous literature. One of the most oft-cited conceptualisations is the typology developed by Schein (1992), which considers culture to be layered in nature: level one consists of observable patterns of behaviour, level two of beliefs and values, and level three of assumptions. Change may occur in patterns of behaviour but if these do not become part of everyday practice the deeper levels are likely to remain unaffected (Mannion et al. 2005). Without changes in beliefs, values and assumptions, behaviour will revert over time to what it was before, in line with underlying assumptions and values that are unchanged. Based on their review of the literature on the clinical application of continuous quality improvement, Shortell and colleagues (1998) suggest that if there is not a supportive culture, only small, temporary, effects will be achieved, with no lasting impact.

Despite the various forms of advice in the literature to consider issues of culture and systems to improve patient safety, the evidence to support this approach is lacking. Essentially, the research simply has not been done to identify the links between systems (in the form of multiple organisational variables) and patient safety. Hoff and colleagues reviewed the literature that examines links between organisational factors, medical errors and patient safety. They concluded that there is no systematic body of empirical evidence to support the proposition that 'organisational variables like teams and leadership make a difference in reducing medical errors or enhancing patient safety' (Hoff et al. 2004: 21).

Given the subject matter and outcomes of these inquiries discussed in this chapter, there is a basic paradox. Those organisations with the greatest potential to benefit are those least able to do so because they simply do not have what it takes to be receptive to change: 'Receptive contexts for change can be constructed through processes of cumulative development but such processes are reversible, either by the removal of key individuals or ill considered or precipitous action.' (Pettigrew et al. 1992: 276).

As an illustration of how long the process of change can take, it is illustrative to consider the case of credentialling medical practitioners. The need for improving standards of credentialling and defining the scope of practice of medical practitioners was recognised in 1996, incorporated in the action plan of the Australian Council for Safety and Quality in Health Care in 2001 and published in 2004 (Australian Council for Safety and Quality in Health Care 2004). State jurisdictions have then taken up the standards in different ways. For example, Victoria produced its own local adaptation of the policy, and by late 2008 was positioned to run a workshop that, amongst other things, identified barriers to the implementation of the credentialling and scope of practice policy. Credentialling of medical staff was an important issue in both the King Edward Memorial Hospital and Bundaberg Base Hospital inquiries, yet twelve years on, work is still continuing to implement a national approach.

A final point about prevention relates to public confidence. Calls for a public inquiry are, in essence, a vote of no confidence in other regulatory mechanisms. The corollary is the importance of making sure that other regulatory mechanisms are understood and are perceived to be effective. Public reporting of the outcomes of other regulatory mechanisms is an essential part of minimising the need for public inquiries.

WHO LEARNS FROM INQUIRIES?

Our description of the impact of the various inquiries was framed around the recommendations arising from each inquiry. Yet the findings of every inquiry clearly have the potential to be generalised to other settings. Indeed, there is a *prima facie* case that one of the potential benefits of a public inquiry is the opportunity for others to learn the lessons.

However, while the implementation of recommendations arising from most inquiries is generally monitored, there is in fact no direct evidence of the impact of public inquiries on day-to-day clinical practice more broadly. One reason is that the findings of public inquiries are typically disseminated passively. This is despite evidence that passive approaches are generally ineffective and not likely to lead to changes in behaviour (Grimshaw et al. 2001). The most common way of accessing the outcomes of inquiries is now via the internet. There may be mechanisms for those working in the organisation that is the subject of the inquiry to be made aware of the outcomes and political leaders and departmental bureaucrats are always briefed. However, for the vast majority of people working in the health system, their main source of information is likely to be the media or accessing the report themselves. More effective spread of the lessons from inquiries is required if they are to make a contribution to improving safety and quality beyond the specific organisation.

CONCLUSION

There is no doubt that Australia, along with countries internationally, needs public inquiries as a response of last resort. They are a visible manifestation of the underlying problem of patient safety and symbolise the failure of strategies to improve health care in a systematic way. The corollary is that most, though not all, of these inquiries could have been prevented had action been taken earlier at lower levels in the responsive regulation pyramid.

All public inquiries have a strong focus on clinical issues but almost inevitably end up spending a great deal of time and effort on organisational issues. The balance between system-level and individual-level investigation is often difficult to achieve, as is the balance between focusing on prosecutorial and systems issues.

There is evidence that inquiries this decade have had a direct impact on the organisations concerned, typically in the form of additional resources, reorganisations and new policies and procedures. In some cases, the changes went much further and had a significant impact on other hospitals. Several have had a direct response at the political and senior bureaucratic level in the form of changes to legislation, new advisory bodies and bureaucratic reorganisations. The impact on some individual clinicians and managers has also been profound.

The empirical evidence has simply not been sought on the impact of public inquiries on day-to-day clinical practice across health systems. The indirect evidence, in the form of literature about quality improvement, change management, the 'black box' of implementation and the dissemination of innovations suggests that public inquiries have little or no impact on the bulk of everyday clinical practice. The links between such practice and public inquiries is tenuous, ad hoc and too distant in both in time and place for any real impact to occur.

The responsive regulation pyramid is consistent with the argument that strategies for change in health care need to be multi-level. What is required is ongoing research into how the different levels interact and influence each other. Public inquiries typically provide detailed information in the form of organisational case studies with the potential to inform both research and practice. However, there are two important caveats. The first is that inquiries do not necessarily apply rigorous methodological standards. The second is that, if the lessons from inquiries are to be learned, they need to be disseminated in ways that are clinically, bureaucratically and politically effective.

REFERENCES

Australian Council for Safety and Quality in Health Care 2003, *Open Disclosure Standard: A National Standard for Open Communication in Public and Private Hospitals, Following an Adverse Event in Health Care*, Australian Council for Safety and Quality in Health Care, Sydney

—— 2004, *Standard for Credentialling and Defining the Scope of Clinical Practice: A National Standard for Credentialling and Defining the*

Scope of Clinical Practice of Medical Practitioners, for Use in Public and Private Hospitals, Australian Council for Safety and Quality in Health Care, Sydney

Bate, P., Mendel, P. and Robert, G. 2007, *Organising for Quality: The Improvement Journeys of Leading Hospitals in Europe and the United States*, Radcliffe, Oxford

Bevan, H., Ham, C. and Plsek, P.E. 2008, *The Next Leg of the Journey: How Do We Make High Quality Care for All a Reality?*, NHS Institute for Innovation and Improvement, Coventry

Bosch, M., Van der Weijden, T., Wensing, M. and Grol, R. 2007, 'Tailoring quality improvement interventions to identified barriers: A multiple case analysis', *Journal of Evaluation in Clinical Practice*, vol. 13, no. 2, pp. 161-8

Brand, C., Ibrahim, J., Bain, C., Jones, C. and King, B., 'Engineering, a safe landing: engaging medical practitioners in a systems approach to patient safety', *International Medicine Journal*, vol. 37, no. 5, pp. 295-302, published online 10 May 2007

Community and Health Services Complaints Commissioner of the ACT 2003, Final report of the investigation into adverse patient outcomes of neuro-surgical services provided by the Canberra Hospital, Canberra, ACT, <www. health.act.gov.au/c/health?a=da&did=10011741&pid=1070942701>, accessed 10 October 2008

Davies, G. 2005, *Queensland Public Hospitals Commission of Inquiry Report*, Queensland Government, Brisbane

Department of Health of Western Australia 2005, *The Implementation of the Douglas Inquiry Recommendations Review Final Report*, Internal Audit Branch, Department of Health, Perth

de Vries, E.N., Ramrattan, M.A., Smorenburg, S.M., Gouma, D.J. and Boermeester, M.A. 2008, 'The incidence and nature of in-hospital adverse events: A systematic review', *Quality and Safety in Health Care*, vol. 17, no. 3, pp. 216-23

Douglas, N., Robinson, J. and Fahy 2001, *Inquiry into Obstetric and Gynaecological Services at King Edward Memorial Hospital 1990-2000: Final Report*, Department of Health, Government of Western Australia, Perth <www.kemh.health.wa.gov.au/general/KEMH_Inquiry/reports.htm>, accessed 3 December 2008

Eagar, K. 2004, 'The weakest link?', *Australian Health Review*, vol. 28, no. 1, pp. 7-12

Ferlie, E.B., Fitzgerald, L. and Wood, M. 2000, 'Getting evidence into clinical practice: An organisational behaviour perspective', *Journal of Health Services Research and Policy*, vol. 5, no. 2, pp. 96-102

Ferlie, E.B. and Shortell, S.M. 2001, 'Improving the quality of health care in the United Kingdom and the United States: A framework for change', *Milbank Quarterly*, vol. 79, no. 2, pp. 281-315

Forster, P. 2005, *Queensland Health Systems Review Final Report September 2005*, <www.health.qld.gov.au/health_sys_review/final/qhsr_final_report.pdf>, accessed 3 December 2008

Garling, P. 2008, *Final Report of the Special Commission of Inquiry Acute Care Services in NSW Public Hospitals*, <www.lawlink.nsw.gov.au/lawlink/Special_Projects/ll_splprojects.nsf/pages/acsi_finalreport>, accessed 20 January 2009

Grimshaw, J.M., Shirran, L., Thomas, R., Mowatt, G., Fraser, C., Bero, L., Grilli, R., Harvey, E., Oxman, A. and O'Brien, M.A. 2001, 'Changing provider behavior: An overview of systematic reviews of interventions', *Medical Care*, vol. 39, no. 8, suppl. 2, pp. 112-45

Health Services Commissioner 2002, *Royal Melbourne Hospital Inquiry Report*, Health Services Commission, Melbourne

—— 2004, *Analysis of The Inquiry held by The Health Services Commissioner 2002, into an Incident at the Royal Melbourne Hospital, Victoria*, Health Services Commission, Melbourne

Hindle, D., Braithwaite, J., Travaglia, J. and Iedema, R. 2006, *Patient Safety: A Comparative Analysis of Eight Inquiries in Six Countries*, Centre for Clinical Governance Research, Faculty of Medicine, University of NSW, Sydney

Hoff, T., Jameson, L., Hannan, E. and Flink, E. 2004, 'A review of the literature examining linkages between organizational factors, medical errors, and patient safety', *Medical Care Research and Review*, vol. 61, no. 1, pp. 3-37

Iedema, R.A.M., Mallock, N.A., Sorensen, R.J., Manias, E., Tuckett, A.G., Williams, A.F., Perrott, B.E., Brownhill, S.H., Piper, D.A., Hor, S., Hegney, D.G., Scheeres, H.B. and Jorm, C.M. 2008, 'The National Open Disclosure Pilot: Evaluation of a policy implementation initiative', *Medical Journal of Australia*, vol. 188, no. 7, pp. 397-400

Iles, V. and Sutherland, K. 2001, 'Managing change in the NHS, Organisational change: A review for all health care managers, professionals and researchers', <www.sdo.nihr.ac.uk/files/adhoc/change-management-review.pdf>, accessed 16 December 2008

Leape, L.L. and Berwick, D.M. 2005, 'Five years after *To Err is Human*: What have we learned?', *Journal of the American Medical Association*, vol. 293, no. 19, pp. 2384-90

Mannion, R., Davies, H.T.O. and Marshall, M. 2005, *Cultures for Performance in Health Care*, Open University Press, Maidenhead

McLean, J. and Walsh, M. 2003, 'Lessons from the inquiry into obstetrics and gynaecology services at King Edward Memorial Hospital 1990-2000', *Australian Health Review*, vol. 26, no. 1, pp. 12-23

Milovanovich, C. 2008, *Inquest into the Death of Vanessa Ann Anderson*, New South Wales State Coroner's Court Westmead, <www.lawlink.nsw.gov.au/lawlink/Coroners_Court/ll_coroners.nsf/vwFiles/Anderson2.doc/$file/Anderson2.doc>, accessed 20 January 2009

Øvretveit, J. 2003, *What are the Best Strategies for Ensuring Quality in Hospitals?*, World Health Organization Regional Office for Europe, Copenhagen

Pettigrew, A.M., Ferlie, E. and McKee, L. 1992, *Shaping Strategic Change*, Sage, London

Schein, E.H. 1992, *Organizational Culture and Leadership*, 2nd ed., Jossey-Bass, San Francisco

Schouten, L.M.T., Hulscher, M.E.J.L., Everdingen, J.J.E., van Huijsman, R. and Grol, R.P.T.M. 2008, 'Evidence for the impact of quality improvement collaboratives: Systematic review', *British Medical Journal*, vol. 336, no. 7659, pp. 1491-4

Shojania, K.G. and Grimshaw, J.M. 2005, 'Evidence-based quality improvement: The state of the science', *Health Affairs*, vol. 24, no. 1, pp. 138-150

Shortell, S.M., Bennett, C.L. and Byck, G.R. 1998, 'Assessing the impact of continuous quality improvement on clinical practice: What it will take to accelerate progress', *Milbank Quarterly*, vol. 76, no. 4, pp. 593-624

Siddins, M. 2003, 'Commentary on the King Edward Inquiry: Lessons we fail to learn', *Australian Health Review*, vol. 26, no. 1, pp. 28-9

Walker, B. 2004, *Final Report of the Special Commission of Inquiry into Campbelltown and Camden Hospitals*, <www.lawlink.nsw.gov.au/special_commission>, accessed 31 July 2004

Walshe, K. and Higgins, J. 2002, 'The use and impact of inquiries in the NHS', *British Medical Journal*, vol. 325, no. 7369, pp. 895-900

Walshe, K. and Shortell, S.M. 2004, 'When things go wrong: How health care organizations deal with major failures', *Health Affairs*, vol. 23, no. 3, pp. 103-11

INDEX

United Kingdom (*cont.*)
health professionals
regulation, 149,
160-1, 163
Healthcare Commission,
221
House of Commons, 55
Medical Act 1858, 144
National Health Service
(NHS), 49, 161
National Institute of
Health and Clinical
Excellence, 64
clinical guidelines, 208
National Patient Safety
Agency, 204
public inquiries, 330,
334
regulation of medical
profession, 144
United States
Agency for Health
Care Research and
Quality, 208, 289, 291
American Health
Information
Management
Association, 56
Centers of Medicare and
Medicaid, 55
clinical practice
guidelines, 79, 85
disclosure policies, 243,
248
Federation of State
Medical Boards, 149
Flexner Report, 149
Institute for Health Care
Improvement (IHI),
86, 208

Institute of Medicine, 55,
64, 86, 194, 237
Joint Commission on
Accreditation
of Healthcare
Organizations, 241,
284, 289
litigation, 254, 256-7
National Committee for
Quality Assurance,
291
National Guidelines
Clearing House, 204
National Institute of
Health, 79
National Patient Safety
Foundation, 204
public reporting of
performance, 289
regulation of medical
profession, 149, 150,
172
Veterans Affairs Medical
Centre, 243
*Uren v John Fairfax and
Sons Pty Ltd*, 257

value-based payment
schemes, 56
values, 65, 126-38
Victoria
Department of Consumer
Affairs, 183
Health Service
Commissioner,
180-1, 322, 323
Medical Practitioners
Board, 174-5
Minister of Health, 322
public health service

governance system,
113-14, 116
statewide emergency
collaborative, 87
Victorian Psychologists
Registration Board, 174
violations, 199-200
vincristine alert, 5, 147
voluntarism, 7, 11-12

Walker, Bret, 324, 329
Western Australia
Department of Health,
321, 322
Minister of Health, 321
whistleblowers, 34, 199,
261, 294, 321
workforce
shortages, 111
health professionals
migration, 157-8
work practices, 201
World Alliance for Patient
Safety, 2, 47, 58
international curriculum
on patient safety, 58
the 'High 5s', 2
World Health Organization,
2, 3, 40, 47, 55, 58, 157,
237
wrong-site surgery, 5, 40,
204, *see also* Correct
Patient, Correct Site,
Correct Procedure
Protocol